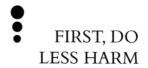

FIRST, DO
LESS HARM

A volume in the series
The Culture and Politics of Health Care Work
Edited by Suzanne Gordon and Sioban Nelson

For a list of books in the series, visit our website at
www.cornellpress.cornell.edu.

FIRST, DO
LESS HARM

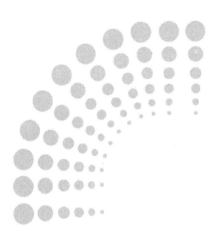

Confronting
the Inconvenient
Problems of
Patient Safety

EDITED BY ROSS KOPPEL
AND SUZANNE GORDON

ILR PRESS
AN IMPRINT OF
CORNELL UNIVERSITY PRESS
Ithaca and London

First published by Cornell University Press 2012

Printed in the United States of America

Library of Congress Cataloging-in-Publication Data
First, do less harm : confronting the inconvenient problems of patient safety / edited by Ross Koppel and Suzanne Gordon.
    p. cm. — (The culture and politics of health care work)
    Includes bibliographical references and index.
    ISBN 978-0-8014-5077-8 (cloth : alk. paper)
    1. Medical errors—Prevention.   2. Patients—Safety measures.   3. Medical care—Safety measures.
4. Hospital care—Safety measures.   I. Koppel, Ross.   II. Gordon, Suzanne, 1945–   III. Series: Culture and politics of health care work.
    R729.8.F57 2012
    610.289—dc23   2011044453

Cornell University Press strives to use environmentally responsible suppliers and materials to the fullest extent possible in the publishing of its books. Such materials include vegetable-based, low-VOC inks and acid-free papers that are recycled, totally chlorine-free, or partly composed of nonwood fibers. For further information, visit our website at www.cornellpress.cornell.edu.

Cloth printing   10 9 8 7 6 5 4 3 2 1

We dedicate this book to the physicians, nurses, pharmacists, researchers, epidemiologists, and others who work so hard to create safe treatment of patients. We also dedicate this book to patients and caregivers who have lived with both illness and patient safety failures.

Contents

FIRST, DO
LESS HARM

Introduction

Suzanne Gordon and Ross Koppel

VIGNETTE 1

A few years ago my wife, Meg, had major surgery at a highly regarded, fully wired hospital. After surgery, Meg was wheeled up to the floor with her assigned room. Computer displays at the nurses' station indicated she had left the post-anesthesia care unit and was now on her floor. I was in the lobby waiting to be told of her room assignment. After about forty-five minutes I became alarmed. I searched the probable hospital floors and found Meg shivering, dehydrated, and alone by the elevators. I ran to the nurses' station down the hallway and asked why she'd been left there so long. They responded that they knew she was being sent up but didn't know she'd been left in the hallway. We hustled her into her room, covered her with blankets, and gave her ice chips. As a scholar of hospital workflow and health care information technology, I understood what happened, but I was still enraged.

Had I not intervened, it's possible that someone would have noticed her. It's also possible that someone would not . . . or that someone would have noticed her and assumed she was calmly waiting for her transportation. (Ross Koppel)

VIGNETTE 2

Joan Smith (a pseudonym) is a nurse at a major American teaching hospital— one that has pioneered patient safety initiatives. She's informed by her manager of a new improvement that allows charting (recording patients' medications and vital signs) in each patient's room, rather than at the central nurses' station. New computers have been installed in each room. Smith is eager to benefit from this improvement, although she finds it odd that none of the nurses was consulted on the placement of these new computers.

She enters one of the newly configured rooms, starts using the computer, and is slammed in the back of the head by the door. Much to her dismay—but perhaps not her surprise—the computers have been placed where the door opens into the room. So if the door is opened while a nurse is standing at the computer, it will whack her in the neck, head, or shoulder. Worse, some of the questions the nurse asks patients are very personal; closing the door is both appropriate and required.

At the next nurses' meeting, Smith points out that the unit's goal of reducing workers' compensation claims will not be aided by the placement of the new computers. More important, she asks why no bedside nurses were included on the team designing computer placement. When there is no response, she sighs and simply states, "Well, there go our compensation claims and our shoulders." As of this writing, the situation has not been addressed.

VIGNETTE 3

The cardiologist T. K. is seeing a patient who needs both a CT scan and an MRI. He uses the Computerized Physician Order Entry (CPOE) system to order both tests and is delighted to find that both tests have very similar ordering templates (user interfaces). Unbeknown to this physician, however, the CPOE system does not actually transmit CT scan orders to the radiology department. A scan is neither scheduled nor administered. CT scans, he later learns, must be ordered via a different computer screen, but there is no indication of this at the time of ordering. For the patient, this means that finding his problem, and therefore starting the needed treatment, is delayed by weeks. The cardiologist did not remember ordering both tests and only reconsidered a CT scan when the patient was in extremis.

Although the saying is attributed to Mark Twain, it was Charles Dudley Warner who said everybody talks about the weather, but nobody does anything about it. By contrast, everyone seems to be doing something about patient safety. Every day our email includes messages announcing a new initiative launched by the Institute for Health Care Improvement (IHI)—one of the leading organizations in the patient safety movement—or a conference hosted by another safety group. Books by patient safety advocates such as Atul Gawande and Peter Pronovost now make the *New York Times* best-seller list. As if to highlight the importance of patient safety, President Barack Obama named the founder of a major patient safety organization, Dr. Donald Berwick, to be the administrator of the Centers for Medicare and Medicaid, although political pressures led to his resignation.

Yet despite more than a decade of highly focused attention on patient safety, anecdotes like those we have related abound. Collected in quantitative studies, these anecdotes paint a sobering picture of the state of patient safety both in the United States and globally. In 2010 several reports from the Agency for Healthcare Research and Quality showed that the rate of bloodstream infections could be reduced dramatically by a series of simple steps (the so-called checklist), but at the same time, that agency reported, such infections had increased by 8 percent in one year throughout most of the nation.[1]

In the same year, two professors from Case Western Reserve published an article in the *Berkeley Technology Law Journal* with even more distressing news.[2] Doctors, the authors, warned, should be wary of the promise of electronic medical records. Software bugs, lack of adequate training in complex technology, incessant warnings of drug interactions with no real threats, and errors that generate the wrong output create significant patient safety hazards for which physicians may be held liable. As other authors, including one of the editors of this book, have pointed out, health care technology may be a bullet, but it does not seem to be the silver one so many experts have promised.[3]

We have been working on this book for over four years. Some of the essays in it were begun that many years ago. When we asked authors for updates, many were able to provide more recent references, but alas, the progress of patient safety was seldom the reason for the updates. Despite the increase in funding and attention, the authors primarily included more recent studies and newer documentation of patient safety's unmet challenges.

Please don't misunderstand our intention. We know there has been movement on patient safety—numerous and important pockets of improvement.

The problem is, as we shall see in this book, that too many of these pockets are isolated, and the sum of the parts does not seem to constitute an impressive whole. Many wonderful initiatives and activities often seem disconnected from, or undermined by, actions taken by the very institutions in which they have been pioneered. Institutions don't just fail to learn from one another; they may not even connect—and learn from—what is going on in one unit or discipline to what is going on in another. Across a single hospital or health system, or throughout a region, or in the entire nation, it often seems that the proverbial one hand not only doesn't know what the other is doing but is deliberately canceling out the other's efforts as well.

Here's a classic example. A hospital participates in a prestigious foundation's initiative on improving care. The project, according to the foundation's website, has done "great work" to improve care on medical-surgical units.[4] Suzanne Gordon is observing on a hospital unit. She sees photocopied yellow sheets—with an image of a traffic sign triangle and in it the words "No Passing Zone" posted on every patient room. What does this mean, Gordon asks. The nurse accompanying her explains that this is an important part of the unit's safety initiative that has been implemented on the unit. Everyone—from unit secretary to janitor—has been told not to go by a patient's room without looking in to make sure nothing untoward is happening. "For example," she explains, "if a frail ninety-eight-year-old lady is trying to climb over her bedrails, you don't just look in, see it, and walk by. You do something about it."

"That's great," Gordon commented and then asked, "Does that apply to physicians as well?"

"Oh, no," she answers, apparently without noting the irony, "only to hospital employees." So the nurse, the janitor, the unit clerk—all have a duty to rescue the patient. But on a unit funded by a leading health care foundation and implemented by a leading patient safety group, the physician, who is supposed to be the captain of the ship/team, is exempt.

Or take the issue of physicians' neckties. We now know that those carefully knotted, handsome cravats, so gracefully dangling over the front of a man's shirt, are the perfect vectors for germs. A male physician leans over a patient to examine a wound or to listen to chest sounds, and his tie brushes against the patient, the gown, the sheets. Now covered in germs, he moves to the next bed and brushes against another patient. And then on to the next. Studies have made clear how harmful this can be—so harmful, in fact, that in 2007 the British National Health Service initiated a "bare below the elbow policy," banning not just ties but long fingernails, jewelry, and lab coats.[5] In the United States, however, ties are still dangling from doctors' necks, lab coats are worn throughout hospitals, and so are jewelry and long nails, even though U.S. hospitals are trying to reduce infection rates.

Patient safety initiatives come and go, some contradictory, many isolated or fragmented by departments or occupations. Some medical services or disciplines are largely ignored. And then there is the disconnect between management and staff, and between management and unions—all important "stakeholders" in patient safety. Efforts requiring comprehensive approaches are introduced in piecemeal fashion; many patient safety programs are unnecessarily entangled with modern health care information technology (HIT), whereas others that could benefit from HIT are bereft of its assistance.

This book is an exploration of why patient safety is advancing at what seems to be an almost glacial pace, despite the often vast and determined efforts of health care workers and managers. A collection of essays from prominent researchers, scholars, and even patients, this book aims to identify some of the gaps in the patient safety movement, the disconnected dots that do not coalesce despite decades of hard work and billions of dollars. It also identifies concerns that have not been integrated into the patient safety discourse or agenda of more established groups.

Although the chapters deal with a variety of issues, a number of themes unite them. The first and most important is the fundamental contradiction between two of the imperatives driving our health care system: safety and cost. This contradiction is perhaps most acutely felt in the United States, where the health care system must address the requirements of many separate insurance companies with differing priorities and patterns of coverage. Frequently patient safety becomes a casualty of the drive to cut health care costs and the accompanying failure to understand that ensuring safety is—in and of itself—a cost-saving activity. The essays in this book illustrate some of the predictable irrationalities of that contradiction. As Rosalind Stanwell-Smith points out in "Too Mean to Clean," and as the chapter by Peter Lazes, Suzanne Gordon, and Sameh Samy makes clear, saving money by outsourcing cleaning often results in dirtier hospitals, more hospital-acquired infections, and the additional costs of those unnecessary illnesses. Further, authors Sean Clarke, Christopher Landrigan, Alison Trinkoff, and Jeanne Geiger-Brown document how increased workload and schedules that prevent clinicians from getting enough sleep increase both errors and costs.

The anecdote recounted by the RN earlier in this chapter depicts the predictable irrationalities that result from the disconnection between cost, safety, and the work environment. The nurse who had her head slammed by the patient room door was on a unit concerned with both patient safety and the cost of worker compensation claims. But no one connected the dots when locating the nurses' computer stations. As a result, as the nurse commented sarcastically, "there go our worker's comp complaints and our shoulders."

Much of the tension between patient safety and the market discourse dominating health care is embodied in the idea of patients as "customers." Patients are not, in fact, customers making informed choices based on full knowledge of their best options. The role and model of professional and caring clinicians is supposed to protect patients from unwise decisions.

But instead we have a marketing metaphor that largely replaces professional autonomy with a concern with salesmanship and misplaced customer satisfaction measures.

The market model stands in contrast to the ethical dynamic at the heart of patient safety. Patient safety begins with the injunction attributed to Hippocrates: the physician (or hospital) should "first do no harm." When, however, doctors, nurses, pharmacists, hospitals, and administrators are obliged to consider their services as competing product lines within their institutions and told to view one another as competitors and their patients as customers, it is hardly surprising that the logic of the market may interfere with the ethics of the healer.[6]

The second theme of this book concerns the place of frontline workers in patient safety discussions and initiatives. At the core of many of these chapters is an analysis of what happens when frontline workers are neither consulted nor involved in the planning, implementation, evaluation, and refinement of patient safety initiatives. Whether they be physicians and nurses who will be using health care information technology, or cleaners who are given insufficient supplies to do their jobs, failing to ask workers to identify safety problems and their remedies represents another hidden problem and cost. Ross Koppel and his colleagues contrast the overwhelming faith in health care information technology with the reality of its use. They discover that lack of on-the-floor observation encourages the creation of software that does not meet the needs of clinicians and often increases the dangers of medication errors in ways that have been systematically ignored, deflected, or intentionally hidden in nondisclosure clauses of vendor contracts. They describe the ways in which software vendors fail to incorporate the often desperate requests of physicians, nurses, and pharmacists who struggle with screen displays that obstruct rather than aid in patient care. Koppel and his colleagues' discussion of the contradictions and inappropriate models underlying patient safety initiatives is echoed in the essay by Joseph Bugajski, a noted authority on IT. Bugajski's sardonic tale of his medical mistreatment involves professional blindness, HIT, foolish routines, and, as the title relates, "the data model that nearly killed me."

Health care settings are messy, often unpredictable, emotional places, and they depend on dedicated workers. Running a hospital is not like running a factory or even a complex power plant; there is no design protocol that will handle all the resulting contingencies. If safety is primarily the province of experts or managers who make pronouncements in public spaces, it nevertheless remains the task of workers who inhabit private spaces.

As Lazes, Gordon, and Samy point out, the failure to consider seriously the input of frontline workers (particularly those low on the health care ladder) is connected to another issue identified in this volume: the impact of status and hierarchy on the safety of patients. On this point, we include Kathleen Burke's brief and insightful essay on how Medicare's rules for administering medication fail to take into account how medication is actually administered in hospitals. When actual work processes are not understood, or when, as Gordon and Bonnie O'Connor argue, some members of the health care team are considered the "mindless" servants of the mindful elite, safety will inevitably fall through the cracks. Similarly, as Gordon writes in "On Teams, Teamwork, and Team Intelligence," even some of the most promising experiments in patient safety are defeated by those who are so concerned about maintaining status hierarchies that they are blind to their implicit but contradictory messages.

As we write the introduction to this book, the world has just celebrated the one hundredth anniversary of the death of Florence Nightingale, one of the first patient safety pioneers. Nightingale was also one of the first "systems thinkers" in health care. She recognized the importance and interconnectedness of every detail of patient care. Nothing and no one was too trivial to command attention and scientific study—from the cleaning of the ward floors, linens, and uniforms, to the food preparation, to the way supplies were maintained.

Nightingale knew that systems thinking isn't just about the big-ticket items; it involves understanding how the components of the system interact.[7] A modern Nightingale would understand that if doctors and nurses have no time to wash their hands, or if outsourced cleaners aren't taught enough about infection control, then they will spread infection from one patient to the next. That is why another concern the authors of this book share has to do with the common but false dichotomy between patient safety and workers' health and safety. Dr. Christopher Landrigan, a renowned researcher and advocate for regulating physicians' working hours, is joined by Alison Trinkoff and Jeanne Geiger-Brown in highlighting the connection between caregiver exhaustion and threats to patient safety. When RNs and MDs are overtired, they are in jeopardy, and so are their patients. Errors go up, and so do exhaustion and stress-related illnesses. Similarly, the skeptical and increasingly cynical nurses we meet in the chapter by Lazes and colleagues are disenchanted with their hospitals' safety efforts because they feel that their concerns about workloads and work safety are ignored, or even attacked. You don't have to be a safety expert to recognize the irrationality of turning health care workers into patients. The chapter by nurse-researchers Linda

Treiber and Jackie Jones unites many of these themes and asks us to consider something that is too often forgotten in much of the discussion of patient safety. That is the impact of errors not only on the patients who suffer from them but also on the nurses and doctors who are links in the chain that led to the errors. Nurses and doctors who are institutionally and/or publicly identified as having committed errors tend to be scapegoated rather than helped. In fact, health care workers are profoundly distraught over any errors they have made. Their careers, their mental—and sometimes physical—health are also casualties of institutions that do not give sufficient attention to the *systemic causes* of patient safety failures but instead rely on overworked staff and hypervigilant clinicians.

The concluding chapter, by Koppel, Gordon, and Joel Leon Telles, presents twenty-seven paradoxes, ironies, and challenges of patient safety. It considers many of the major reasons why it is so difficult to ensure the unharmed passage of patients through health care facilities—and why our efforts are so frequently contradictory or misdirected. As they note, even the concept of "avoidable" errors is a contested terrain of economic, professional, ideological, ethical, and even epistemological disputes.

The catalogue of disconnected dots mentioned earlier is certainly not exhaustive. Nor are the issues we tackle. Every discipline or occupation could have its own chapter. We do hope that these twelve essays stimulate a much-needed discussion.

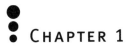

CHAPTER 1

The Data Model That Nearly Killed Me

Joseph M. Bugajski

In 2009 the U.S. government appropriated about $38 billion for health information technology and to create a program to digitize and network health information.[1] The appropriation law also defines rules for some health information standards and systems. It does not, however, explain how to test the validity of the information used by those systems. I argue that these prescriptions for a Nationwide Health Information Network (NHIN), though necessary, are insufficient.

During the last week of January 2009, a faulty electronic networked health information system nearly killed me despite its being run by two advanced, state-of-the-art medical facilities. This will come as no surprise to health care IT experts because health information is inherently complex, medical science develops extraordinarily rapidly, patient interactions are intensely personal, and the number of data types and sheer volume of health care data explode prodigiously with new tests, instruments, and treatments.[2] Because the purpose of an NHIN is data exchange, and data exchange requires a good model of the data being exchanged, and rapidly changing data make modeling intensely difficult, an NHIN is at worst infeasible and at best an extraordinarily difficult undertaking.[3]

My near-death experience at one of the best tertiary medical centers in the world, equipped with modern electronic health information systems, illuminates the chasm between the NHIN vision and its reality.

Treatment Saga

My ordeal began on Sunday, January 25, 2009. I returned from church, ate breakfast, and sat down in my favorite chair to read the paper. Within an hour, my lungs were causing me so much pain that I had to lie down. Two hours later I had a 104 degree fever, a not-working-so-well emergency asthma treatment regimen, and a tortured conversation with my by then very concerned allergist. I was on my way to urgent care. My wife reluctantly agreed to drive me to the clinic affiliated with my allergist's office rather than a closer-by clinic, because, I entreated, the farther-away, affiliated clinic would enter the attending doctor's report and any test results into my electronic health record for my allergist to review on Monday morning. (Okay. Low blood oxygen was messing with my brain, but it seemed a good idea at the time.) Thus, day one of a near-death experience began.

Urgent Care

The nurse who escorts me into urgent care asks me for my doctor's name. I tell her my allergist's name. The nurse argues that she wants to know the name of my primary care physician. Of course, that information is in my electronic medical record, which she can readily access. The nurse next requests that I relate my medical history, which information is available in my electronic health record (EHR). Next, an attending physician asks for my doctor's name—no, not my allergist, my internist—and tells me to please relate my medical history. Never mind that (a) I provided this information to the nurse only moments ago, (b) I can barely breathe, (c) I have horrible pain in my lungs, (d) I have a high fever, and (e) the requested data already are in my electronic health record. Perhaps, I think, these professionals must verify my data—regardless of whether or not my brain wants more oxygen. I explain to the nurse and doctor that my allergist, who is a specialist in allergy and immunology, and who also has a Ph.D. in pulmonary medicine, wanted me to receive certain treatments. The attending physician at urgent care says that I may have pneumonia. I say that I also have severe asthma. She smiles politely and walks away.

By and by the attending physician requests an X ray and a blood test. I ask for pain relief medication (the correct prescription is in my electronic health record). The doctor prescribes two Tylenol tablets, which do nothing for the pain. Hours go by. The X ray shows no pneumonia, says a radiologist. The attending doctor orders an intravenous antibiotic to help me deal with the infection and asks if I feel better. I say, "No, not really." Do I want a breathing treatment? "Yes, that would be good." I am sent home.

During my visit to urgent care, starting about 1 PM and continuing until 7 PM, my respiration is double to triple its normal rate. My lungs are bags of pain that trap CO_2. I have a high fever. I want to die. Despite the existence of a well-maintained electronic health information record in a state-of-the-art health information network, I am not treated for asthma aggravated by a lung infection as my medical history clearly and unambiguously indicates I should have been.

Doctor's Office

I cannot sleep during the night following the visit to urgent care. I am unable to breathe without intense pain. My respiration rate remains much higher than normal. But my fever has broken. First thing in the morning, I call my allergist's office. My allergist's nurse returns my call around 2 PM. She says that the doctor wants to see me at 4:30. He believes that I am still in serious trouble. My wife collects my medications (bless her, because later these would keep me alive) and drives me to my doctor's office.

My allergist and his nurse do not take my medical history. I lie on a gurney in an examination room, hooked up to monitors and supplemental oxygen. My doctor listens to my lungs as I labor and cough my way through a few breaths. He observes my respiration rate. He waits awhile. He repeats these observations thrice. Around 5:30 my allergist says that I am too sick to return home and he wants me admitted to the hospital for continuous observation. I object. He replies that I may die if I go home. His nurse calls for an ambulance. No, my wife cannot drive me a mile and a half to the hospital—the doctor says this would be too dangerous.

Ninety minutes pass before the ambulance arrives. My allergist spends the intervening time preparing a four-page memorandum giving my medical history, my current condition, and a recommended treatment plan. He also telephones the admitting physician at the emergency room, where I am heading next, to discuss my medical issues. My allergist then entrusts this information to the ambulance attendant.

ER and ICU

Once I am in the ambulance, the attendant asks me to give my medical history, including allergies and medications. This information he enters into a multipart form. When we arrive in the ER at the medical center affiliated with a world-renowned university, someone behind a desk calls me "asthma" then tells the ambulance attendant to park me in a hallway. The attendant delivers his report, oral and written, to the triage nurse, who by then is examining me. The attendant tells the triage nurse that he brought a written report from my physician for the admitting doctor to read. The nurse instructs the attendant to deliver his reports to a person behind a nearby desk. She says the information will be put into my chart.

I remained in the ER for twenty hours before being admitted to the hospital. Throughout my stay, I was hooked up to network-attached monitors that incessantly sounded alarms to which no one responded. I was asked eleven times to repeat my medical history, medication, and allergies to as many different medical professionals. Seven doctors who saw me each asked similar questions. Five of the doctors were never to be seen again. All the doctors mumbled something about putting their findings into the hospital's EHR system. Later I learned from the nurses that most did not do so. No one read my allergist's detailed report about my condition and health history.

I was moved from the ER to an ER holding room for admitted patients, back to the ER, to and fro to other departments for tests, then finally to an ICU. I was visited by nurses and technicians who pushed laptops mounted on wheeled sticks (COWs—computers on wheels). They checked my vitals; asked me questions about my history, medications, and allergies; and entered findings into the hospital's electronic medical record using the laptops mounted on wheeled sticks.

I asked every nurse and doctor who met me for medication to relieve the intense pain from my lungs, and was told I would receive it. Each claimed that he or she would note the order in my electronic medical record. No one did until about fourteen hours after I arrived, when, during the middle of the night, one thoughtful ER nurse finally found a doctor to authorize giving me the oft-approved but never delivered pain relief medication.

Data Lost and Not Found

No one in the ER or, later, the ICU, knew about, or could find, my allergist's memorandum describing my medical history, current medications, and treatment plan. My wife eventually called the allergist's office to obtain a fax copy for the ICU. No one ever mentioned reading the fax copy, although an ICU nurse confirmed its receipt. The list of persons who denied knowledge of the memorandum included the on-site doctor (the "hospitalist"), who represented the same clinic as my allergist. The hospitalist could view my electronic health records on-line from the hospital, but she ignored this rich source of vital information about my condition, preferring instead to come to her own (unbiased?) conclusion.

One heroic medical professional, the first nurse I met in the ICU, worked to create a consistent record of my condition, allergies, and medications in the hospital's electronic health information system. She spent over an hour searching for previously entered data, correcting errors, and moving or reentering data. She argued with one doctor whose concurrent access to the hospital's system blocked my nurse's access to my information. She called the hospital's pharmacy repeatedly to get my medications delivered. She met and called doctors several times. She even persuaded one doctor and a pharmacist to come to my room to resolve data errors in person. Despite these heroic efforts, I never received the correct medications during my stay. Indeed, my wife sneaked one of my inhalers into my room. After I used it, I finally began to recover.

A Near-Death Experience

At one point during my battle with illness and electronic health care data, the only asthma medication that had kept me alive began to wear off. I knew that if I did not receive the right dose within an hour or so, my condition would deteriorate rapidly and I would die. This critical information I had repeated nine times to doctors and nurses, who recorded it in my electronic health record. They promised that I would receive the medicine when it was time. That time came and went. My lungs began to scream with pain. My respiration rate accelerated. My breathing became more labored. I was crashing. I begged the doctor who next stopped in to check my condition for her help. She said she would authorize the prescription. The heroic ICU nurse stopped by my room, checked my electronic records, but could not find the prescription. She then ran to find a doctor to authorize my medicine. She succeeded. I received the medicine. I lived.

During the time I was hospitalized, I forced myself to remain coherent so that I could correct errors whenever medical professionals provided "prescribed medications" or came to run tests. Figure 1 illustrates my experience. I twice received food to which I was allergic, both times after a doctor "recorded" a list of my food allergies.

Needless to say, I was exhausted from labored breathing, a lung infection, pain, tests, effort expended to correct data model errors, energy wasted giving my medical history, and lack of sleep. Several times I stopped fighting. I relaxed. I thereby slowed respiration to my normal rate. This made my blood oxygen saturation rate drop precipitously, which in turn triggered monitor alarms—to which no one responded. (I learned later from a nurse's assistant that alarms always sound in the ER and the ICU, which is the reason no one pays attention to them.)

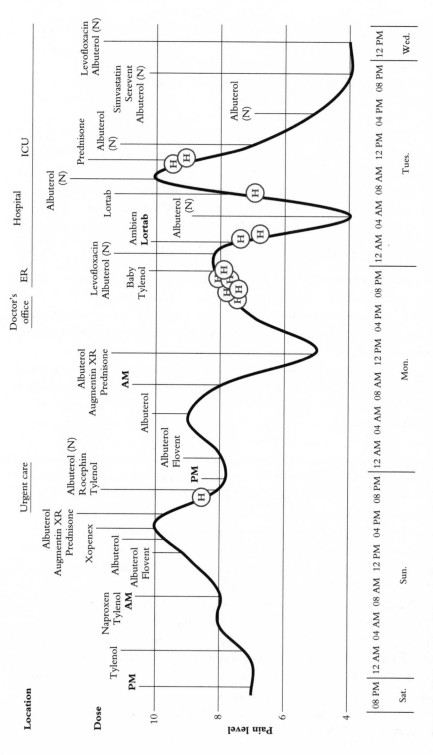

FIGURE 1. Asthma-pneumonia episode chronology. The chart shows the pain level, dosages of medication, and histories taken (H) for the author over five days by location. Daytime medications: Allegra, Nexium, Lisinopril, Omnaris, and Optivar. Nighttime medications: Simvastatin, Omnaris, and Optivar.

I finally understood the problem everyone was having when the heroic ICU nurse explained what she was doing while working with the hospital's electronic health records system. That in turn explained why so many caring, competent, knowledgeable, and talented medical professionals behaved so strangely when interacting with patients. It was because they were fighting a horrible data model. It was that data model that nearly killed me.

Electronic Health Information Systems

Medical personnel at urgent care and at the hospital who interacted with me all used a version of the same electronic health information system (the "system"). It became clear that everyone was fighting that system. Indeed, observations of their performance revealed that they wasted perhaps two fifths to three fifths of their time trying to make the system do something useful for them. The system prevented the medical professionals from fulfilling their duties rather than helping them.

Since my hospital stay, literature research and conversations with medical professionals around the world have confirmed that electronic health information systems are mostly broken. For example, I interviewed medical professionals, health care IT experts, and my allergist. They confirmed my sickbed analysis. Indeed, several experts said that they longed for handwritten charts once more hanging from the foot of every patient's bed.[4] My analysis argues for a less reactive response. The industry requires a careful analysis of the strengths, weaknesses, opportunities, and threats (SWOT) associated with building a national health information network. If the nation simply accepts the NHIN vision while health care IT vendors collect some of the $38 billion stimulus bounty, individuals and businesses will pay higher medical costs, patients will receive inferior care, and medical professionals will lose precious time fighting IT systems instead of delivering better care.

Killer Data Model

Poor data model design deters medical professionals from delivering quality care. Conceptual data models capture information requirements from medical practitioners' perspectives.[5] In contrast, IT professionals only vaguely understand medicine.[6]

There are three types of data models: conceptual, logical, and physical. Logical data models express information requirements from a technical design perspective (for example, schema for relational database management system [RDBMS], schema for extensible markup language [XML] documents, or formats for health insurance claims [a message model]). Logical data models fail if conceptual models are wrong, if errors occur in the transformation of the conceptual model into the logical model (forward engineering), or if logical design is faulty.[7]

The root of the problem I experienced with health information systems is a bad data model. Evidence supporting my claim includes these observations:

- Incoherent database design isolates patient information from one department to the next and from one organization to the next. This wastes time and increases errors because medical personnel must enter patient information into a unique view of the system that corresponds to user identity and department. This prevents one medical professional from seeing patient information input by another medical professional.
- Patient information is easily lost inside the electronic records system.
- Hard copy patient information becomes dissociated from the electronic record.
- Neither the system design nor the data model in this case suited the health care professionals' work patterns. They spent considerably more time performing record searches and data reentry than they spent interacting with me, the patient.
- No master data management (MDM) was in evidence. Producing a consistent record of me as a patient required the ICU nurse to copy data from multiple database views into the inpatient record.
- Records of admitted inpatients are treated differently by the system than are records of outpatient or ER-only patients. No information about my medical history gathered during a prior visit to the same ER was available to my doctors or nurses.
- Nurses and doctors do not have ready access to formulary listings. As a result, they wasted much time searching for information about my daily medications. Access to lists of medications in the system is limited to those at the hospital pharmacy.
- No support existed for recording chronic allergies differently from allergies to ambient sources and foods. Lists of allergies were not available in drop-down menus, although these are well known to allergists and drug companies.

The root cause of these problems is the failure of IT system architects to capture (health care) business requirements correctly. There also is no evidence that anyone ever produced a reliable conceptual data model. The problem occurs commonly. Too often, system architects simply gather lists of requirements, then they ask their favorite vendors to quote the price for a product. This is non-architecture and system non-design. Rarely do architects request information architecture.

Fault also rests with independent software vendors (ISVs) whose products fail to support the requirements of end users: real doctors, nurses, technicians, and pharmacists. Instead they build products to a marketer's or a developer's best guess about end users' requirements. It is easier to rush to market with a product that "looks good" to IT people but horrifies end users. This seems to have been the case with the electronic health information system used by the clinic and the hospital that treated me.

Another common problem is that useful conceptual data–modeling tools do not exist. This broad challenge to the industry makes the best data modelers' task more difficult as they work to create conceptual models, then validate those models with end users. Without good tools, information architects and data modelers often use technical elements to represent business concepts. This leads to problems with forward engineering because health care (business) concepts are mixed with data design technology artifacts. One group, HL7, has been working to develop a health care data model.[8]

IT security professionals in the medical industry appear to be reluctant to deploy document authentication and encryption for users. Many commercial health information systems can produce Adobe Acrobat versions of doctors' reports. These reports could be authenticated through the use of Adobe technology and transmitted to another physician via email encryption programs. The patient might even certify such transmission of his or her information by using electronic systems. This simple practice might have enabled admitting doctors to see my allergist's memorandum in their in-box instead of requiring paper copies to pass from one person to the next until they become lost.

Clearly, the most serious problem is the lack of a consistent data model across departments and providers. This wastes time and increases errors.

Unreliable Information

Poorly articulated data models engender disbelief in system data among end users, who see data inconsistencies in competing entries about patients, their symptoms, their illnesses, and data entered by different physicians and nurses who cared for the patient. This problem was in ample evidence in the eleven full histories taken by every medical professional who checked my condition.

If externally generated information history is difficult to integrate, particularly if that information is not in the form used most frequently by medical professionals in the receiving organization, then there is a propensity to misplace that information. Witness the lost memorandum from my allergist. That document was misplaced shortly after its confirmed delivery to the ER. Its loss dramatically reduced the quality and effectiveness of my care.

Other problems arise when doctors can arbitrarily block nurses or other doctors from completing data entry tasks. Such issues delayed provision of medications appropriate to treating my ailment (such as pain relief medication). Because information was not shared between departments or between the hospital and the clinic, each doctor felt obliged to build a diagnosis, and each nurse had to gather my data anew.

Bad Systems

Clearly, the networked monitors with alarms sounding so frequently that no one believes they mean anything is a serious design problem. Operating inconsistencies among systems and apparatus that increase the rate of false alarms lead to errors in patient care management, some of which are potentially fatal.

IT does provide an event-driven messaging technology to deliver data and manage workflow for doctors and nurses who need to review patient and treatment information. Too much of health care professionals' time is lost in tracing test results and gathering information about medications. These unnecessary activities dramatically increase error rates that lower the quality of patients' care.

Recommendations

A national health information network, while a laudable vision, requires massive data integration engineering at a scale never before undertaken by the IT industry.[9]

The only way to achieve the vision of reliable information transfer requires narrowing the scope of work to demonstrable and doable tasks that can be executed in a finite amount of time. NHIN proponents should not be fooled by IT vendors telling (false) tales of magnificent data exchange capabilities possible with their heath information system development. Instead, those proponents should call upon the best system and data architects to report for duty. Send these people to meet with doctors, nurses, test technicians, pharmacists, and hospital and clinic administrators. Have them learn what practicing medicine really means. Tell them to do these things:

- Build a business (medical information system) requirements model.
- Create a conceptual data model and information architecture.
- Validate these models in a public forum, as HL7 does, those used by open standards organizations such as OASIS, Object Management Group (OMG), Worldwide Web Consortium (W3C), and others.
- After the models are validated, create formal requests for information (RFIs) for vendors.
- Heath information technology vendors can respond to the RFI so you can see whose system matches those requirements.
- Seek hospital and clinic volunteers to test the new systems.
- Find the best matches to requirements and submit to the winning vendors a request for proposal (RFP) to build and install the first systems at the volunteers' facilities.
- Narrow down the list of vendors and send them a request for a quote or proposal to decide who will win the initial integration trial between two medical institutions and between two departments in each of those institutions.
- Establish criteria for success and measure vendors' achievements relative to that target, not one of their making.
- Be sure the vendors work for the volunteers and not for the government. A health information system is needed that meets their unique requirements.
- Integrate the systems. Pay the winning vendors a bonus for early completion.

The National Health Information Network will remain a pipedream unless and until IT professionals learn how to build systems and data models that meet end users' requirements, that is, models useful to medical professionals. My experience with an urgent care clinic and a major hospital convinced me that in the United States, it will be a long time before there is a consistent data model capable of recording a patient's health information, let alone a data model capable of accurately and reliably transmitting that information from one health care institution to another. Much of the groundwork required to achieve the NHIN vision remains undone. The $38 billion–plus allocated by the American Recovery and Reinvestment Act for a health information network will be squandered by IT vendors and hospital administrators long before the nation has a viable network unless the industry acts rationally to establish a program of development that is free of vendor and administrative greed. Take it from a person who found breathing quite difficult, and who nearly died because of a failed data model: Do not hold your breath waiting for a national health information network to appear.

Epilogue

Nearly one year after I posted a version of this article on my personal blog, the health care system continued to be plagued by data inefficiencies and inaccuracies because of insufficient priority being placed on building standard data models. For example, on a visit around that time to her primary care provider, my wife had some X rays taken. Another provider at a different location needed to access those X rays, but because of the lack of a coherent, shared (physical) data model, her X-ray image formats were not readable outside the system that created them. This incompatibility delayed moving forward with the treatment plan prescribed by her physician, and its solution required a second costly examination procedure that would generate serviceable images.

Dozens of health care and IT professionals have commented on my original blog post, both to validate and to express shared concerns about the realities of failed health information systems. Although disagreements were voiced, they related to medical issues associated with my treatment and not my data analysis.

Research I performed since writing of my travails revealed similar problems extant for all national health information networks, both planned and under construction. The root cause of interoperability problems for a national health information network is inadequate or nonexistent data models. Fortunately, data-modeling problems, while difficult, are solvable. For example, data-modeling work could proceed for a single medical subspecialty with limited scope for data transmission requirements. This is a narrower objective than promising to build a national health information network, and a substantial effort by experts at data standards bodies to create a narrowly defined model is feasible.

I hope that articles like this one and others in this book will help health care leaders learn the value of addressing systemic data-modeling issues like those that affected my care. Data-modeling improvements will prevent problems like those I experienced from becoming more commonplace.

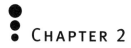

CHAPTER 2

Too Mean to Clean

How We Forgot to Clean Our Hospitals

Rosalind Stanwell-Smith

> The greater part of nursing consists in preserving
> cleanliness.
>
> —Florence Nightingale, *Notes on Nursing*, 1863

In April 2010, the centenary of the death of
Florence Nightingale, a nurse came before the British Nursing and Midwifery Council for having told an elderly bedridden patient to clean up his
urine spillage. Handing him a mop and bucket, she reportedly said, "Here
you go, you can mop it up." Finding her guilty of misconduct, the council
nevertheless ruled that her fitness to practice at a major London teaching
hospital was not impaired. The media were quick to connect this story to
deaths in another English hospital associated with tales of dirty wards and
soiled sheets going unchanged and also to a recent government commission
urging nurses to take better care of patients.[1] Such stories are not restricted
to the United Kingdom: there is general concern in the United States and
other "developed" countries that hospitals are not as clean as they should
be—nor as clean as they were in the past. Florence Nightingale would be
horrified, having emphasized throughout her career the necessity for hospital
cleanliness and the responsibility of nurses in maintaining it. The duty was
not theirs alone but a supervisory role that still largely persists, though now
perhaps eroded and certainly undermined. Unions for cleaning staff attribute the cause of this undermining to the policy of contracting out cleaning
services with insufficient budgets, as well as to poorly trained staff. Another
underlying trend, not as frequently cited, is the declining importance of environmental hygiene as a clinical topic. Once the chief focus of public health,

along with control of infection, "hygiene" now ranks very low among the targets for hospital performance. Examining the historical development of "hospital hygiene" and shifts in the public perception of cleanliness helps to explain how our hospital cleaning services have reached their present state. This chapter also examines some of the modern dilemmas and the relationship between cleaning, infection, and health care.

The Rise and Fall of the Sparkling-Clean Hospital

> It may seem a strange principle to enunciate as the very first requirement in a Hospital that it should do the sick no harm.
>
> —Florence Nightingale, *Notes on Nursing,* 1863

> Over 12% of hospital liability claims are associated with infections, injuries and other conditions that patients contracted in the hospital itself. It's what some are calling "dirty hospital syndrome."
>
> —Free Legal Advice website, 2010

Medieval hospitals were charitable refuges for the sick poor, and this was still much the case by the nineteenth century. Anesthetics, Listerism (use of antisepsis), and the humanizing role of nurses championed by Florence Nightingale transformed these places into all-purpose medical institutions, but other influences, such as the need to care for soldiers and sailors injured in war, also gradually established cleanliness at the center of hospital care. The development of hygiene, cleanliness, and health care did not follow a neat, linear progression through the ages, although in the early days of public health as a profession it was often portrayed as doing so. This was largely due to the triumphs of nineteenth- and early-twentieth-century sanitary advances, leading to airy hospitals with tiled walls and a strong smell of carbolic disinfectant, underpinned by drains, sewers, and clean water supplies. So hygiene, originally a classical term for general health and well-being, was narrowed in scope, first to scrubbing brushes (Florence Nightingale ordered three hundred of them as soon as she and her team arrived at Scutari during the Crimean War, 1854–1856);[2] then becoming a term almost synonymous with disinfection. The drive for better cleanliness *preceded* the establishment of the germ theory, for the previous prevailing philosophy of the "miasmatic" spread of infectious disease held that "miasmas" present in stale and fetid air contained noxious vapors and poisonous particles from decomposition of organic matter.[3] Thus a clean, pleasant-smelling environment meant the absence of miasmas and infection. Moving air and flowing water were thought to be safe. The germ theory of disease came many years later and was not linked to hospitals' original focus on cleanliness. Ironically, many doctors and nurse leaders resisted the germ theory of disease because they felt it would detract from cleaning efforts.

Improved means of ventilation in nineteenth-century hospitals, such as high ceilings and open windows, were inspired by the miasma theory, in turn harking back to ancient temples of health, spas, and that eighteenth-century fashion, favored by Benjamin Franklin and many others, of "air bathing," although most people wore clothes to take their recommended daily outdoor exercise. While the poor succumbed from infection in overcrowded, filthy early hospitals, the rich visited spas and inhaled fresh breezes, though they too were vulnerable to infection, since the mode of transmission was not understood. The miasma model of disease transmission dated back to the work of the Hippocratic school from around 300 BC but was not formally developed as a theory until the early eighteenth century.[4] The opposing theory, that many diseases were contagious, was voiced in the eighteenth century and first explicitly stated by Fracastoro in the sixteenth century.[5] Early microscopes, from the late 1600s, also encouraged the idea that there were many things too small for the naked eye to see. Focusing on miasma, however, had the additional advantage of averting costly quarantine measures, so was strongly supported by political and economic groups.[6] The debate about the role of environment and the potential role of microbes waged throughout the nineteenth century, even after the discoveries of Pasteur, Koch, and other microbiological pioneers. Florence Nightingale, like many of her contemporaries, was not enthusiastic about the discovery of bacteria as a cause of infection: while grudgingly accepting the existence of microbes toward the end of her career, she also feared that the germ theory would lead to complacency and a decline in sanitary standards.[7] She championed the "pavilion" hospital design, which originated in eighteenth-century France and was introduced to England in the mid-nineteenth century. The guiding "pavilion principle" was to improve ventilation and thus reduce mortality by diluting or removing miasmas: the design allowed a greater degree of separation and segregation of patients and activities.[8] When Nightingale referred to sanitary reform, she included cleanliness but was most eager to increase hospital ventilation and light. She believed that smallpox could be bred in the stagnant air of a closed room and that bad sanitation caused the newly discovered bacteria.[9] While these beliefs were wrong, the obsession with fresh air and cleanliness in hospitals by the turn of the twentieth century was indubitably helpful for infection control, especially as there was very little effective treatment before the antibiotic era: "From a practical point of view the miasma theory, although eventually discredited, led to important public health interventions."[10]

Florence Nightingale might have observed that the obverse also applied: the establishment of the role of microorganisms in the transmission of infectious disease, followed by the development of antimicrobial drugs and vaccines, may also have sowed the seeds of complacency about hospital cleaning. It became clear in the early twentieth century that "no amount of ventilation could kill germs,"[11] so hospital architecture evolved into the labyrinth of windowless corridors and rooms familiar to us today. Demographic analysis of the causes of death rates and population trends focused on nutrition and hazardous exposures rather than on the contribution of poor hygiene, this topic being thoroughly outdated by the 1970s. The "March of Hygiene" embraced by the late-nineteenth-century reformers thus petered out, not least because the concept of hygiene had been tainted by the new discoveries. The ancient model of hygiene included the effort to eliminate sickness by purification, removing those bad miasmatic odors. When rediscovered and developed in the seventeenth century as a protection against plague, elimination of bad odors by cleansing became a cornerstone of science.[12] The aftermath of the removal of that miasma cornerstone, and the subsequent crumbling of the hygiene edifice, is still with us today, reflected in relatively little research and low priority for cleaning, despite protestations of its importance from governments and health care managers.

Cleaning was of course not eliminated in the decline of the scientific relevance of hygiene. Cleaning products are a major industry, with replacement of unpleasant odors by sweet smells an interesting vestige of the miasma theory. Nor have infections disappeared, and the mid-twentieth-century optimism surrounding antimicrobial agents and vaccines has been shaken by the discovery of new infectious diseases and the reemergence of old ones. The cleaning emphasis has shifted from scrubbing and disinfecting every surface from ceilings to bedposts, to concentrating on places where microbes might be gathering, such as the surfaces of instrument carts and food service areas, as well as on personal hygiene such as hand washing and the use of protective, disposable clothing. Toward the end of the twentieth century, this shift was also associated with concerns about the overuse of disinfectants and cleaning agents, leading to the "Are we too clean?" debate and the "hygiene hypothesis," proposing that exposure to some types of microbes in early infancy is beneficial to the development of the immune system, with low or no exposure possibly causing allergic disorders.[13] Such debates were not intended to support perceptibly grubby hospital floors or a cut in cleaning staff, yet they may have contributed to a new zeitgeist with regard to cleanliness, not just encompassing the idea that cleaning can be overdone but also allotting it a lower priority in the highly technological modern hospital, where targets involve patient outcomes, not sparkling-clean walls and floors. The result has been questions about why, where, and how frequently we need to clean both high–and low–infection risk areas in our hospitals. Once something has been questioned, it cannot be long before budget managers examine how it can be reduced. This has occurred in hospitals, leading also to the possibility of contracting out specified levels of cleaning, as well as reports and surveys addressing public and health staff concerns about perceived drops in cleaning standards and their contribution to the "superbugs" that now stalk health care facilities.

In response to repeated concerns about hygiene and cleanliness in hospitals, as well as rising levels of antibiotic resistance in hospital infections, a "Matron's Charter" was published for England in 2004, aiming to strengthen the authority of nurses in maintaining cleaning standards. The reference to "Matron" was a nod to widespread public respect for this role since the Florence Nightingale era, though it was abolished in the UK in 1966 and replaced by complicated tiers of nursing and nonclinical managers. In reintroducing the title "Matron" into this hierarchy, the aim was to give cleaning authority back to a senior nurse. The secretary of state for health summed up the principles of the charter as "cleanliness is everyone's responsibility, not just the cleaner's," with much emphasis on all staff getting involved in keeping hospitals clean. It contained a statement reminiscent of Florence Nightingale: "A clean and tidy environment creates a virtuous circle of good practice—a dirty one encourages an attitude of sloppiness and neglect."[14]

While there has been little research and therefore sparse evidence of the influence of a virtuous circle for cleaning in hospitals, this statement draws on sociobehavioral research into what motivates people to clean up an environment or respond to hygiene improvement initiatives. The effectiveness of health-related behavior change programs is hard to prove and may depend on using local research, locally appropriate channels of communication, and repeated interventions over an extended time. So nationally issued platitudes about being clean and tidy may not do the trick. We know from research into graffiti and street litter that people are more disposed to alter their environmental behavior if they receive repeated feedback,[15] and also that the environment and pollution are ranked high by the public in surveys of important issues for governments, at least in the UK.[16] These surveys do not get into specific issues such as dirty hospitals, although there is no doubt that it is both a public and a media concern. Behavioral research suggests that other factors must be included before people become more willing to care actively for the environment, such as self-esteem, belongingness, self-efficacy, personal control, and optimism.[17] To this list we might add belief systems about whether a contribution will make a real difference. In the present context, do staff, patients, and visitors believe that environmental cleaning will have an impact on hospital infection—and do they believe this enough to contribute actively to the process? At this point, we should consider the rationale, in the post-Nightingale era, for why we clean hospitals.

Why Hospitals Need to Be Cleaned

> It is difficult to defend high levels of hygiene when there is little scientific evidence to support cleaning practices.
>
> —S. J. Dancer, "Mopping Up Hospital Infection," 1999

When the Department of Health (DH) in England announced a costly deep-cleaning program for 1,500 hospitals in September 2008, it was roundly attacked.[18] Health service managers were skeptical that this would cut infection rates, the very reason why it had been proposed, while academics questioned the scientific evidence base and accused the government of pandering to populism. Microbiologists weighed in with the information that the deep-clean effect would last only a few weeks. Even the cleaning companies, which stood to profit from the program, argued that better funding for day-to-day cleaning would be a preferable policy. The deep-cleaning initiative had been prompted by the relentless spread of antibiotic-resistant bacterial infections and outbreaks of infection, such as methicillin-resistant *Staphylococcus aureus,* (MRSA), *Clostridium difficile,* and vancomycin-resistant *Enterococci.* In some ways, the concept of "deep cleaning" recalls the Nightingale era, involving wall washing, dismantling and cleaning of beds, and cleaning behind radiators and light fixtures. Instead of the late-nineteenth-century method of cleaning with copious quantities of hot water and pungent disinfectants, the process uses high-tech equipment such as ultrasonic machines, steam cleaners, and hydrogen peroxide vaporizers. There are several points of interest in this policy and its reception: first, that cleanliness had reemerged as a way of combating epidemics; second, that understanding about the role of cleanliness appears to have become a bit confused, as though a one-time scrub of everything would suffice to ward off those invisible microbial invaders (if only); and third, that if there were funds for this exercise (£63 million, around $80 million), why had they not been used to maintain a higher level of cleaning on a regular basis?

It was all a lot easier before evidence-based practice. This is not to denigrate the progress due to an evidence-based approach in examining treatment efficacy. The relationship between hospital cleanliness and hospital infection is harder to investigate, not least because of uncertainty about how to define cleanliness in a health care setting and the role of the staff, patients, and visitors in spreading infection. The lack of a generally accepted evidence base on cleaning and infection risk is central to the current dilemmas about hospital cleaning.

The evidence that infections can be acquired in hospitals is not in dispute. For example, an audit report for the British National Health Service (NHS) in 2000 estimated 100,000 nosocomial infections annually, costing approximately £1 billion to treat and associated with fifteen thousand deaths.[19] It was estimated that a third of these infections were preventable by infection control; a later government report revised the figure upwards, to 300,000 cases a year while also claiming large reductions in MRSA and *C. difficile* infections following various infection control initiatives.[20] The *Chicago Tribune* investigated infection-related deaths in the United States, claiming that cleaner facilities, instruments, and hands could prevent 75 percent of the estimated 103,000 annual deaths from hospital infections.[21] The *Tribune* investigators also reported evidence of inadequate training of cleaning staff and progressive cuts in cleaning budgets. With this plethora of things to blame—training, cleaning of buildings and of instruments, infection control work, hand washing—the evidence base table of factors is already groaning with uncertainties and measurement quandaries. So the British government's quick solution of deep cleaning becomes more understandable. Yet it would seem that splurging on deep cleaning, instead of increasing education, cleaning staff, and easier-to-clean facilities, is possibly the least evidence-based approach. There is evidence for reducing infection risk by improving "basic" cleaning; for example, a seven-year-study in the United States found that it reduced levels of nosocomial *C. difficile*.[22] The interventions comprised a set of "aggressive infection control measures" covering isolation and precautions policies, the use of disinfectant and antibacterial soap, and other factors, as well as cleaning. It is interesting to note that "mandatory" monthly education sessions were instituted for health care workers, but cleaning staff did not attend, their training being left to environmental service supervisors. There have been several other studies demonstrating how cleaning can help interrupt the chain of infection.[23] Most studies concern the broad topic of infection control measures, confounding estimates of the contribution of cleaning alone, for infection control must include cleaning of various types, although the broad textbook definition of infection control does not necessarily encompass mopping the floors and other mundane cleaning tasks:

Each hospital has many procedures and policies which attempt to reduce the chances of hospital infection occurring, but the extent to which these policies are effectively carried out on a day-to-day basis varies greatly between different hospitals or different areas in the hospital. Relevant procedures include those carried out for the sterilization and disinfection of contaminated items and disposal of infected rubbish or linen, and aseptic techniques in the operating theatre and in the wards for procedures such as changing wound dressings, urinary catheterization and setting up an intravenous drip; the "source" isolation of highly susceptible patients, preferably according to an agreed policy; the education of staff in hospital hygiene; good staff health facilities; the adequate use of the clinical microbiology department for the precise bacteriological diagnosis. An essential administrative requirement for the effective control of hospital infection is an active infection control team.[24]

A perusal of other current infection control definitions showed that cleaning, other than that regarding surgical instruments and aseptic technique, is conspicuous by its absence. In a few published studies the role of what we may term "general environmental cleaning" can be disentangled, epidemiologically, from an assortment of other measures. For example, attempts to contain the spread of MRSA in an English hospital by stringent infection control measures were not successful until they were supplemented by doubling the cleaning hours and allocating responsibility for the cleaning of ward medical equipment.[25] In a hospital outbreak of MRSA in Scotland, increasing cleaning times from a paltry two hours daily in a surgical unit also halted the spread.[26] Infection control teamwork and efficient cleaning are both labor-intensive, but it has been observed that good cleaning is achievable, whereas enforcement of hand washing and good antibiotic prescribing are not.[27]

A 2007 historical analysis of the changing meaning of hygiene over the ages identified the emergence of personal hygiene as a major influence in modern society.[28] So it is not surprising that people dismayed by the perceived careless approach to cleaning in hospitals, and all those "superbugs," should seek personal hygiene solutions to "dirty" clinical environments. In 2009 a Scottish primary care physician reported the increasing use of "hygiene packs" for those going into the hospital.[29] For around £16 ($21), patients or their anxious relatives could purchase a pack containing soap, lip balm, fabric spray, surface wipes, body wash, and illustrations about how to use them. Their popularity seemed to rest in part on the sense of giving people more power over their immediate surroundings, a "zone of protection," even if the floor and bedside lockers looked as though they could use a good cleaning. Critics pointed out the lack of any evidence for their efficacy, while supporters argued for the psychological benefits and claimed that this type of pack provided a reminder of the importance of behaviors such as hand washing and cleaning surfaces. On this basis, it could be argued that the packs did not go far enough: Why not include toilet paper, to account for the mysterious absence of toilet rolls (as well as soap) in many hospital toilets and bathrooms, perhaps because these items are often unfortunately pilfered by mean-minded people; or because there are not enough house-keeping staff to keep them topped up? Why not add facemasks to the pack, to don when there seem to be body fluids or noxious aerosols in the vicinity? Personal pillowcases—and, let's face it, your own pillow untouched by other patients—would seem useful items in this "personal protection zone" approach. Silver-threaded pajamas to ward off infection are available, but sadly not your own member of the cleaning staff to disinfect problem areas constantly, such as the alarm buzzer, patient console, bed frames, radiators, and door handles. The company responsible for the leading hygiene pack on sale in the UK was forced to change its advertising after receiving complaints, removing the phrase "essential for your wellbeing." The underlying lack of confidence in hospital cleanliness, which had brought the company sales of around ten thousand packs a month, was broadly ignored.

The renewed public interest in hospital cleanliness is related to the publication of hospital infection rates and news of major outbreaks of nosocomial infection.[30] Several countries have been publishing rates for some time, though only recently with readily available details of which hospitals are best or worst on these rates. In the United States, legislation in 2005 required publication of rates of hospital-acquired infection (HAI), leading to the increasing availability to the public of rates in their local facilities. National figures are startling enough—for example, over 100,000 cases of HAI (9% of inpatients), associated with five thousand deaths, in England in 2000 and around 2 million HAI cases annually in the United States between 1990 and 1999—but they are also increasing.[31] Much depends on definitions and quality of surveillance, so it is possible to claim a decline for some infections or in some patient categories, or to argue that increases may be related to greatly improved ascertainment with compulsory and more comprehensive reporting. With the rising use of central venous lines and catheters and prolonged survival of seriously ill people, one might expect an inevitable increase in infections, or so the official line goes. Initially, these publicized figures and rates led to calls for more infection control staff, especially as surveys showed that these were below recommended levels in many hospitals.[32] In a follow-up to its 2000 report, the National Audit Office for England highlighted concerns in 2005 about "patchy progress" and "a distinct lack of urgency on issues such as cleanliness and compliance with good hand hygiene."[33]

The DH for England published a report in 2004, backed by legislation and a new code of practice for the prevention and control of HAIs, with ambitious targets for the reduction of infections particularly associated with hospitals, such as *C. difficile* and MRSA.[34] Reporting on good progress with targets overall, particularly *C. difficile,* in 2009, the National Audit Office concluded that the £120 million spent on control of infection in the previous three years, including the £63 million "deep clean," had saved an estimated £141 million to £263 million in treatment costs.[35] Nevertheless, there is still considerable skepticism about whether spending on cleaning is the answer. In the 2004 English DH report, the role of cleaning in infection control appeared to be sidelined as part of making a "good first impression," "just like a clean hotel," in other words, mainly as an issue of public perception:

> Cleanliness and infection control are closely linked in the public mind, but there are important distinctions to be made. Cleanliness contributes to infection control, but preventing infections requires more than simple cleanliness. Cleanliness produces a pleasant, tidy, safe environment that makes us feel better; however, the scientific evidence that the environment is an important contributor to infection rates is not always clear cut.[36]

This was supported by a study examining hospital cleanliness ratings and rates of MRSA. Researchers in the north of England reported in 2006 that they had been unable to establish a link between hospital cleanliness and lower rates of this infection, commenting: "Programmes that target standards of hospital cleanliness alone are unlikely to succeed in lowering MRSA infection rates. A high standard of hospital cleanliness is certainly a goal worth achieving. However, it is not helpful for trusts [hospital administrations], and specifically infection control teams."[37] The annual infection control report for hospitals where this research was conducted nonetheless reported that, while there had been progress in delivery and monitoring of environmental cleaning, "further work is still required to ensure that timely and effective cleaning of patient care equipment occurs. Accessibility to out of hours cleaning services needs to be improved."[38]

The hospital cleanliness surveys used by these researchers were based on visual assessments, which may not be sufficient to determine appropriate levels of cleaning. A study to evaluate hospital cleaning regimes reported in 2000 that 76 percent of surfaces in an operating room and a hospital ward were unacceptable after standard cleaning, as demonstrated by microbiological methods and ATP (adenosine triphosphate) bioluminescence, although only 18 percent were rated unacceptable when judged by visual assessment.[39]

With hospital infection control budgets being squeezed, one can understand the reluctance to identify spending more on environmental cleaning as preferable to, say, funding more infection control nurses or hand washing initiatives. But when hospital infection control teams try to improve environmental cleaning, they encounter a particular difficulty. Many of these services have been separated from any direct clinical management, and a large proportion of cleaning work has been contracted to outside firms. The chair of the Infection Control Nurses Association in the UK commented with classic understatement that it was "quite surprising" to discover shortcomings such as cleaning cloths and mops going unwashed from day to day and that training requirements for cleaners were often cut from contracts to save costs. The UK government Committee on Science and Technology observed that with cleaners not being responsible to a ward nurse, "instilling high standards and pride in the job is more difficult" and referred to "penny pinching" by contractors as a possible cause of falling hygiene standards, among other factors such as policies to maximize bed occupancy, failure to isolate infectious patients, and the perennial problem of inadequate hand washing. On a visit to the United States, this committee learned that these problems are not confined to the UK. One member of the National Institute of Allergy and Infectious Diseases (NIAID) told them that there was a general breakdown in hygiene, infection control, and public health programs. The committee recommended that "purchasers and commissioning agencies for hospital services should put infection control and basic hygiene where they belong, at the heart of good hospital management and practice, and should redirect resources accordingly; such a policy will pay for itself quite quickly."[40] This was the only recommendation pertaining to cleaning. As with so many reports, it bundles together infection control with basic environmental cleaning; and the optimistic claim of the policy paying for itself has been contested, as we have seen, by some researchers and by government departments. But at least the issue of external contractors was raised. We next need to consider whether "contracting out" is the problem in cleaning up our hospitals.

Contracting Out

Catering Staff to Fill In for Axed Hospital Cleaners amid MRSA Fears

—headline, *Evening Times* (Glasgow), April 9, 2010

Nurses have called for hospital cleaning to be brought back in-house to tackle hospital infections.

—BBC news, April 29, 2008

In the glory days of hospital hygiene, there was no concept of "outsourc-ing," contracting out cleaning to companies that offer attractive cost savings. Cleaning contracts in the UK have been outsourced since the 1980s, with a rising trend that is difficult to estimate as this information is not centrally collated: it was estimated at around 30 percent of UK hospitals in 2005;[41] and slightly higher in 2008, at 40 percent, by the Cleaning and Support Services Association, which represents British hospital cleaning firms.[42] The increas-ing use of "multiservice contracts" covering cleaning, laundry, catering, and so on makes precise figures elusive. Outsourcing of cleaning services in U.S. hospitals started earlier, but with a similar increase to that in the UK as a result of cost pressures in the 1990s, as well as a perception that cleaning, along with services such as food and transportation, are outside the "core competency" areas of hospital administrators, and therefore outside contracts are suitable, even preferable.[43] Concerns about high staff turnover and poor performance have led a few hospitals to return to in-house "ward domestics." But with complicated chains of command, "in-house" does not necessarily mean a revival of the good old days with nurses having clear authority for cleaning on their wards. While visiting an elderly relative in the hospital, I noticed an unsightly mess of paper and fluid on the ward floor: another patient had called for help in getting to the toilet, but with no help arriving had been un-able to get there in time. The nurses had covered the urine with the paper as they had to wait for a "cleanup squad" to clear it up. The mess was still there an hour later. But are examples like this due to outsourcing, to poor manage-ment and low priority for cleaning, or to the competitive tendering process, which possibly encourages a sacrifice of quality for cost, whether or not an in-house service wins the contract? Private cleaning firms have claimed that standards would be no better with a return to "in-house" cleaning; and when asked to comment on a report that nurses had called for hospital cleaning to be brought back in-house, the DH for England replied that infection rates did not differ between hospitals using outsourced versus in-house services.[44] Health service researchers have countered this with evidence for the link between cleaning and infection control, supporting a view that government ministers are reluctant to compare longitudinal data for cleaning standards and infection rates, and to recognize the link with contracting out to the lowest bid.[45] British nurses seem confident that in-house is better, however; for example, a nurse told their annual conference in 2008, "I have worked in hospitals which used private firms and the dirt was there for all to see."[46]

Studies of contracted-out cleaning present a rather confused picture of whether outsourcing is the real problem. Monitoring of a private cleaning service at Denmark's National Hospital showed that quality of cleaning had improved over a four-year contract, while also saving 43 percent over the in-house costs.[47] Generally higher levels of cleaning performance were also reported for competitive tendering of hospital cleaning in Sydney, Australia.[48] In another Australian study of three hospitals, the cheapest contract bids achieved improved service for less cost in two hospitals (one using an in-house service) but serious deterioration of service in the third.[49] A UK report from Patient Environment Action Teams (PEATs) in 2004 rated hospital cleaning as "poor" more frequently in hospitals cleaned by private contractors (fifteen of the twenty-four were rated poor).[50] PEATs were set up in 2000 to do annual inspections of NHS inpatient health care sites, giving scores for areas such as food, cleanliness, and infection control. More recent reports suggest improvement, with only nine sites (1 percent of those surveyed) being rated as poor and three as "unacceptable" in the environment category, which includes other factors such as décor and lighting.[51] The UK, with its state-funded National Health Service, has to show value for taxpayers' money in a number of ways, but the rise of resistant bacterial infections has resulted in calls for a more generous budget for cleaning. An independent report for the trade union representing the largest number of cleaning staff reviewed literature on outsourced cleaning and concluded that while it was intended to raise efficiency by giving more choice of suppliers, this rhetoric of choice disguised its opposite, "with the imposition of a single model of service provision—one that may cut costs but is unable to focus on quality."[52] Unions, of course, have an agenda where the associated problems of pay and staffing levels are concerned, but the report argued that the disadvantages of outsourcing include other issues:

- Difficulties in drawing up contracts in "complex practical situations" such as hospitals, for example, in specifying all eventualities, thus providing little incentive to go beyond levels specified; also the difficulty of monitoring performance and adjusting levels of service as needed.
- Lack of information given to hospital managers because of the commercial sensitivity of data held by outsourced companies, so that quality and value are hard to assess—including the reported high levels of absence due to sickness for this type of work.
- Inflexibility that may not allow, for example, for rapid enhancement of cleaning during an infection outbreak or for modification of a job description beyond the narrow role specified in the contract.
- Difficulties of imposing sanctions: penalty clauses are of little use if performance is hard to measure or if sanctions would damage relationships with contractors or with other types of service, where there is a multiservice contract.

- Separation of the cleaners from the rest of the health care team. By definition, outsourced cleaners are outsiders who may have little interaction with clinical workers and who may feel they have no role in patient care or that they are important in the associated control of infection.

Following a serious salmonella outbreak in a Scottish hospital, clinical staff pointed to long-standing concerns about the quality and frequency of contract cleaning: the contract had been renegotiated, but prior to the outbreak, staff had not been able to get the cleaning inadequacies addressed.[53] Inflexibility of contracts seems a fair point, but rigidity of working routine is not confined to private contracted workers; publicly funded services, too, have long acquired the reputation for too many "Jobsworths" (as in "It's more than my job's worth, guv"), or for complacent attitudes toward quality and efficiency stemming from public-sector job security. It is also easy to see how the regular salaried staff may find agency, temporary, and other outside staff a convenient scapegoat when things go wrong, as in a hospital epidemic. The rate of absence due to sickness in hospital domestic staff is higher than for other staff groups, running at 7.6 percent, compared with 4.2 percent for all UK employees.[54] Indeed, one of the perceived advantages in contracting out hospital (and other building) cleaning in the 1980s and 1990s was providing more reliable service; but an audit of absence in Wales indicated that ancillary hospital workers lost 8.1 percent of contracted hours through sickness,[55] suggesting that it is the job, rather than who employs the workers, that is the real problem. One clue is the point about separating cleaners from the clinical staff, so they neither attend team briefings nor take part in training and social activities organized by hospital staff. Another concern is the social or language divide that may exist between the health care team and the people who come in to clean. The divide may also include immigration status. In November 2009, managers of a British cleaning company were arrested for allegedly employing illegal immigrants and also for pocketing the wages of former workers after they left. Their company supplied more than 43,000 cleaners to NHS and private hospitals around Britain.[56]

What the Cleaners Say

> Why don't those journalists writing the newspaper articles, and claiming that our hospital is dirty, ask the obvious question about how many staff there are to clean it?
>
> —Housekeeper in English hospital, *Cleaners' Voices*, 2005

In response to the "Matron's Charter," which highlighted perceptions of poor cleaning, a trade union commissioned a series of interviews with cleaning staff and their managers in December 2004.[57] While the union's opposition to outsourcing was clear, probably influencing the selection of cleaners' views in the report, the words of the staff themselves suggested a more deep-rooted problem in the organization of cleaning services. For example, one worker commented, "It's quite obvious that there is no common culture of hygiene or awareness of infection risks. The problem runs from top to bottom," citing problems such as operating room staff and doctors "swanning around," taking meals and breaks in their surgical scrubs, or nurses wearing their uniforms off-site. Others complained that they were not included in discussions about infection problems, such as the need for more thorough cleaning during an infection outbreak or alert. Lack of respect for or interest in their work was another frequent theme, for example, in this poignant comment from a ward assistant: "On the wards, sadly we are still looked upon as being something under the shoe, so we are only allowed to speak when we are spoken to."

Other views in the same vein included "Some nurses are a problem, they just think they are above you. You are a domestic and you are not as good as them," and "Many of them [nurses] have never done any cleaning work themselves, and don't seem to realise how much effort is involved." (The latter would never have been the case in the Nightingale days!) The dislocation in modern hospitals between nursing care and cleaning was an inevitable consequence of increasingly specialized and highly trained nursing, but with the result that cleaners are cynical about calls for a team approach to hospital cleanliness:

> We are continuously being told we are part of a team. But you have people, other members of staff, walking down the stairs who will spot a scrap of paper of something lying on the floor, and instead of picking up, they ring and demand that one of us has to stop what we are doing and go to collect it. Surely a cleaner hospital should be everybody's job, and the team that we keep hearing about has to work together?

The cleaners also felt that they were put at risk by not being told about infectious cases: "We've had TB and scabies cases, and nobody has told us anything, have they? We've had the lot. It's as though they don't care about domestics, while they get all gowned up before they go in. We can take our chances." Many commented on reduction of staffing for this work, which again seems to be part of the general squeezing of hospital care budgets in tough economic times, rather than something than can be blamed solely on competitive tendering: "They have cut us down, cut us down during this contracting out, so when they brought us back in house on the bare minimum, and it's all down to money."

"Teamwork" as far as the cleaners are concerned, may involve simply doing a wider range of tasks because of these cuts, as this male domestic commented: "It has got worse. They used to have a cleaner in the evenings. If you were lucky. But if not, you had to do the bins, mop the floor and serve the food, too."

Long-established policies to reduce hospital stays and maximize bed occupancy have also had an effect on cleaning efficiency: "The hospital is packed every day of the week, every week of the year, giving us no chance to do any deep cleaning or anything like that. So wards are left with just the basic cleaning and that's it."

There were frequent comments about being expected to accomplish in one hour what should reasonably take three, as well as poor cover for sick days or leave. While a cynical view would be that this is what one would expect cleaners to say, the lack of staff is supported by government surveys, for example, by the auditor general for Scotland, who reported that staff time available for cleaning fell below planned levels in a quarter of wards surveyed in 2002, while the time for monitoring was below planned levels in a third of the wards.[58] Performance indicators for sick days, turnover, and vacancies were not in place in half the hospitals surveyed. The irony of "planned levels" of cleaning is that on occasion, cleaners have been told that they were working too far *above* the level, or "too clean." One can sympathize with the exasperated comment: "Too clean? How can you have a hospital that's too clean?"[59]

In-Sourcing Cleaning

> Healthcare associated infection has in the past not been as high a priority for action as some other aspects of health care.
>
> —Liam Donaldson, Chief Medical Officer for England, UK Department of Health website, 2003

As Florence Nightingale might have commented, with severe disapproval, it may seem a strange principle to enunciate that a hospital can be too clean. Yet this is what specifying standards of cleaning may imply, and it is what cleaners say they are told. Reports of dirty hospitals and views of the public and clinical staff suggest that we have evolved quite a muddled approach to cleaning our hospitals. From pavilions of air, light, and cleanliness, those advanced nineteenth- and early-twentieth-century hospitals, we seem to have progressed to increasingly technical environments where the role of the mop and bucket has little prominence. Infection control within hospitals has become sophisticated and enshrined in policies, but with so many factors to consider, it is not surprising that basic cleaning of the hospital environment has little priority. Worse, it is largely outside the remit of infection control teams. Cleaners have indicated that they want to be considered part of the team, but there are education, patient confidentiality, and other barriers to including them in all discussions, so realistically, is that going to happen at more than a token level? With hospitals struggling to update infection control training for frontline staff, we've also learned that training may be conveniently dropped from contracts for cleaning, whether in-house or out-sourced. Putting cleaning firmly back into the control of the clinical staff on wards and surgical units seems to be an excellent solution. There is just the megalithic management structure to sort out. In difficult economic times, nursing and medical posts have been cut along with cleaning budgets, putting clinical staff under ever more pressure, so one can understand why many just leave the cleaning staff to get on with their work and don't communicate much with them. The equality rhetoric of our times has not yet solved the problem of making people feel equal and part of a team when their mundane work keeps them apart: "never the twain will meet," as a ward assistant expressed it.[60] These jobs are low paid, with little respect from co-workers and the added disincentive of an infection risk about which cleaners have little knowledge or training to protect themselves. If "integrated health care" is to include cleaning staff, the focus should not be so much on outsourcing and competitive tendering, for all its possibly negative effect on standards, as on revaluing the cleaning work itself.

The other theme arising from the hospital cleaning debate is that we have forgotten not just how to clean hospitals but why. If the scientists cannot agree about the contribution of environmental cleaning to preventing infection, then there will be no progress in cleaning up hospitals. The politicians and others controlling the budgets need to receive clear messages. If various opposing factions present cases for more infection control staff, hand washing leaflets, isolation facilities, and other worthy issues, cleaning will always be the overlooked "Cinderella." This theme of why we should clean hospitals is closely linked to our success in dealing with infectious disease in general. Although there are still some serious, relatively untreatable infections lurking in hospitals, there has been a general decline in the fear of infection—for have we not sorted out, in the wealthier parts of the planet at least, cholera, typhoid fever, typhus fever, smallpox, and other traditional scourges of our populations? This makes infection at once something eminently manageable in the public eye but also disproportionately scary when a new, incurable infection such as HIV emerges. Health care personnel are not immune from this combination of complacency about hand washing and cleanliness, even in high-risk areas, and seemingly fatalistic helplessness when faced with new infection hazards or outbreaks. When, while investigating an outbreak on a liver transplant unit as a trainee infection epidemiologist, I observed to a doctor that staff hardly ever washed their hands between patients, I was told, "Quite honestly, infection is the least of their problems." Campaigns on the importance of hand washing may have changed the way this opinion might now be expressed, but not the underlying attitude toward the importance of controlling infection. Compliance with hand washing is outside the scope of this chapter: suffice it to say that it is still a major issue in infection control and that since hands touch so many potentially contaminated surfaces, environmental cleaning surely has a key role. In outbreak investigations and research projects over the years, I have been struck by how often infections have been seen as not preventable, as somehow an inevitable occurrence in hospitals. It is only around a century and a half since deaths from infection were simply to be expected, with pioneers of hand washing and antisepsis initially mocked. Infection control specialists and their teams are changing the complacency in these better-informed times, but few seem to be fighting for the cleaners. Whether we are truly more enlightened, given our approach to hospital cleaning, remains debatable.

The underlying beliefs about the effectiveness of environmental cleaning are important because of their persistent influence on behavior—and priorities. Even if people are convinced of an impact on health, bringing about changes in health-related behavior has been described as a complex and uncertain exercise.[61] The "Matron's Charter" contained this admonishment: "Cleanliness can be catching. All staff should work tidily and clear up after themselves. . . . Even the best cleaner cannot be everywhere at once."[62] Cleanliness can be catching? This interesting take on the debate turns the old theories of hygiene upside down: in an era in which many no longer believe that dirty environments lead one to catch infections, we seem to need to recall virtuous past ways and exhort teams to clean up hospitals, while there is uncertainty in government and scientific circles alike as to why we should do this. This is in part due to the replacement of the miasma model, which led to widespread cleaning to eliminate sources of dirt and odor, and by the germ theory, which has redirected the march of hygiene toward attacking microbes with antibiotics and avoiding them via sterile procedures. It would appear that we lost the cleaning paradigm when we disproved miasma, although the icon of Nightingale, the lady with the scrubbing brush as well as a lamp, is still used in policy documents regarding health care infection: "No risk is more fundamental than the risk of infection. Florence Nightingale understood this when she published 'Notes on Nursing' . . . and placed great emphasis on the importance of hygiene, cleanliness and standards of care."[63]

Meanwhile, cleaners and their unions are cynical about "virtuous circles" of health care staff doing more to keep the hospital environment clean and are particularly cynical about the parsimonious cleaning budgets, which gives an ironic note to the "Matron's Charter" plea that cleaners cannot be everywhere at once. It seems unlikely, from the comments made by cleaners, that staff are acting on the questions posed in that charter, for example, "Do you pick up odd pieces of litter?" and "What could you do to make it easier for cleaning staff to do their job?" The charter's aim that "cleaning staff will be recognized for the important work they do" with nurse administrators making sure "they feel part of the team" has been rebutted by the trade union view that this means a lot more than knowing cleaners' names and inviting them to staff social gatherings, two of the recommendations in the charter.

The trade union's claim that outsourcing or contracting out is the real problem is worth considering, although with clinical jobs under threat in the pursuit of further health service economies, it seems unlikely that the number of "in-house" cleaner posts would increase if the contracting system were to be stopped or radically overhauled. Treatment costs can only increase with the rise of aging and vulnerable populations, so hospital cleaning has to be weighed against which treatments could be curtailed to provide the funding. In the UK and other countries with comprehensive state-funded or otherwise subsidized health care systems, there are far more complaints about the rationing of expensive treatments than about dirty hospitals. If any government dared to put to the vote whether people wanted more treatment funding or spotless hospitals, few would vote for the latter, although this kind of choice is very hard for either the public or the media to consider. So cleaning continues to be "demand led" in the sense that there is a flurry of activity after a publicized outbreak or epidemic, as in the "deep clean" exercise in England, with little priority given to cleaning in between these events. We have not forgotten how to clean our hospitals as much as we have forgotten why this should be a prime aim. Yet the costs of cleaning are very modest in comparison with some costly and, on scientific evidence, not very effective treatments. Therefore, better environmental cleaning of hospitals is probably affordable; and hard-pressed health care staff should not be urged to subsidize the meager cleaning budgets by pitching in with litter collection and the like. Of course they should be clean and tidy themselves; and any initiative to improve those sloppy, neglected environments should be welcomed, particularly if it involves a larger and better-motivated housekeeping support staff. With increasing microbial resistance making antibiotics less effective, there is some hope that environmental cleaning will reemerge as a vital part of infection control, a "core competency" that should be nurtured. Meanwhile, the conclusion has to be that we have become "too mean to clean" our hospitals, and we have also forgotten the hard-fought battles that established why we should do it.

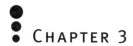

CHAPTER 3

What Goes without Saying
in Patient Safety

Suzanne Gordon and Bonnie O'Connor

> We were always told to be nice to the nurses because they have so much more contact with patients—and they can make your life difficult if you're not.
>
> —Internal medicine physician
>
> I feel like there's a gap between doctors and nurses communication-wise. . . . I feel like the nurses are busy; they're running around. They're not friendly to each other and they're not friendly to us either. I don't know if it's the nature of the work or the culture they're working in. I have no idea. It makes me wonder.
>
> —Internal medicine resident
>
> Why should I go out of *my* way to fill in her [knowledge] gaps when *she* [the MD] can't be bothered to be there and do her job in the first place? Bitch.
>
> —Senior bedside nurse, inpatient wards

Since its inception, the patient safety movement in the United States has focused on easily quantifiable indicators whose incidence can readily be compared over time and among venues. Consistently missing from the general discourse and implementation planning is any systematic study or integration of a wide range of sociocultural and organizational issues that largely defy quantification and that can significantly affect efforts to protect patients. Included among these are intraprofessional and interprofessional hierarchies and turf battles; interprofessional antipathies, competition, and fundamental misconceptions; linguistic incompatibilities and other interprofessional communications barriers; and poor (if any) conflict management.

Exploring each of these critical areas illuminates why progress in actually keeping patient safety at the forefront of health professionals' attention all day, every day, has been so difficult and at times so halting. Problems in dealing with these issues also help to explain why health care has thus far remained largely untouched by the kinds of safety enhancements that have been so successful in other high-risk industries, where they are applied equally to systems and to personnel. An early model is the aviation industry, which, since the late 1970s, has developed and implemented a now universally required skills training and safety quality assurance program called crew resource management (CRM).

Crew Resource Management

Hospital discussions of patient safety often mention the cultural transformation that occurred in aviation between the late 1970s and early 1990s through the mechanism of crew resource management.[1] In analyses of numerous airline crashes, it became clear to researchers, regulators, airline owners, pilots, and other stakeholders that very basic human errors, rather than equipment malfunctions or gaps in technical proficiency, were responsible for the majority of the crashes. Primary among these were "preoccupation with minor mechanical problems; inadequate leadership; failure to delegate tasks and assign responsibilities; failure to set priorities; inadequate monitoring; failure to utilize available data; failure to communicate intent and plans."[2]

Analysis of these problems revealed that most were the result of inadequate communication, lack of role clarity, and normalization of role interdependence, as well as a tacit acceptance of the "un-challengeability" of the captain. To deal with this problem, airline researchers and social psychologists collaborated to create crew resource management, initially called cockpit resource management.

From its inception, one of CRM's primary targets was the traditional steep hierarchy in aviation. In a culture in which the captain of the aircraft was king, pilots widely believed that if you were a "good stick" (that is, if you had excellent "stick and rudder skills"), you not only would not make mistakes but also would inherently make a good leader.[3] Researchers found that captains would dismiss the concerns and safety observations of their first officers or flight engineers as insubordination. In turn, first officers and flight engineers were so hesitant to point out errors and oversights to their captains that they sometimes literally "went down with the ship" rather than speak out urgently or assertively about a safety concern. Few heeded the questions and concerns of flight attendants or passengers, whose information, by virtue of their low status in the hierarchy of expertise, was presumed by definition to be uninformed and non-critical. That open communication could be a crucial safety feature, and that deference could kill, were ideas that were completely off the radar. Indeed, one might say that a stereotypical view of communication in aviation pre-CRM was that it consisted of a captain issuing an order and someone below him saying "roger and out."

Over the course of three decades, and on the basis of systematic social-psychological research findings in studies the industry itself commissioned, the CRM personnel training programs evolved to include not just cockpit but cabin crew members, and sometimes ground crew and staff, and thus became known as crew resource management. The principal goal of this training has been to reduce the frequency and minimize the effects of human errors in aviation. To do this, human factors researchers and others conducted numerous studies in an effort to understand how errors happen and how crews can react to prevent, manage, and contain them when they inevitably do occur. One clear obstacle to safety is poor communication. CRM teaches teamwork organizational and operational skills, as well as skills in communication, negotiation, and conflict resolution. Robert T. Francis, a former vice chairman of the National Transportation Safety Board, and before that a senior official at the Federal Aviation Administration, succinctly described the changes in the commercial airlines industry as a result of CRM. Before CRM, he said, the culture in the cockpit was "'I'm the captain. I'm king. Don't do anything; don't touch anything; don't say anything. Shut up.' Now it's, 'I'm the captain, please tell me if you see me making a mistake.'"[4]

In the interest of safety, hierarchy has been not eliminated but rather flattened, so that anyone, of any rank, may speak freely and without fear of reprisal when she or he has a safety concern. The effect on aviation safety and culture has been tremendous, with the number of airline crashes dramatically reduced.

Obvious parallels between the hierarchical structures and multidisciplinary staffing of both aviation and health care have led physicians, administrators, nurses, and many others to learn more about aviation and other high-risk industries. CRM techniques have been applied in individual hospitals and in specific high-risk settings: anesthesia, operating rooms, emergency departments, labor and delivery suites, and intensive care units. As yet there is no industrywide application. For example, in recent decades medical and nursing schools have placed much emphasis on, and devoted increasingly significant curriculum time to, the crucial issue of effective communication. Trainees have received instruction in delivering bad news, dealing with "difficult" patients or families, the particulars of informed consent, cross-cultural awareness, and empathic interactions with patients and their family members, among other topics. Models of communication in medical and nursing training are still largely dyadic, however, and most of the formal training is focused on communication between provider and patient. Nurses and physicians in training of course also learn the expectations and requirements of communicating patient information with others in their own professions through notes and sign-out formats, and acquire fluency in the languages and modes of expression of their particular professions. But there remains a significant gap: effective communication *among* the health professions on an ongoing, daily basis. In the United States, there is currently no routine or systematic inclusion of training in interprofessional communication and interaction in nursing or medical schools. Few curricula include even one or two joint education sessions for nurse and physician trainees, although many topics are common to both professions' education, and for most, their entire professional lives will require constant daily interaction.

When medical students receive skills training or evaluation in the now universally accepted method known as the OSCE (objective standardized clinical examination)—clinical scenarios that employ trained actors playing "standardized patients" who (purportedly) behave identically with every trainee—the focus of the exercise is on the student's skill in eliciting the "patient's" narrative, concerns, and key diagnostic or medical management data. We know of no documentation of OSCEs that include roles for physicians together with nurses, physical or respiratory therapists, or other health care personnel who might convey crucial information about or insight into the "patient's" condition, or whose educational or skill-testing focus is on communication and interaction between physicians and nurses. In the more recently introduced use of simulation training (or "SimCenters") in medical education, simulated urgent or emergency patient situations do include nurses, but the focus of the training remains on appropriate clinical skills and physician responses to the medical demands of the "patient's" situation. There is typically no explicit training or debriefing discussion devoted to appropriate interprofessional communications—even in the service of the patient's best interests. There is similarly little training in interprofessional communication and negotiation in schools of nursing. The sole exception is the running of practice "codes" or resuscitation efforts, in which all trainees are taught the requirements of specific roles and positions, including "calling out," or repeating instructions, for verification before actions are taken that will affect the (real or simulated) patient.

When it comes to working nurses and physicians, few of the veteran clinicians whom we have interviewed over many years have been taught even the most basic details of the nature, requirements, workloads, or scheduling patterns that govern the work lives of those with whom they will share the care of patients and interact daily for the balance of their professional lives.

With very few and recent exceptions, neither profession is trained in shared communications protocols, terminology, or styles.

Suzanne Gordon has elsewhere described doctors and nurses as intimate strangers who often seem to be engaged in a professional form of parallel play at the bedside.[5] As one nurse at a major northeastern teaching hospital observed, "[The doctors] do their thing and we do ours."[6] To date, neither profession is routinely educated about or trained in the nature and requirements of teamwork. Although health care is full of references to "teams," this usage typically refers to aggregations of people assigned to a particular unit, task, or roster of patient(s) during a specific time frame (for instance, "the care team," "the transport team"). Actual safety-directed *teamwork* requires much more: the deliberate and mindful creation of a jointly trained group of professionals with specifically identified individual and interactive roles; a distributed set of skills that serve a common purpose; a collaborative work style; and shared and explicit goals, information, terminology, plans and protocols, and feedback or correction mechanisms. In spite of the isolated and episodic introduction of CRM approaches in a range of health care institutions in recent years, and a proliferation of consultation and training businesses specializing in applications of CRM to health care, there has as yet been no industry-wide or even hospital-wide movement in health care to adopt this very effective form of safety enhancement and error management.

Hierarchies in Health Care

Intraprofessional Hierarchy: Scenario 1

In a medical school committee meeting attended by administrators, faculty, and representatives of each student class, a third-year student recounted an "embarrassing moment" during the previous semester when, on one of her clinical rotations, she had made a significant physical finding crucial to the patient's proper medical management, which had not been noted by the attending physician. The student was distressed because she, as a junior person, could not fathom how to report her finding without implying that the attending physician had missed it—that is, made an error. Making this known to others involved in this patient's care seemed somehow unwise, if not actually impermissible. She was in a quandary: if she reported her finding, a senior physician might be embarrassed; if she failed to report it, the patient could suffer. (She resolved this dilemma by suggesting that her finding was probably a misinterpretation, thus letting the senior physician be the public arbiter of its accuracy and significance.)

The few non-physicians on the committee did not understand how this could be a problem. They presumed that *what* was discovered would naturally be of greater significance than *who* made the discovery.

The physicians and the other medical students in the room, by contrast, all reacted with sotto voce utterances such as "Yikes!" and "Oh, man!" that expressed both their empathy with the student's anxiety and their ratification of her experience as an alarming situation and a genuine dilemma. Having been schooled (however informally) in the fine points of functioning within and carefully maintaining the medical hierarchy of rank and "face," they understood that it can be dangerous for a junior person to trump a senior physician. A few senior physicians on the committee contributed their own "horror stories" about similar experiences during their training years. All appreciated that the dread of "showing up" a senior physician-mentor competed for trainees' attention with pointing out findings relevant to patient care and safety.[7]

This event occurred before an audience of only four medical students. Nonetheless, these soon-to-be doctors learned an important and indelible lesson: it is dicey for a junior person to know more than, show more clinical skill than, or appear to disagree with a senior physician. Only in the most painstakingly diplomatic, even self-effacing way could a junior person reveal that she or he had made a finding that a senior physician might have "missed." Conversely, they learned that if a senior physician makes an error or misses something significant, especially if "even a medical student" could have seen it, this is a truly shameful lapse.

These medical students learned that—rhetoric about patient safety notwithstanding—it is as important to be as vigilant about "messing up" in the management of power relationships as about making mistakes in clinical practice. Failing to maintain the face-saving and deference of the medical hierarchy could, they believed, lead to a reprimand by the administration for poor professionalism, poor performance evaluations or lukewarm letters of recommendation by offended faculty members, and other disadvantageous consequences.

At least since the 1999 publication of the Institute of Medicine's report *To Err Is Human*, some hospitals—or departments and specialties—have expended a great deal of energy to dispel the pervasive "culture of blame" that has made honest reporting—and subsequent analysis and prevention—of medical error prohibitively dangerous to one's career trajectory and job tenure. These steps, and their implementation in such venues as monthly morbidity and mortality (M&M) conferences, in which preventable errors and near misses are candidly discussed without assessment of blame or levy of penalty, are absolutely essential to patient safety. They make it possible to analyze the chain of events that may lead to error and identify one or more procedural steps in which system improvements or other interventions may "trap" and reverse significant errors in their formative stages.

Yet our physicians in training are still learning in no uncertain terms (that literally "go without saying") the risks and dangers they face if they make indelicate missteps as they climb the professional ladder. These young doctors in training are aware of their vulnerability to retaliatory behaviors by embarrassed or offended senior physicians, and they are not necessarily mistaken in their sensitivity to it. This lesson is part of the "hidden curriculum" in medical school.[8] In order to make patient safety truly the primary concern of physicians in training *at all times*, these aspects of the hidden curriculum need to be explicitly addressed in medical school and residency, where many professional attitudes and focal points of worry are initially forged.

The patient safety movement has not yet penetrated this level of concern, which continues to plague residents, fellows, and junior faculty in academic medicine. Most will (we hope) come down on the side of the patient. But for some, this hierarchical code of honor and its (real or imagined) sanctions against "violators" will sometimes interfere with that all-important goal. Nursing is equally prone to this problem. Nurses who leave the bedside to travel up the professional hierarchy are notorious among their former peers for taking sides against them when questions of conduct or similar conflict arise. Indeed, one of the mantras in nursing is that "nurses eat their young." Those who are newer to the field, or lower on the totem pole, are well aware of the risks of giving offense, and weigh them in the balance against other compelling concerns.

Interprofessional Hierarchy: Scenario 2

A nurse in a critical care unit at a major academic medical center was discussing an urgent patient safety issue with a resident. She identified a question requiring further clarification and remarked that she would ask "[First Name]," the attending physician, for more information. The resident at once interrupted to chastise her for referring to a senior physician by his first name rather than by his title and last name, and firmly insisted that physicians should always be addressed or referred to as "Dr. [Last Name]." (He pointed out that it is expected and acceptable for a physician to address a nurse by his or her first name, without professional designation or title, but never the reverse.) The resident was so exercised about this issue that he failed to focus on the patient safety matter under discussion.[9]

The asymmetry of address which this resident insisted on maintaining is one of the hallmarks of differential social status that is recognized in virtually every known culture: those holding higher status are accorded a more elaborate and typically honorific form of address than persons of lower status. In many languages this kind of status relationship is signaled by the use of formal terms of address—the *vous* (versus *tu*) in French, *usted* (versus *tu*) in Spanish, or *Sie* (versus *Du*) in German. In English, which has no formal or informal variant of the pronoun "you," status and deference are most commonly expressed by the use, or not, of last name and title, or the use of first name versus surname.[10] The resident's conflation of this type of overt articulation of status with proper professional decorum was emotionally fraught, and it displaced—indeed effaced—his concern with the patient about whose needs he was being briefed. We cannot know whether he would have been less concerned about this form of address if he'd known that the nurse and physician—both veterans of this particular critical care service—had a professional relationship of many years' standing in which the use of first names was the norm. In any case, he never asked.

This example is hardly an isolated one. The history of the relationship between doctors and nurses is one of nonstop struggles over self-definition, professional control, and dominance in the arena of the hospital. In the mid-nineteenth century, the hospital became contested terrain between the newly burgeoning movement of scientific medicine and the newly secularizing movement of nursing reform and professionalization.[11]

Influenced by nineteenth-century class and gender relations, medicine constructed nurses as servants (handmaidens) or even as tools of the doctor. Certainly they were not to be consulted about elements of patient care, any more than one would consult a scalpel about making a surgical incision: the very notion was ludicrous.[12] The model was emphatically one of command and control, and contained no concepts remotely akin to consultation or collegiality. Like the captain who declared himself to be king, and in whose realm no one was to do, say, or touch anything without his express authorization, the physician was constructed as the captain of a ship for which he had full responsibility and which he alone could comprehend and steer. Just as in aviation, the legacy of these historical attitudes in medicine affects new efforts to create genuine, functional teams—ones that share goals and information and deliberate together about how to create better outcomes.

Opposition and Invisibility

Thinking Alone: Scenario 3

A nurse was caring for a patient admitted with abnormal liver function. While she was at the patient's bedside, the attending physician came in to report the results of an MRI. Without asking the nurse to leave the room and talk to him for a moment so he could brief her on the results, the physician approached the patient and told him the MRI had revealed suspicious spots. To the "team" this suggested a possible malignancy. (Translation to patient: cancer.) The patient burst into tears. The attending soon left the bedside. The nurse did not follow him out and only revealed much later that she was deeply concerned about the encounter. She felt "blindsided" by receiving the information along with the patient. When questioned about this incident, the internist could not understand her concern. What was wrong with telling the nurse and patient at the same time? After all, he'd discussed the patient's condition with the "team," that is, the medical students and residents.[13]

How is it that physicians can be unaware of the absence of key care providers from critical patient care discussions? How is it that nurses can fail to ask for critical briefings from doctors? How can members of either profession fail to comprehend the consequences of these omissions for patient care and professional communication? These questions have some fairly straightforward answers.

During their education and training, both in medical school and in their residencies and fellowships, physicians are endlessly reminded that they hold ultimate responsibility for everything that happens to the patients in their care. In today's litigious climate, physicians are continually warned to be hyperaware of their risk of malpractice litigation. Many believe that when such suits are filed, it is primarily the physician (*me!*) who is in the crosshairs. The constant reinforcement of this "buck stops here" message makes physicians feel not just that they "own" their responsibility for their patients but that they must also "own" their patients in order to fend off potential disasters. They may fail to recognize that other health professionals involved in the patients' care also feel and share both moral and legal responsibility for patients' well-being and for treatment standards and outcomes. They may well be unaware that nurses too bear legal responsibility and liability for their actions and risk suspension of their licenses for malpractice.

The extreme vigilance that creates a heightened sense of both responsibility and vulnerability for physicians may also lead them to ignore the fact that other professionals—like the hospital nurses who are available to them on any given shift—have experience, knowledge, and insight about patient care. Jerome Groopman, in his 2007 book *How Doctors Think,* describes his first night on call as an intern as "being on call *alone,* responsible for all of the patients on the floor as well as any new admissions."[14] Alone? Where were all of the nurses, many of whom, without doubt, had several years' experience in caring for patients (and all of whom, with the exception of the very newest hires, would have had more experience than a first-night intern)? They were probably available for consultation and assistance at a moment's notice. Indeed, the hospital could not have functioned without its nurses, who are on duty 24/7. In this narrative, the intern's bacon (and a patient's life) is saved by the sudden appearance of a senior physician, whom Groopman characterizes without irony as a deus ex machina.[15] The clear, if unspecified, message of this narrative is that "alone," for Groopman, meant without other doctors scheduled to be on the premises, and that other doctors are the only ones whose presence actually "counts."

Similar examples abound in the medical literature, whether recounted in physicians' narratives of anxiety and seizing up "under fire," or unwittingly revealed in titles like that of an article in the *Journal of the American College of Obstetrics and Gynecology* decrying home births attended by midwives: "Unattended Home Birth." (*Who* isn't there?)[16] This perspective of physicians parallels what Steve Predmore, vice president of safety operations at JetBlue, reports of pilots pre-CRM. Because pilots had been completely unaware that many other employees had knowledge and expertise, which they could use as a resource, they truly thought that they, and they alone, were responsible for *everything.*[17] If the knowledge of what other health care professionals know and do is invisible, it is easy to understand why little communication may exist between the ranks, why physicians, as "captains," feel so responsible and so vulnerable, and why patients may suffer from this significant misunderstanding.

Nursing as Not-Medicine

While nurses complain vociferously about this kind of medical exclusion, they do not hesitate to return the favor or to aggravate communication problems. If the historical trend in medicine has been to turn nurses into servants, tools, or (more recently, and with scant difference) "physician extenders," nurses tend to construct doctors as elitists who are self-serving, arrogant, and uncaring. Doctors are portrayed as being so narrowly focused on the scientific and the quantifiable that they routinely miss what is most important not only to patients but also to nurses, who view themselves as patients' advocates and special champions.[18]

A critique and diminution of medicine has become a centerpiece of the recent construction of nurses' professional identity.[19] Medicine is viewed as a discipline that fails to serve the needs of the "whole" patient. As a result, since the early 1980s, nursing has cast itself as the professional antidote to a misguided medical model that focuses on diseases to the exclusion of those who have them—making the patients invisible as people—and that consistently undermines the efforts of nurses to deliver "holistic patient care."

In the service of this ideology, nurses often choose symbols and slogans that advertise nursing as "the caring profession" or "the heart of health care," as if the "the" were in emphatic capitals and italics.[20] One implicit message in these self-portraits is that doctors have no heart or do not care about patients as people. Many doctors find this posture very alienating. As one surgeon commented: "If the nurse is the patient's advocate, what does that make me? The patient's enemy?"[21] This tacitly exclusionary rhetoric can be a significant deterrent to collegial relations and teamwork. Nor is this message or its enactment in the clinical setting restricted to physicians. A physical therapist who no longer works in hospitals observed:

> One of the things I hated most about working in hospitals was the tension with nurses. You'd enter a room and the nurse would instantly assume you were there to do some kind of harm to the patient and she had to protect the patient from you. I don't know who tells them this. But I think every nurse learns on the first day of nursing school to believe that nurses are the only ones who care about the patient.[22]

Mandatory Unintelligibility

It is well established that clarity and transparency in communication are critical to effective teamwork. Such clarity is lacking in health care settings in great part because, for decades, nurses have been firmly instructed—both in their professional education and in their workplaces—to refrain from using "medical language." This proprietary language has been reserved for physicians because its use, in some circumstances, constitutes diagnosis, a function and a privilege reserved by law, as well as by long and carefully enforced custom, to physicians only.

Social or legal constraints on the use of certain linguistic forms by some groups while permitting them to others have long been recognized anthropologically and sociologically as markers of in-group versus out-group status.

This social indicator function is another reason why medicine (or any profession) is keen to control and limit access to its language of professional discourse. Under penalty of disciplinary action, nurses have been enjoined, for instance, from saying or noting in a patient's chart that that the patient "has developed an infection." This is medical-speak. In 2002 an oncology fellow at Boston's Beth Israel Deaconess Medical Center insisted that a nurse should report to her the *signs and symptoms* of a urinary tract infection but should *not* state to her the conclusion that a patient had a urinary tract infection. That would be to make a diagnosis, which, she observed, was her job. "The nurse would never do such a thing," she asserted proudly.[23] Depending on the hospital, nurses must report in descriptive terms the symptoms that led them to their suspicions, or describe them in a written nursing note, and leave it to the doctor to apply the label or reach the diagnosis. Similarly, nurses have been schooled not to make direct recommendations to physicians, nor to suggest to a doctor what they think is wrong with the patient: this is not their place. Both physicians and nursing managers reinforce these lessons by reprimanding or disciplining nurses who violate the linguistic—as well as the behavioral—norms of status and deference. Moreover, nurses can lose their professional licenses if accused of "practicing medicine without a [medical] license," which includes making medical diagnoses. This penalty for "practicing medicine" (as opposed to practicing nursing) is explicit in every state's Nurse Practice Act.

As a result of these pressures, nurses and doctors are segregated not only by the power of diagnosis, prescription, and treatment but also by access to language. Since doctors and nurses have historically used different languages to describe the same problems and events, each has developed its own professional lexicon and forms of discourse. For nurses, this discourse is known as "nursing diagnosis," and it allows them to discuss significant patient findings without trespassing on medical turf. In some hospitals, nursing diagnosis is the language in which nurses chart their professional activities in the official written record as well. This separate and unequal language—in which nurses can safely express their conclusions about a patient's status and annotate their particular concerns regarding the patient's condition and care—virtually ensures that physicians will not understand what nurses are talking about or, at the very least, will be prompted by obvious linguistic cues to dismiss its relevance and informational value.

Use of nursing diagnosis is thus an inherently conflicted process: both not-medicine in its restricted terminology and range of specific concerns, and emulating medicine in title ("diagnosis") and form (analysis of patient data and observation to arrive at a diagnostic conclusion). Nurses are obliged by hospital and interprofessional circumstances to be bilingual—fluent both in the language of nursing diagnosis and in the terminology of medicine, in which physicians' orders are received, documented, and interpreted for implementation. Physicians, as the higher-status group in hospital culture, have neither the mandate nor the felt need to become conversant in the language of nursing. The *flow* of communication remains essentially unidirectional, since the *language* of valid communication belongs to only one of the two professions. Juxtaposed to the rarified argot of medicine, the language of nursing diagnosis seems unsophisticated, even unlearned; barred from access to medical shorthand, it resorts to circumlocutions that sound irritating and foolish to get-to-the-point physicians.

Residents in one Ivy League academic medical center dismissed nursing notes in their patients' charts as "not worth spending the time to read," explaining that they were "way too wordy" and "never say anything useful."[24] In another large urban academic hospital, nursing notes are kept in an entirely separate chart from the one used by physicians to record patient progress. (In a perhaps unconscious symbolic statement, the physicians' charts are dusty gray-blue notebooks, while the nursing charts' binders are a subdued rose color.) Many physicians *do* routinely ask nurses to tell them about relevant observations, changes in patient status, and so forth, but they do not generally read the nursing notes, which one junior faculty physician dismissed as "noncontributory" to essential patient care. Neither the residents nor the faculty attendings present at a discussion in this hospital of strategies for improving interprofessional communication had any inkling that nurses had actually not been *permitted* to use the language they as physicians would have preferred, respected, and found authoritative; nor could nurses use the same shorthand forms (such as SOAP—subjective, objective, assessment, and plan—notes) for communicating their clinical impressions and recommendations.[25] As this hospital made its transition to electronic medical records, two *separate* electronic systems were put in place for physician and nursing entries to patients' records, thus further ensuring the separation of the two professions' assessments, plans, and activity records, and reinforcing, by making them now physically invisible to doctors, the sense of irrelevance to patient care of the nursing notes. At initial deployment, not only were the two systems not linked electronically (an ongoing state of affairs), but also physicians could not even gain entry into the nursing note system because they had not been issued password access.[26]

The lack of a common language and communication medium—or at least of mutual professional intelligibility—both creates and sustains friction between nurses and physicians, and the cumulative irritation runs in both directions. Nurses resent having their knowledge and competence shrugged off by physicians, while doctors resent having to "wade through" written chart notes that do not come succinctly to the point with respect to patient data and the treatment directions they may indicate. What can be done to bridge this gap? Some hospitals in the United States have been introducing a communication protocol called SBAR, adapted to health care from its original application in the safety-critical environment of nuclear submarines.[27] (The acronym SBAR stands for the crucial steps in the communication exchange: clear identification of the *situation*, its *background*, and the speaker's *assessment* and *recommendation*.) The purpose of introducing SBAR to nurses and physicians is to create a shared stepwise protocol, and a set of terms and expectations, for exchanging crucial patient information.

A typical format for SBAR training demonstrates flawed communication scenarios and how the application of the SBAR protocol can be used to correct them. Of necessity, the scenarios depict interactions between physicians and nurses in which members of each profession are at various times shown to "blow it." Unfortunately, the successful implementation of SBAR may be compromised if the complex history of interdisciplinary tensions is not taken into account in the planning stages. Thus, in some hospitals where SBAR has been introduced to mixed audiences of nurses and physicians, there have been some unanticipated reactions. Many representatives of both professions have become defensive when the instructional scenarios depict a member of their discipline as the person who failed to communicate well. Rather than viewing the scenario simply as a teaching tool, they have responded to it as an unfair depiction—and even as scapegoating—of their particular discipline. Interprofessional antipathies have surfaced fairly openly in some training sessions. When, at one hospital, physicians expressed their belief that doctors didn't "really act like that," nurses insisted that actually they did, and often. When nurses felt that they were being shown in a poor light, the physicians responded that the nurses could dish it out all right but couldn't take it. At least one group of residents, when later asked what they had learned in the training session, replied, "We learned that the nurses hate us."[28]

Nurses have also expressed some anxiety at the SBAR requirement of stating their assessments and recommendations unequivocally and directly to physicians. Almost all of them have heretofore been expressly instructed *not* to do this very thing. Many are openly skeptical that doctors would be receptive to this approach, and some exchanged comments about particular attendings with whom they felt that this certainly would not work. For many, these reactions overshadowed the content of the training, whose basic message and rationale could not later be easily summarized.[29] Hospitals would be well advised to address these tensions, both in communications training of this and other types and in the active introduction of shared communication protocols in clinical settings. Otherwise the Great Professional Divide, and the traditions of mutual skepticism, mistrust, and defensiveness that help maintain it, are likely to undermine the bridge to patient safety that communications training is intended to create.

Organizational Obstacles

Managing Difficult Colleagues: Scenario 4

A twenty-two-year-old nurse one year after graduation was caring for a patient awaiting surgery in a teaching hospital in Boston. The young nurse was concerned because her patient, who was supposed to have surgery the next morning, was still on blood thinners. She contacted several different doctors to inquire about stopping the Coumadin, to which each one replied that the woman was not "my patient." Finally, in the middle of the night, she located the physician of record. This doctor, however, immediately began to yell at her for waking him up. The next morning he stormed into the unit and, in front of a handful of attendings, nurses, and other patients, screamed: "If I had a gun, I would shoot you! You are never to call and wake me up again! You woke up my wife and she couldn't get back to sleep!" When the nurse manager of the unit heard about this exchange, she backed up the young nurse. The charge nurse, however, informed the tearful young woman that the harsh reprimand she had suffered was her own fault.[30]

Nowadays all medical and nursing students have some degree of training (however small) in how to manage the "difficult" patient or family member. But—in keeping with the dyadic provider-patient model of communication employed in health professions education—there is little if any attempt to teach students (or veteran professionals for that matter) strategies for dealing with difficult *colleagues*. Yet difficult and unprofessional colleagues abound in one's own and other disciplines, and their behavior patterns have serious effects on morale, staff retention, and the kinds of interprofessional communication that affect patient safety. In the nursing literature, studies of abusive treatment of nurses by physicians document this problem.[31] Few, however, document the problems of, for example, "the chief resident who asks a junior resident to return his book to the library in the middle of a rain storm,"[32] the attending who makes sexual advances on or verbally humiliates an intern, the nurse manager who denigrates the intern or systematically humiliates the recently graduated new nursing hire.

Another level of complexity is added when problems that junior personnel experience are "kicked upstairs" to their organizational seniors. The attending physician is asked to resolve a problem between a junior and a senior resident; a charge nurse or nurse manager is asked to handle a problem between two bedside nurses, or between a doctor and a nurse. Unfortunately, most of the senior clinical personnel have no more training in negotiation, conflict resolution, or dealing with disruptive staff members than do their juniors. On top of that, they are being called on to mediate or to adjudicate when they are one, two, or even more steps removed from the original problem or conflict. Unable to coach the principals adequately or to draw upon the conflict as a teaching opportunity that can lead to collaboration, these senior staff members frequently end up dismissing or suppressing the problem in order to "smooth over" the conflict, or they resort to punitive disciplinary actions as a way of "closing" the issue.

These non-solutions perpetuate existing problems, and their deleterious effects often leave collegial interactions and communications. nurses (and others) far less likely to seek future consultations with a doctor about important patient care issues if the particular doctor has previously been testy or verbally abusive. Studies of nurse-physician relationships report that many nurses have left a unit, a hospital, or even the profession because of unresolved problems with abusive or difficult physicians.[33]

The range of entrenched impediments to optimal patient safety that we have outlined here can be grouped into two broad categories of human factors. The first includes those having to do with interrelations of profession (linked by historical circumstance to gender and often to social class), status, modes of communication, and long-standing cultural traditions of mutual tension and even antipathy. The second comprises those having to do with human capabilities and limitations in the face of duration, demand level, and intensity of a kind of work that requires continual precise attention, rapid analysis and decision making based on an enormous but often incomplete set of continually changing data, and resultant action of enormous consequence to others whose health and well-being, whose very lives, are at the mercy of those whose duty it is to act on their behalf. Health care, like other safety-critical industries, needs to address realistically both of these broad sources of risk to safety and invitation to error, which are inherent in human enterprises. The successes of other industries in this regard have all involved forms of teamwork and communications training, of which CRM is the primary and most thoroughly researched example, together with regulatory restraints on workload and work hours to promote safety and minimize error. This is an approach we strongly endorse for heath care as well.

The work of the University of Texas human factors research group, widely applied in the continuous evaluation and refinement of CRM over more than twenty-five years, has demonstrated repeatedly that that errors *will occur* in complex operations; that catastrophic outcomes rarely result from single errors but rather arise from sequences of related errors; and that error can be *managed,* and its consequences contained, through consistent use of well-rehearsed teamwork skills. This research has also shown that—widespread personal convictions to the contrary notwithstanding—stress, fatigue, emotional states, and other individual factors *cannot* be set aside by acts of will and *do* affect performance.

A study published in the *British Medical Journal* in 2000, comparing attitudes of pilots (all trained in CRM) with those of health care professionals in surgical specialties and intensive care units, revealed some discomfiting findings. Physicians were far *less* likely than pilots to acknowledge that error is inherent in their professional activities while being *more* likely to deny that either stress or fatigue contributed to error in their fields. Sixty-seven percent of medical respondents (attending physicians, nurses, fellows, and residents) believed that "true professionals" can leave personal problems behind when working (rising to a high of 82 percent among surgeons), and 70 percent stated that their decision-making abilities were just as good in medical emergencies as in routine situations. One third of ICU staff respondents did not acknowledge that they made errors at work, and over half said that they found it difficult to report or discuss errors in their professional settings because of concerns about reprisals to oneself or others. Reports on effectiveness of teamwork varied by status of the respondent on the "team."[34] This finding alone is not surprising (although it is disturbing), since perceptions of the effectiveness of teamwork in strongly hierarchical settings can be expected to vary by one's position along the power gradient, which will correspond with one's capacity to issue orders, exert influence, or exercise a significant voice.

Human factors research demonstrates that attitudes toward stress, hierarchy, teamwork, and error are predictive of performance, and of the abilities of individual professionals to manage threats and errors in a team environment.[35] And—contrary to the general presumption in health professions education—this same research indicates that attitudes *are* actually relatively malleable to training interventions. The attitudes of health professionals should ideally come to mirror the turnaround that Robert Francis described among senior pilots after the successful implementation of CRM: "Please tell me if I'm making a mistake." This astute reframing of "the captain's orders" allows all team members to express themselves freely on critical matters of safety and does not appear to challenge those in command when errors (including their own) are brought to their attention.

Effective teamwork does not imply egalitarianism, but it does imply collegiality, trust, shared and mutually intelligible communications, and a focus above all else on a common goal—in this case patient safety. Teamwork does require leadership, as well as clarity of function in all roles, and a very "flat" hierarchy with respect to communication. In the promotion of safety, communication must be clear and direct, and must cut across rank and role; *anyone* must be able to state or pursue a valid safety concern without fear of reprisal. Subordinates in rank are thus encouraged to practice what Gordon calls assertive followership, raising questions or objections whenever patient safety appears to be at risk of compromise. Many experts have pointed out that for teamwork and communication to function, and to contribute optimally to error management in health care, cultures of blame must change. Dealing with errors nonpunitively increases error reporting and creates some of the necessary conditions for the post-error analysis and learning that are essential to future error management (for example, the M&M report). At the same time, error must be reconceptualized throughout medical and nursing training and employment so that—as an enormous body of empirical research has made clear—it is understood to be *inherent* in the human enterprise. This should be part and parcel of the evidence-based practice of medicine.

If they are to attain their transformational goals, efforts of this magnitude cannot be undertaken casually, quickly, or intermittently. These are not once-and-done interventions or staff development workshops. Aviation committed to the CRM concept and to achieving and maintaining its goals with the aid of serious social-scientific research in communications, human factors, and error detection and management. The way was not smooth. Many pilots in the early years of CRM dismissed the model and its core component of safety-oriented communication as "touchy-feely," as a sort of "charm school," or as an industry attempt to erode the captain's authority. Most believed (indeed, hoped) that it would be a passing fad, and few took it seriously at the outset. But airlines demonstrated that they were in it for the long haul. Airline companies, working with a variety of experts, continued to refine the method and its messages with stringent data gathering regarding its effects and outcomes on personnel; on communications effectiveness; on error prevention, management, and containment; and—most important—on crashes and near misses.

In time, once-skeptical pilots began to be won over, as the evidence for the effectiveness of CRM practices grew, noting that whatever their prior sentiments about the program had been, "you couldn't argue with the facts."[36] Along the way, researchers also discovered that effective teamwork and communication yielded additional "positive effects such as . . . increases in morale, job satisfaction, and efficiency."[37] Over the decades it has now been in use, and under continual evidence-based refinement, CRM has radically altered pilot and personnel expectations, socialization, knowledge, skills, and work patterns.

Similar changes are badly needed in health care, and they are needed systemwide. The example of aviation illustrates that this can be done—*and* that it requires a sustained effort over time, and must be accompanied by both exploratory and evaluative research that contributes to the design, implementation, and ongoing refinement of the training program. One-shot workshops, short courses, or occasional (even annual) lectures cannot accomplish the objective of teamwork, communications, or error management training. These are complex sets of professional skills and need to be taught with the seriousness of all other critical clinical skills, and likewise reviewed and renewed on a regular basis across the active professional life.

For CRM to be successful in non-aviation venues, it must be carefully and appropriately adapted. In its own environments (the many branches and subsets of aviation), CRM is not formulaic; it is continually adapted and modified on the basis of ongoing research and direct experiences. Its transfer as a model into health care can most emphatically not be formulaic either, in spite of great pressures in health care environments to encapsulate complex and nuanced nonquantitative information into an algorithmic or mnemonic cognitive style. David Musson and Robert Helmreich suggest that CRM adaptations for other industries and settings must be developed within those specific organizations or industries, with active input from frontline personnel. "Hospitals must be willing to share experiences, training materials, and lessons learned in an open forum for scholarly debate and feedback from practical experience.[38] Training programs need to focus on specific sets of skills and behaviors, and must be updated continually with teaching scenarios and lessons learned from actual events and operations. They should use role play and "high-fidelity simulations" among their training techniques and incorporate actual errors into the training and learning process. This allows adult learners the opportunity to rehearse techniques for debriefing and analyzing mistakes, and to apply their findings to designing situation-specific prevention and error management strategies. These skills and behavior training programs are most effective when introduced at new employee orientations, and as part of initial training experiences— which also suggests that this training should begin early in health professions education. The content needs to be "normalized" by being introduced in conjunction with already recognized professional skills training, and should be practiced and evaluated alongside more technical skills. Recurrent practice and regular, formalized refresher trainings are essential to the maintenance of these key skills.

Teamwork and communications trainings, like other patient safety enhancements, must also take place in the context of efforts to regulate work hours and workload. Fatigue and sleep deprivation are now incontrovertibly documented to increase not only error rates but also the kinds of compromised judgment, slowed reaction times, and communications failures that make error both more probable and more difficult to manage. Similarly, excessive workloads severely compromise the ability of staff to make time to engage in critical communications that both anticipate possible threats and provide for rapid and effective responses when errors occur. People who are exhausted or overtaxed tend to be irritable, to lack the ability to perceive and interpret subtle signals; and they try to curtail, rather than pursue, conversations that require their attentive participation and could prove critical to patient outcomes. Regulation of all health professionals' work hours, whether originating within the ranks at any level or at the local legislative or federally mandated levels, is one measure that can ameliorate this significant challenge to patient safety. Implementation of evidence-based safe staffing levels and workloads for nurses and other professions is another.

Only sustained and well-coordinated changes on this scale can truly bring about the "paradigm shift" that the U.S. Agency for Healthcare Research and Quality (AHRQ) recommends for health care systems.[39] Teamwork training and safety-based workload and work hours limitations, when properly implemented, do—over time—change professional and organizational cultures and expectations. Changes in practice both promote and emerge from changes in attitudes, and the cycle is sustained by positive feedback loops between the two. In aviation, pilots and crew accept limitations on their consecutive duty hours as the safety measures that they are. Pilots are now specifically recruited with an eye toward their enthusiasm for teamwork and their team leadership and team management abilities; their initial and ongoing maintenance of certification requires successful completion of CRM training and regularly scheduled, updated refresher courses (for commercial airline pilots, every six months).

The same could and should be done in health care. Physicians, nursing leaders, hospital administrators, and the public should be able to be confident that in hospitals and other health care settings, "pilots and crews" are communicating systematically and effectively; that they are emphatically on the same team; that patients' safety is at every moment more important to every actor than saving face or maintaining status or guarding turf, and that the great technical prowess of the American medical system will not be compromised by lack of will to tackle this imposing—but manageable—organizational challenge.

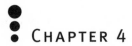

CHAPTER 4

Health Care Information Technology to the Rescue

Ross Koppel, Stephen M. Davidson, Robert L. Wears, and Christine A. Sinsky

It's late in the nightshift. A new doctor uses the hospital's computerized physician (or provider) order entry system (CPOE) to choose the appropriate dose for a medication she has prescribed only occasionally. In her hospital, as in many others in the United States, this CPOE has been installed, at great expense, to improve patient safety and prevent medication errors. She finds the medication on the screen. The doses are displayed in a stack from top to bottom: 5 mg, 4 mg, 1 mg, 3 mg, 2 mg. She assumes the display reflects dose preferences, indicates common doses, or obeys some other logic. She therefore selects the 5 mg dose for the patient, assuming it's the usual choice.

In fact, this doctor's assumption is wrong, and because of that, so is her choice of dose. The dose listing is based on alphabetical order, not on any logic associated with medical practice or anything scientific. In the English alphabet *five* precedes *four*, and *four* precedes *one*, and so on. With this medication, 5 mg may be an extraordinarily high dose, prescribed only after weeks of the usual doses.

Why would this happen? Because somewhere deep in the software code, the default listing for numbers is alphabetical. To change the dose listings for thousands of medications would require drug-by-drug reprogramming, which would be very expensive. Also, the reprogramming would be quickly superseded by new formulary offerings, for example, a 1.5 mg dose, or sustained-release doses, or liquid formulations.

The resolution, we are told, will come with the next version of the software, which will default to numerical rather alphabetical order. That way, when a new dose or formulation is offered (which occurs frequently), individual reprogramming will not be required. Unfortunately, the new version of the software won't be in place for another year or two.

A nurse is using the barcode scanner to ensure correct administration of a patient's medications. The patient has a barcode on his wrist bracelet, and each of his medications also has a barcode. The patient is to receive 10 mg of drug X. The pharmacy has sent up two packages, each of 5 mg. The nurse scans the patient's ID wristband and then repeatedly scans the packages. But the computer barcode scanner won't accept the two packages because it was "expecting" one 10 mg tablet. As a result, it alerts the nurse to an error. She must either override the computer alerts or deal with the pharmacy and the physician to alter the order.

Part of the problem is that the computer's error message is not as helpful as the nurse would like because it did not tell her what was wrong about the dose or why. She's not sure if the dosage was too low or too high, or in the wrong form (for example, pill versus liquid versus suppository). Often the scanning fails because the barcode label is wet, crinkled, torn, or smudged. Sometimes it's covered by another label reminding the nurse to scan the barcode. Is it also possible that the medication is generating an alert because it should be given at a different time. Perhaps it's for another patient?

As noted, this problem was caused by the computer program, which will accept only the one 10 mg package and cannot accept the two 5 mg packages sent up by the hospital or nursing home pharmacy.

If the nurse overrides the computer alerts, which is done in about 15 percent of such cases, she will also need to enter the information manually into the computer record of medication administrations. If the system had worked the way it usually does, the nurse could have relied on the barcodes to feed the drug administration data into the patient's record automatically. Because of the alert problem, however, the nurse must spend an additional five or ten minutes sorting out the reason for the computer rejection, overriding it, and manually entering the information. And with the manual process there is the risk of a transcription error. She now also has less time to devote to other patient care tasks.

Medical practice is beset by many woes. The most frequently reported are inefficiency, loss of patient information, fragmented information (failure to integrate medication information and treatment plans within a single record as well as among several health care providers), inadequate patient safety, exorbitant costs, staffing shortages, misallocated staff, and redundant tests and procedures. And that's only a few of the items on a long list of problems. The solution most often proposed for these difficulties is computerized information systems, commonly called health care information technology (HIT).

We find, however, that hailing HIT as health care's panacea is premature. We do not discount the dramatic benefits these systems offer and will continue to offer as they evolve. Rather, we seek to consider the roles of HIT within the entire health care system, including the social, physical, and existing technological environments into which new HIT is placed— generally a frenetic hospital where workarounds are the norm, nurse and technician staffing levels are often inadequate, and patients are sicker than ever before.

Ironically, these HIT systems provide more data, more test results, and more information in settings that offer less time to read that information and even less to think about that information. Counterintuitively and counterproductively in these time-pressured settings, accessing, integrating, and responding to information in HIT systems can require an order of magnitude more time.

Furthermore, understanding the successes and challenges of HIT means we must appreciate the market forces that drive those who develop, sell, implement, and evaluate these remarkably expensive and complex computer systems. Market forces are also involved in structuring (and sometimes restricting) the search for solutions to both the underlying problems and the side effects of the technologies themselves.

Sometimes, of course, the problems are simple: There is a lot of very dumb software in use that could be fixed by a software engineer in a few hours but has not been fixed.

Before we continue, allow a very brief introduction to three technologies that are key to the promised web of high-tech salvation:

1. The *electronic medical record (EMR; also called electronic health record, EHR)* is the digital version of a patient's chart, containing all diagnoses, tests, notes, treatments, and history. EMRs enable physicians and patients to maintain a coherent, complete, and omnipresent medical record.
2. *Computerized physician (or provider) order entry (CPOE)* systems allow physicians and other health care professionals to enter medication orders directly into a computer system, avoiding handwriting errors and speeding the prescription to the pharmacy.

3. The *clinical decision support system (CDSS) or decision support system (DSS)* provides information to physicians or nurses when they order or administer medications, for example, warning that the proposed dose exceeds the normal range or the patient is listed as being allergic to a proposed drug. These systems guide physicians and nurses to ensure that medications are ordered and administered in a correct and timely fashion.

In addition, these technologies promise to reduce costs and labor, and eliminate unnecessary services, tests, and procedures.

Many of the promises of HIT have been fulfilled. Every day, electronic medical records are viewable from any point in health care facilities that have them, as well as from any linked physicians' offices. EMRs can combine the many hundreds of tests, documents, orders, medications, and nursing notes. CPOE and CDSS help physicians order medications with much less ambiguity than with paper prescriptions. CPOE medication orders also reach the pharmacy much faster than do paper prescriptions (although it's often faster to write a prescription on paper).

The Wizard and the Curtain

A vast array of impressive reports sing the praises of HIT, which many consider the key to improving quality, patient safety, and efficiency.[1] This almost ubiquitous chorus of veneration and yearning comes from academics, public officials, vendor groups, business groups, and civic groups.[2] Enthusiastic support comes from the left and the right, from physicians and nurses, from pharmacists and hospital administrators, as well as from business leaders and some unions. Much enthusiasm is sincere and concerned with patient safety and efficiency; much is orchestrated by the HIT industry.

Not only is there vast enthusiasm for HIT, but also its spread is presented as manifest destiny, temporarily slowed by lack of financing, reluctant physicians, and unfocused legislative support.[3] In recent years the number of firms developing and selling various applications has mushroomed. There are, for example, over three hundred to four hundred makers of EMRs alone at this writing.

To encourage health care providers to buy these systems, a plethora of private- and public-sector initiatives have developed. One such inducement is the federal HITECH Act of 2009, which allots $19.2 billion to help hospitals and doctors buy these systems and another $30 billion to encourage their use. There are even payment reduction penalties for medical facilities that are slow to buy and use the technology. The private inducements come from organizations including the Leapfrog Group (a group of the five hundred largest purchasers of health care, that is, big U.S. companies), Bridges to Excellence (BTE),[4] and Doctor's Office Quality–Information Technology (DOQ-IT).[5] The Healthcare Information and Management Systems Society (HIMSS) sponsored scores of IT bills and legislative efforts in every state, paid lobbyists and "government relations" experts, ran dozens of workshops to train industry leaders in "advocacy," and "sought federal and state subsidies to underwrite the work of the free market in developing and installing HIT products."[6] The lobbying by the vendors and IT professional societies produced spectacular results. The foxes are not just guarding the henhouse; they have designed it for their use.

The problem is that many of the promises of HIT are not supported by available evidence.[7] Not only is HIT slow to diffuse throughout the health care delivery system, but also when it is implemented, its accomplishments are often disappointing. Some technologies have significantly improved particular functions in settings where they have been introduced, but in the process have created problems elsewhere in the patient's record or treatment planning. All too often we see the triumph of marketing over sensible software development and the success of vendor implementation strategies over caregiver needs. Frequently, purchasing decisions are made by those without sufficient clinical involvement, such as CFOs and hospital board members. No matter who makes the decision about HIT purchases, the constant message of the industry's lobbyists—that HIT equals safety and cost savings—is the basso continuo of this marketing effort. Here are three statements from a strategy paper for a major vendor about the creation of regulations to ensure that hospitals and doctors buy the company's software and use it to achieve minimal use levels (called the "meaningful use" criterion):

> The higher the regulatory burden placed on vendors, the greater the advantage is to incumbent vendors. Therefore, it is a critical time to influence the direction of regulatory decision regarding "meaningful use." . . . [Our company] should invest resources . . . and partner with other incumbent firms to lobby the government to raise the regulatory hurdles as high as possible.

> [Our company] should influence policy makers to [increase] the meaningful use bar. . . . [A high bar] would also erect significant barriers to entry for new firms and encourage small, less technically capable and financially limited firms to exit the market.

The message to government officials must not appear to be for the purposes of establishing barriers to entry, rather, it must suggest that *meaningful* cost savings and quality improvements cannot be achieved without a high standard of "meaningful use."[8]

More concretely and empirically, when one looks behind the curtain of optimism that dominates conference proceedings, vendor claims, and large parts of the scientific literature, one finds that the number of HIT applications actually in use is remarkably modest.[9] Until recently, the diffusion of HIT among hospitals and physicians' offices advanced at a snail's pace. In 2009, EMRs and CPOE systems were only found in about 10 to 15 percent of U.S. hospitals and physicians' offices, with most only used for a fraction of their stated capabilities. After the introduction of government economic incentives (and disincentives for laggards), however, the number of implementations more than doubled, according to 2011 government and American Hospital Association surveys.[10]

As earlier (2009), when one examines the number of hospitals or physicians using even one fifth of the EMR functions, the rate of acceptance is even far less robust.

If one insists on the (reasonable) stipulation that to be considered successful, the CPOE system or the EMRs must also contribute to the quality and efficiency of patient care, then the numbers and ratios of successful implementations are considerably smaller. If the requirement of satisfied users is added to that, the numbers shrink still further. The most common concern one hears from primary care physicians is that they are spending two hours on EMR documentation from home every night. But the catalogue of this dissatisfaction is increasingly appearing in professional journals, some of which are publishing an increasing number of studies that document disappointing results following implementation of a variety of HIT applications—a topic we shall visit shortly.[11] Most commentators also fail to acknowledge that the promises of these still elusive technological salvations are over thirty-five years old.[12]

The Research Literature and Day-to-Day Practice

Electronic Medical Record (EMR)

From the time of Hippocrates, doctors have been taught to look carefully at patients as they explain their symptoms and answer questions about their condition. Even the movement and tension in a patient's hand as she moves over or touches an area in pain can provide clues to the type and severity of an illness. Alas, EMRs or EHRs (the digital version of a patient's chart, containing all diagnoses, tests, notes, treatments, and history) and computers can inadvertently interfere with this connection. One observer watched while a young woman patient spoke with her doctor. The doctor sat at his desk facing the computer. The young woman sat to his right, slightly behind the desk. The doctor was intent on simultaneously questioning his patient and recording her remarks in the computer. Unable to type while looking at her, he kept his eyes glued to the screen as he continued to ask questions, which he addressed to the screen rather than the patient. The observer saw what the doctor missed while he typed information into the EMR: (1) indications that the patient was sometimes being facetious (a common occurrence among teens); (2) the indications of doubt when she answered a question; and (3) a flicker of withholding while she vaguely responded to a more sensitive question about her sexual activity. Miscommunications or failures to perceive cues that would lead to further probing can lead to unfortunate consequences.

Of course, physicians are not always attentive to patients' nuanced communication even when writing notes on paper or dictating into a machine, but at least these did not set up such a difficult barrier between doctor and patient as a computer keyboard and screen. EMRs require a lot of the physician's attention because they contain elaborate checklists, menus and submenus, pull-down screens, boxes, and reminders that require the doctor to pay close attention to the screen. Nevertheless, if the patient is on certain medications, the EMR will remind the physician to order certain tests. If the patient has a chronic disease, the EMR will remind the physician to ask about symptoms, treatments, and medications. If the physician checks off several risk factors for some illness, a submenu of options may emerge. These may be beneficial functions, but they require the physician to attend to the computer, and perhaps be less observant of the patient—as was the case reported by the observer in this instance.

Another problem with EMRs is the limited view they provide of a data field. As a colleague writes:

> In our outpatient EMR, the screen set-up allows me to see only four of a patient's medications at a time. Three quarters of the computer screen is wasted on duplicate, low-priority information. (The same navigation choices are inexplicably displayed on the left-hand side and at the top, leaving only one quarter of the space for clinical information.) My brain cannot look at a list of fifteen medications through this thin slot and integrate the information, especially when the diabetic

medications are not grouped together and cannot all be seen at once. All of the primary care physicians in our organization print a portion of the medical record for each patient visit to compensate for this problem.

Chaudhry and colleagues in 2006 published a systematic review of 257 articles on EMRs, some of which also include DSS.[13] Their sample of studies was drawn from a much larger set, most of which failed to meet the methodological criteria the authors establish to justify confidence in the results. After culling the relevant research, they found that 25 percent of the studies came from just four large medical institutions or systems, each of which reported results from "the incremental development over many years of an internally designed system led by academic research champions . . . [which] is unlikely to be an option for most institutions." These are called homegrown systems. While studies from these institutions "demonstrated the efficacy of health information technology for improving quality and efficiency," the magnitude of the benefit was often small even when it reached the level of statistical significance.[14]

In other words, of the many EMR systems examined, only those from four large institutions seemed most likely to produce useful results. All of those systems were developed in-house, over long periods of time. Yet when implemented, these systems also often failed to produce more than small improvements in care or efficiency.

If we apply these lessons to other institutions, or even to physicians' offices, the data are hardly encouraging. Chaudhry and colleagues report that "the relevance of these studies to the probable experience of most doctors and hospitals is uncertain." Since doctors and community hospitals cannot afford to spend decades and millions of dollars developing homegrown systems, they "are likely to purchase off-the-shelf EMRs." Indeed, they make an even stronger statement: "Published evidence of the information needed to make informed decisions about acquiring and implementing health information technology in community settings is nearly nonexistent."[15]

It is therefore not surprising to read accounts like this one from an internist:

A patient was hospitalized after spinal trauma. As the patient was treated, his condition slowly improved. To complete the daily EMR record, however, his physicians cut and pasted the previous notes day after day. The patient's recorded neurologic exam didn't change from the first day, despite the fact that he couldn't walk when he was admitted and was fully ambulatory at discharge. The medical record becomes

cluttered with meaningless or inaccurate information, repeated endlessly so that it takes ten times longer to read and to find the relevant
information.

Electronically cutting and pasting previous medical notes introduces
another source of error since bits of sentences can be lost each time someone
cuts and pastes. In a process that oddly parallels cancer growth, the cutting
and pasting of previous notes loses essential information (DNA-RNA) while
it enlarges the size of the patient's record and can add to the amount of inaccurate and unwanted information (a tumor).

If the physician is focusing on medical history, then chronology is
the clinically relevant organizational scheme. If the physician is focusing
on medications, then organ system is the medically useful organizational
scheme. Often the most appropriate order is determined by the presenting
problem. If a physician is evaluating a patient for shortness of breath (SOB),
it is important to be able to ascertain quickly that that patient recently had a
total hip replacement—and thus is at high risk for a pulmonary embolism.
If, however, that patient has a list of twenty-three events and entries, the hip
replacement will be buried within it and is easily missed. The technology
that would permit the physician to structure the information in the most
appropriate format could be easily provided but seldom is.[16]

Many EMR developers design systems that do not reflect the way medicine is practiced, producing a mismatch that generates conflict and endangers
patient safety. For example, in one system, reported by one of the authors
(Ross Koppel), the physicians rejected the programmers' templates underlying the EMR.[17] In that system, physicians were obliged to enter a diagnosis
as part of the initial EMR screen. But often patients are admitted to the
hospital precisely to determine the diagnosis—usually via tests and observations. After several months of complaints, physicians demanded, and received,
changes in the templates.

There is another reason—beyond the obvious logic—why the physicians
were wise to seek changes in the template. Information entered into EMRs
often lives on far beyond the immediate purpose. A practitioner may enter
a diagnosis just to start the intake process moving, with every intention of
correcting it once better information is known. But the tentative digital
information might well become part of many other permanent records,
influencing the patient's treatment, insurance, and life options.

One primary care physician offers a chilling example of the digital persistence of misinformation. Upon returning from a conference, a physician
saw a patient who had been cared for in the interim by a trusted colleague.

She was stunned to see that the EMR reported new and totally unexpected diagnoses. What happened? The colleague treating the patient had ordered some reasonable and appropriate tests. But the computer system required all physicians to enter one or more diagnoses to justify the tests. The colleague had entered a few diagnoses that would allow the tests, ones he knew were not exact fits for the patient but would permit him to order the needed lab work quickly. Unfortunately, the computer system auto-populated most of the patient's past and current record with the new and inaccurate information. Had the patient's long-term physician not noticed the errors upon her return, the patient's record would have been permanently and wrongly changed.

Missing data or erroneous data are almost guaranteed in systems like those in common use today, as this physician's account suggests:

> Yesterday I printed out the results section of our hospital EMR on a patient who had been in the hospital eight days to illustrate the poor display of data. It took 215 pages. That is, the data were displayed on 215 screens, which the physician has to scroll through to get all of the information. The patient was not in the ICU, and his care was of average complexity. This is unmanageable.

> I fear referrals from fellow physicians with EMRs. Instead of getting a coherent paragraph about the patient's relevant condition, I'm sent dozens to thousands of pages of text, gibberish, copy-and-paste redundancies, and lists of tests and medications. I must go through this mass to find the few relevant items I need.

It is not surprising, then, that the diffusion of EMRs has already been recognized as a major challenge.[18] As noted elsewhere in this book, in 2009, only about 14 percent of physicians in ambulatory practice had an EMR with capabilities approximating those defined by the HIT Adoption Initiative.[19] Physicians with EMRs also complain that the specificity of EMR checklists is sometimes maddening and counterproductive. If a physician suspects a possible stomach cancer in his patient, he will refer the patient to a specialist for evaluation of the abdominal symptoms. But some EMRs do not allow such a request. The referring physician is obliged to scroll through a list of scores of different stomach cancers to pick one. As one internist remarks, he has no idea what kind of stomach cancer it is, or even if it is stomach cancer. He very much suspects it is, but he has neither the experience nor the tools to make that determination. He has not encountered many of the types of cancer listed since medical school. Worse, as suggested earlier, the physician realizes that if he checks off one type of cancer, that information might well appear as a more certain diagnosis in many other documents rather than as an effort simply to refer the patient to a gastroenterologist.

Another danger in this example is that if the physician selects one type of cancer (his best guess), he will probably send the gastroenterologist down the wrong initial path. While we assume that the gastroenterologist will discover the correct diagnosis, the unintentional misdirection will probably cost time, money, and maybe even the patient's health or life. As the referring physician exclaimed: "What would it cost them to include an option that read, I'm rather sure it's stomach cancer, but I don't know what kind it is, and if I knew what kind it is I'd probably be a gastroenterologist and not an internist."

Computerized Physician/Provider Order Entry (CPOE)

Computerized Physician (or Provider) Order Entry (CPOE) systems, enabling physicians to prescribe medications directly via computer, were heralded as a breakthrough that would eliminate medication prescription errors. CPOE promised a long list of benefits, including the end of handwriting interpretation problems; faster access to pharmacies; fewer errors associated with similar drug names; easy integration into medical records and decision support systems; drug–drug interaction warnings; identification of prescribing physicians; ability to avoid specification errors, such as trailing zeros; data available for immediate analysis; and significant economic savings.[20] Despite these many heralded advantages, a more complex picture of CPOE systems has emerged in the last few years. Consider the following examples.

House staff (hospital interns and residents) using CPOE to order medications are often uncertain about patients' medications and dosages because they can't see all of the patients' medications on one screen, with some listings requiring dozens of screens for each patient.[21]

Several CPOE systems require the doctor to enter certain information before he or she can continue with the work of entering medication orders. This is called a "forced field," such as when the doctor must enter the patient's weight into a computer before ordering a medication. Say, for example, that the doctor wishes to order Tylenol, which is not especially dose-specific to an adult's weight. The doctor has seen the patient a few times and estimates her weight at about 150 pounds, but in reality, under the covers, the patient actually weighs 185 pounds. The doctor is not certain, but the weight is not important for prescribing Tylenol. Unfortunately, that estimated information is now on the patient's record. Now, say the next doctor is a nephrologist, for whom the weight may be critically important. That nephrologist has no idea that 150 pounds is a guess, and makes delicate adjustments of dosage and schedule based on the listed information.

Several children's hospitals have been fighting with vendors over the number of decimal places allowed for dosages. That is, dosages of all children's medications are based on weight. The algorithms that calculate the dose may also include the child's age and degree of impairment or infection. For adults, rounding the dose to one decimal place is usually fine. The difference between 48.4 mg and 48.5 mg is insignificant. Alas, for a 2.4-pound baby, the decimal places may need to be extended to three or four digits to avoid overdosing or underdosing. Pediatricians report that HIT vendors have been slow to accept this need despite its obvious value.

A study by Koppel and colleagues of one widely used CPOE system documented twenty-two different error-increasing aspects of that system.[22] That work generated a firestorm of protest because it highlighted some of the possible flaws of HIT. In the ensuing years, however, about three dozen studies were published that reinforced those findings. Han and colleagues reported a doubling of infant mortality after the introduction of a CPOE system.[23] Introduction of a CPOE system into a tertiary children's hospital apparently reduced bedside nurse-physician interaction about critically ill infants. Nurses therefore had fewer opportunities to provide feedback that sometimes led to medication changes. CPOE procedures also altered communication between transport teams and the emergency room. Prior to the introduction of CPOE, the transport team radioed the ER so it could order medications and complete admission forms before a patient's arrival. When CPOE was launched, medical transport staff had to provide patient information in the ER. Treatment was delayed until after the ER staff entered the data into their computers. (And in short-staffed and overcrowded emergency rooms, these data entry tasks may be further deferred.)

Resulting delays and reduced interaction among physicians and nurses may have contributed to higher mortality rates. Nebeker and colleagues likewise found high rates of adverse drug events (ADEs) in the highly computerized Veterans Administration system.[24] Shulman and colleagues conducted a classic before-and-after study of the transition from paper to CPOE system.[25] They found that CPOE was associated with fewer inconsequential errors than paper-based systems but also with more serious errors.

Ash and colleagues, Campbell and colleagues, and Aarts, Ash, and Berg have found unintended consequences from CPOE systems to be the rule rather than the exception.[26] David Bates, one of the most respected advocates of CPOE, has written about his own experience: "After implementing CPOE, we routinely tracked errors and problems that were created and made thousands of changes to the original application. If I had one thing to 'do over' in our CPOE implementation, it would be to have devoted more resources to this area—it is just impossible to 'get it all right' at the outset, because the processes involved are so complex."[27] He adds that, while HIT is "an extraordinarily powerful tool" it is "only a tool, and . . . for it to have the desired impact socio-technical factors must be considered and addressed."[28] Nemeth and Cook agree: "Error is [often] a *consequence* of interaction with IT systems. . . . The core issue is to understand healthcare work and workers."[29] And although "healthcare work seems to flow smoothly," the reality is "messy." Therefore, future "progress in healthcare IT systems relies on scientific data on the *actual,* not the perceived, nature of day-to-day operations."[30]

To maximize the benefits and minimize the unintended consequences requires arduous and ongoing vigilance and effort. Even a "perfect" CPOE system must constantly adapt to changes in other IT systems, staff, protocols, medications, patient populations, and utilization of interior space. The inherent risk-reward tradeoff requires continuous attention to both patient safety and efficient medical care delivery.[31]

Sending and Receiving: An Uncertain Link with Unknown Implications

Another aspect of CPOE and digital communication has received little attention even though it has profound implications for patient safety, workplace morale, and teamwork.[32] That is the belief that if an order has been electronically submitted, then it was received and acted upon. As anyone recognizes who has ever sent an email that was lost in the oceans of spam or in the depths of recipients' in-boxes, such faith is not always rewarded. While we realize that someone we are speaking to may not be listening (perhaps because he or she is a teenager), we have visual and other clues to indicate whether the message was received. With digital communication, there are no immediate clues. Even an automated response that such communications were received is not a confirmation of information transfer. As researchers have repeatedly demonstrated, physicians frequently assume that if an order has been submitted (or an email instruction has been sent), the nurses have received and executed the order.[33] The nurses, however, may not have received the order; or they may be working on other tasks, distant from a computer screen. The error is compounded when the physician then assumes that the patient's most current lab results or vital signs reflect the newly ordered medication or treatment, for example, that the most recent blood pressure readings manifest the effects of a recently ordered medication.

There is a related myth that if a piece of information is in the computer, it is simultaneously and magically in the physician's head. Historically, it has been the hospital's responsibility to call a physician about a significantly abnormal result. Traditionally, physicians relied on the hospital staff to notify them when a test was abnormal and to understand the speed with which that datum should be conveyed. Nurses used their experience and skill to decide when to call the physician. Now these results are often not seen by the physician (or perhaps by anyone else) in a timely fashion. Now the hospital staff seldom call physicians with this information, apparently thinking that if a result is in the computer, the physician will just know it. But doctors cannot spend the entire day reviewing all of the screens for all of their patients to find an abnormality.

While CPOE and other forms of digital communications are clearly efficacious, and no one would seek to limit orders to only face-to-face communications, these types of "assumption errors" are constant. Moreover, replacement of team discussions and oral communications in general has not been sufficiently explored to determine whether there are serious consequences for either patient outcomes or health care workers' morale. As noted, the study by Han and colleagues, which found a near tripling of infant mortality in the transfer unit using CPOE, suggested that one possible cause might be reduced physician–nurse communications because orders were electronically submitted. But the study did not discuss the implications for nurses' job satisfaction. Work by Harrison, Koppel, and colleagues clearly reveals the need to study workflow in relation to new technology.[34] When the implications of using HIT are studied, it seems reasonable to add workplace morale, nursing turnover, and job satisfaction to the issues under consideration. It may also be reasonable to add physicians' irritation at spending an additional two hours each day doing what they consider clerical data-entry tasks.

Building on Imperfect Foundations: Decision Support Systems and Evidenced-Based Medicine

Decision support systems (DSS) are software programs to remind or warn physicians about drug-drug interactions, dose limits, allergies, best practice guidelines, and "order sets"—groups of drugs that often work together. They are usually add-ons to CPOE systems.

The logic of DSS is impeccable. With the use of IT, dosage guidelines and warnings are supposed to reflect the latest and best research. So if some combination of medications is found to work better than, say, some old standby, DSS will provide up-to-date information exactly when the physician is ordering the relevant medication(s). Similarly, if a previously standard dosage has been shown to be higher or lower than needed, DSS will also help physicians make the best choice. The use of the best and most recent medication guidelines is part of "evidenced-based medicine" (EBM), the use of research-based practices to improve patient treatment and reduce adverse drug events. It builds on the ability of information technology to inform clinicians about the best advice learned since they went to medical or nursing school.

In theory, decision support systems are a great idea. In reality, they generate frustrations more consistently than any other form of HIT. Physicians quickly become enraged at the constant reminders associated with many of the medication orders they enter. Imagine that you are a physician specializing in infectious medicine and you order antibiotics all day. With each order of many antibiotics, you are reminded that they interact with other medications. Perhaps the system reminds you to monitor your patient carefully. Or imagine that there are some weak studies which show that most medications might interact with Tylenol, and most of your patients are on Tylenol. You nevertheless receive warnings about Tylenol interaction dangers with 85 percent of your medication orders. These frustrations produce what is called "alert fatigue," which occurs when physicians ignore the warnings or even bypass them before they fully form on the computer screen. The data on alert fatigue are stunning: most studies show that 80 to 96 percent of alerts are ignored and overridden by physicians!

In one study of three hundred overrides of DSS alerts, the researchers found that *all three hundred were medically correct.* That is, the physicians did not err in ignoring the DSS alerts, but rather they made appropriate decisions in overriding them. From the physicians' perspective, all of the DSS alerts were wrong (or at least unhelpful) and generated a lot of make-work. Here is a typical comment from a physician:

> More often than not, the alerts are nuisance pop-ups, either telling the physician the obvious or advising on something clearly inconsequential. This morning I was discharging a patient from the hospital and converting a prescription for meclizine to an outpatient prescription. It took five minutes! One of the screens included the warning of a drug-drug interaction between IV saline and orally administered meclizine. It did not state what this interaction was. It is clearly a false warning as there is no contraindication to IV saline and orally administered meclizine. In addition, this patient was going home without any IVs.

In terms of patient safety and hospital operations, the alert process often requires time and work, generates no value, and may cause harm by diverting scarce resources away from other important clinical activities.

A study by Metzger and colleagues found that DSS detected only 53 percent of all medication orders that would have resulted in fatalities, and anywhere from 10 to 82 percent of orders that would have caused serious adverse events.[35] Drugs prescribed for a wrong diagnosis were caught only 15 percent of the time (that is, in cases in which the computer already had the patient's record and could "know" that the drug was inappropriate), and drugs that were wrong for a patient of a given age were intercepted only 14.1 percent of the time.

DSS alerts are ideally based on the latest research, and no one could be against "evidenced-based medicine." The problem, however, is that the research is often conducted with carefully selected samples of patients so that researchers can observe the effects of the medicine or treatment without additional interference from other conditions. The flaw is that hospitals are full of elderly patients suffering from multiple organ system problems, with a long list of co-morbidities. Therefore it is often a great leap to apply findings from a study under "ideal conditions" to the fragile patient; that is, a medication that has been shown to be effective for a particular type of liver problem may dangerously strain the kidneys of elderly patients. So the physician must then balance the DSS information with the various vulnerabilities of the real patient in front of her.

As can be immediately imagined, physicians must constantly deal with these messy tradeoffs, and the utility of EBM-generated guidelines is mitigated by the complex challenges of the sick patients. This mix of clear-cut research with the messy reality of medical practice means that DSS guidance is often not fully applicable; physicians' reactions to alerts and recommendations reflects not only alert fatigue or professional pride but also a considered understanding of the complexity of medical care. Moreover, there are as yet unknown implications of the use of DSS recommendations for medical students and residents who have grown up with these systems and have never practiced medicine without them.

Alert and Order Set Wars

In addition to the alert fatigue difficulties with decision support systems discussed earlier, selecting among the specific alerts or medication recommendations is usually a source of conflict within hospitals and can itself be a cause of medication error. Here the discussion shifts from the individual physician to the social interactions among hospital departments or among hospitals. Differing sets of dosage recommendations and differing thresholds for alerts (for example, the dosage at which an alert fires) can themselves increase the possibility of errors. How can this happen? Because DSS alerts are so often disliked, so often ignored, and yet so potentially helpful (and life-saving) that considerable professional energies (read: committee meetings) are devoted to the creation of each hospital's (or each department's) set of warnings. One physician or department may insist that 30 mg should be the highest permitted dose for a particular drug. Another group may feel that up to 35 mg is acceptable. Often the disagreements reflect honest and understandable differences based on different physicians' past experiences, the types and ranges of patients typically encountered, or alternative interpretations of "best practices." In general, committees of physicians in each hospital determine the sets of alerts, reflecting a three-way tension among physicians' irritation levels with the alerts, the known incidence of overriding or ignoring the alerts, and genuine efforts to stop adverse events and help clinicians make wise choices.

Tradeoffs

The results are of course compromises and tradeoffs. Hospitals with a powerful central authority structure or with extraordinary levels of cooperation tend to institute a single hospital-wide (or hospital system–wide) set of rules. This route enables physicians and physicians in training to deal with the same set of triggers and reminders while forgoing the advantages of sometimes appropriate adaptations to each subgroup's desires. By contrast, untamed customization metastasizes into a patchwork of alerts and dose thresholds that promote alert overrides, inconsistent guidelines, and medication error. (For a more complete explanation, see the section on the implications of medication error from DSS.) Before choosing sides, however, one must consider the even more complex reality of how the systems are installed and addressed.

The Typical Installation Process

The vendor selling the DSS software (which is usually linked to the CPOE system) installs the DSS structure either without any rules or with a standard software package of drug alerts based on dosage levels, known drug-drug interactions, and so on. If the CPOE system can interface with patient information on a digital record (such as an electronic medical record), the DSS will probably also warn prescribing physicians about known drug allergies. The DSS will generally also include "order sets," that is, groups of drugs that are usually prescribed together to address frequently encountered medical conditions, for example, a recent heart attack, or diabetes, or any one of hundreds of other conditions. The order sets may give specific dosages—or a range of dosages—with each medication. Sometimes the order sets offer options, such as suggestions that one prescribe medication A, B, and C plus either D or E.

What happens? Within a few hours after the DSS is installed, the physicians become enraged at the constant and quickly ignored alerts. Alert fatigue takes minutes to develop but the irritation continues. Reactions to prepackaged order sets become a flashpoint. Medication combinations and dosage levels may not match the local practices; specialists might insist that the order sets do not reflect new findings about this or that drug.

The hospital usually reacts by stopping the DSS or allowing only the most obvious alerts (perhaps warning physicians about sixfold overdoses or against prescribing large doses of blood thinners when the patient is about to undergo surgery). Order sets, likewise, are stopped until they can be reviewed or redeveloped by in-hospital committees of physicians.

The Triumph of Professional Autonomy Over Rational Planning

Committees of physicians negotiate which medications will generate warnings and alerts and the types of alerts. Those same committees also negotiate the order sets for each disease or condition. In each hospital, thousands of professional hours are devoted to these processes even though most of the medical conditions and medications are almost identical to those addressed in thousands of other hospitals. That is, it often appears that each hospital is independently negotiating its own version of medication guidelines for each type of illness and condition—even though there are available libraries of recommendations and treatments accessible via the Internet. And while one might applaud the localized focus of care and the amount of thoughtfulness, experience, and passion evident in these meetings, it's also evident that they take a tremendous amount of time. Perhaps more important, these hospital-specific committees and decisions may negate or at least mitigate the concept of internationally and scientifically derived "best practice" advice and findings.

The Implications of Medication Errors Increased by DSS: Diversity and Its Discontents

Because of the processes we've just discussed, DSS alerts and order sets often differ from hospital to hospital, or even among units in the same hospital. In hospital A, the order set for treatment of a heart attack will include, say, five medications each at a suggested dosage. In hospital B, two blocks away, the order set for treatment of the exact same heart attack will include, say, four medications, two of them different from those at the neighboring hospital, and some at different suggested dosages.

Likewise, DSS alerts will fire for very different drugs and drug combinations in different hospitals or departments. Far worse, accepted upper- or lower-dose parameters will differ by wide margins from institution to institution.

These differing alerts and order sets increase the risk of medication errors for a number of reasons:

1. Many young physicians, interns, and residents prescribing a medication with which they are unfamiliar use the alerts as "bumpers"; for example, if the alert fires for "too high dosage," they lower the dosage to something that stops the alert.

2. General dose warnings are notoriously difficult to establish because patients may have a wide range of medical conditions, previous exposures to that medication, co-morbidities, and sizes (weights).

3. Perhaps more dangerous, many young physicians, interns, and residents will prescribe a dosage assuming that alerts will fire if there is a problem. As we have seen, however, hospitals differ on which medications are linked to DSS warnings. Many interns and residents rotate among several hospitals in the course of their training and work, and many physicians practice in several hospitals. Inconsistent limits and guidelines—or their existence at one hospital but not at others—can be confusing and lead to errors. Thus doctors who expect alerts if they order lethal dosages or incompatible medications may receive no warnings whatsoever. Relying on DSS when there may be none is therefore especially dicey.

4. Assuming that DSS alerts for allergies are in place, many physicians will not bother to look up listed patient drug allergies because the DSS usually warns of them. Again, variations among hospitals and departments may alter the types or existence of warnings.

5. One possibly ironic protection is that most alerts are overridden anyway—many before they even fully appear on the screen. (The cursor is "pre-placed" on the "OK" box before the alert is read.) Of course, the flipside is that crucial alerts may well be ignored.

6. Order sets are written for specific diseases or conditions. We have found, however, that busy residents will refer to a quickly available order set for guidelines on dosages. Alas, that dosage, designed for a

specific disease and treatment strategy, may not be appropriate for the disease the resident is addressing.

Decision Support Systems: In Sum

In theory, DSS is a remarkably useful information tool for clinicians. It provides guidance and warnings just at the point when the physician is about to order a medication. (DSS can also provide advice and alerts to nurses as they prepare treatment strategies.) If DSS did not exist, we would want to invent it. DSS has undoubtedly prevented thousands of adverse drug events (ADEs) and hundreds of deaths. In practice, however, it's hard to implement for all of the reasons we've enumerated. We assume that DSS will improve as computer systems are better able to integrate more of the patients' information, and more nuanced algorithms are devised that incorporate a patient's complex conditions. We hope that some institutional body of medical professionals will establish meaningful and consistent rules for alerts and order sets. The current system of order set wars, endless alert-setting meetings, and frequent fatigue-inducing warnings is not ideal. It makes little sense that physicians practicing a few blocks from one another should receive very different treatment guidance for identically sick patients.

As with all HIT, decisions about DSS alerts and order sets reflect the usual battles of departmental politics, economic power, professional prestige, and bureaucratic maneuvering. Unlike with many forms of HIT, however, improving DSS is less likely to require significant changes to work processes, hospital architecture, or social systems. To this extent, it holds promise for significant improvement as the technology is developed.

What to Do? Understanding Why HIT Problems Are Not Addressed, from Corporate Marketing to Clinicians' Making Do

If, as we have suggested, HIT is insufficiently responsive to the needs of health care professionals, the question is: Why? Why is HIT unduly cumbersome and unnecessarily error enhancing? We proposed fourteen reasons for the persistence of faulty HIT and for the slow pace of improvement and adoption.

1. Workarounds are the norm, not the exception, in hospitals. Clinicians are resourceful, and the medical ethos of "getting the work done" often obscures problems with the software.

2. Problems are difficult to locate in the matrix of work arrangements, the built environment, linkages to other technology, and different levels of training and tenure. It is often hard to determine if the problems with HIT are due to links with other programs, the microwave tower across the street, and/or the legacy of anger over a previous HIT implementation. Is it understaffing of nurses? The insensitivity of the geeks in the technology office? Technophobic doctors?

3. The methodologies, research tools, and resources needed even to perceive problems are often scarce in the hospital setting. Finding and correcting HIT problems requires the full range of research techniques and data sources. Believing standardized reports or vendor specifications is generally unwise. (See the stories from the hospital earlier in this chapter about the reporting system.) Koppel and colleagues' study of CPOE employed several techniques: surveys, observations, focus groups, shadowing of physicians and nurses, one-on-one interviews with many different kind of staff, expert interviews (with IT and hospital leaders), and shadowing of pharmacy personnel as they used the system.[36] Koppel and colleagues' study of medication barcoding administration used all of these methods plus analysis of almost half a million scans of patient IDs and medication IDs, vendor interviews, review of vendor specifications, and interviews with dozens of hospital and IT leaders from throughout the United States.[37]

4. Belief in technology often prevents users (and everyone else) from even seeing its limitations. Staff are told to trust the technology. To admit you are having problems with the software or technology implies that you are the problem. Few wish to be seen as technophobes, so there is a barrier to users' even articulating the problems with HIT in their environment. Doing so may give the impression that they are not technologically savvy. In some hospitals, nurses' enthusiasm for newly implemented HIT—no matter if the HIT is great, awful, or both—is considered in their evaluations. They face real disincentives to commenting on the emperor's new clothes.

5. Vendors recite the mantra that the next version of the software (which costs several million dollars) will fix the problems. Promises can also blunt frustration for surprisingly long periods of time. We all want to accept these promises.

6. Although the next versions of the software will probably solve several of the identified problems, they will also introduce new problems that may take a while to emerge and to understand.

7. Vendors' policies on modifications serve as deterrents to making repairs and improvements. That is, large vendors require that the *entire*

customer base—national or global—must agree to a change in the program or even to a screen interface. For example, if clinicians at fifty hospitals identify a serious problem, the vendor will insist that those clinicians must convince the rest of the customer base that the specific change is needed. But other customers are focused on other problems that are perhaps more salient to their work. The vendors in response to this seemingly democratic and technocratic process espouse non-action as the best action. The vendor is off the hook. It may incorporate the requested change in the next (and more expensive) version of the software. In the meantime, the customers are left with difficult or even dangerous problems. What is equally frustrating is that no one seems to be responsible for the problem, and no one is even allowed to fix it because the software is the property of the vendor, merely on lease to the hospital. As one colleague stated: "I can get everyone at my hospitals to agree that our CPOE should display the name of the patient and the medication, but I need to convince the customer base that this is the priority or it won't get done." It shouldn't be the job of clinicians to get the system fixed. When the AC doesn't work here, I refer it to maintenance, whose job is to get it fixed." Vendors, of course, are faced with myriad requests for fixes. Using the customers as screeners is potentially a good idea and certainly not inherently manipulative. While it does enable vendors to slow or derail demands for repairs or improvements, we have no idea if this use of customers to retard change is an unintended or intended consequence.

8. Often, clinicians working with HIT experts go native. That is, doctors and nurses are unintentionally co-opted away from their previous focus on healing to the intricacies of bandwidth, server capacity, and screen refresher rates. Within a few months on the implementation team, many doctors and nurses sound more like engineers than clinicians. They often find it difficult to maintain their clinical priorities in the face of the newfound wonders of the technology and its management. This tendency to lose clinical focus helps explain the poor fit between what the software does versus what the clinicians need. This misfit of medical work practices compared to the logic embedded in the technology leads to a constant cycle of workarounds and demands for customizations for each practice setting. Each alteration in turn generates myriad "unintended consequences," which require additional adjustments.

9. It's remarkably hard to fix HIT while it's being used in the hospital. Neither hospitals nor vendors can afford major errors when patient

safety is always on the line. Even downtime for repairs is dangerous in a 24/7 institution.

10. The market both creates and restricts innovation and responsiveness. Dominant HIT corporations and individual entrepreneurs are constantly developing new or improved applications. But the large corporations do not want to disenfranchise their installed base (the existing customers) with advances that may be incompatible with their existing programs. Real customization, as we have discussed, makes updates a nightmare—with the need to reconfigure each hospital's new versions. New, small innovators may offer specialized products (for example, HIT to track pediatric ER dermatologic cases), but these, alas, further balkanize the market and contribute to incompatibility across HIT systems. Instead of achieving the digital nirvana of total data sharing (interoperability), the market too often extends the digital Tower of Babel. There are earnest efforts to create interoperability, but they face a Wild West ethos of individualism and resistance to regulation. Surprisingly, much of the HIT market is built on a foundation of what economists call "imperfect information"—an irony for an information technology industry, and an impediment for the health care industry. As we have argued, any understanding of the successes, challenges, and prognoses of HIT must incorporate the market forces that develop, sell, implement, and evaluate these remarkably expensive and complex systems.

11. The high initial and continuing costs of HIT are also a barrier to adaptation and innovation. From the perspective of the hospital administrator or medical practice manager, much of the benefit of HIT accrues to payers and "the health care system," not to the organizations that buy the technology. Moreover, the purchase price of an HIT system is only a fraction of its total cost. If an integrated system for a large hospital costs, say, $120 million, the hospital will spend three to five times that amount on implementation, redesigning work processes and information channels, training, and linkages with other systems, both human and technical Most of those costs, it should be clear, are on people, not hardware or software. Although software is the most plastic of technologies, administrators too often treat the software as frozen but the social systems and professional practices as infinitely malleable.

12. Often, too, back office functions, like billing and insurance, drive the clinical and work processes. Many of the software programs used in clinical practice are part of large suites of programs that generate bills, insurance statements, internal accounting records (for example, charg-

ing the pharmacy for the pills, assigning funds to the X-ray department for its services). Altering a clinical part of the program (for a clearly good reason) can be delayed or denied because it requires complex or undesirable changes in the many other parts of the program. The IT serves several masters, of which medical care is only one.

13. Several of the problems with HIT fall in the spaces between professional departments. Thus, for example, information loss or delays between the pharmacy and nursing departments may not be the focus of the IT systems with which either group works. The problem may be in the faulty linkages between the two systems—and thus no one's direct responsibility.

14. Woefully insufficient attention is paid to the social costs of HIT use. As we have seen, many aspects of these technologies may increase workers' stress and work time even while facilitating other tasks. Annoying medication alerts, which must be read and overridden, increase the time required for ordering drugs even though they sometimes prevent mistakes. When a referring physician must scroll through dozens of subtypes of possible stomach cancers instead of just writing "examine for possible stomach cancer," HIT does not speed her work. Nurses often complain that the implementation of complex HIT systems, without adjustments in staffing, means that they have two patients to care for: the patient and the computer. Asking nurses to reenter data from one computer system to another is neither efficient nor a wise patient safety move. Nurses, who must print out the lists of medications, check them off as they administer them to patients, and then enter that information again in the computer, have developed a workable solution that may facilitate billing, pharmacy records, and essential patient records. But it is not necessarily faster than the old paper-based system for the nurses. Physicians complain that they are now the ward's typists in addition to being secretaries and file clerks.

These explanations are neither exhaustive nor mutually exclusive. Vendors and others argue that HIT has not made more inroads because of lack of government funding and physician resistance. Government funding is now abundant as a result of the HITECH Act and other ARRA (American Recovery and Reinvestment Act) stimulus funds. Physician resistance was always a red herring, reflecting far more about the cumbersome software than about doctors' views of technology. The various vendor societies and others succeeded in redressing that governmental "failure" with a daily stream of enthusiastic reports and millions of dollars in additional lobbying.[38] Others claim that HIT is already superb but will continue to benefit from additional funding and from reduced physician resistance. Almost all agree that shared data standards are required, but each corporation is reluctant to give up its proprietary software codes and intra-company networking abilities.

What to Do? Specifics

Some of the problems of HIT can be addressed immediately and will produce fast and positive results. Hospitals buying HIT systems from vendors should read the contracts with great care. They should use their lawyers and experienced HIT people to craft contracts that require repairs to patient safety problems with the software. They should insert contractually specified penalties sufficient to ensure vendors are responsive to the needs of clinicians and of patient safety. Identification and rectification of problems should be spelled out clearly: Who defines a problem? Who is responsible for fixing it? When must it be fixed? Who pays for the fix? We know EMR vendors who classify their repairs as "enhancements" and therefore bill the customers for them. There are websites devoted to tales of vendor intransigence and ineptitude.[39] They should be read closely. Hospitals sharing similar vendor systems should create their own communication channels, in addition to user groups hosted by the vendors. Here are our recommendations:

- Efforts to find HIT problems should include investigation of the technology, the tasks, the organization, the patients' issues, and the environmental circumstances. Seeking to increase staff compliance with HIT use protocols is helpful, but making the technology compatible with the hospitals' work processes is more useful.
- All HIT implementation requires meticulous attention to its actual use in situ. Multidisciplinary teams should be used to review both qualitative (for example, observational) as well as quantitative data.
- Evaluation and implementation teams should work with technology vendors to align hardware, software, user, policy, workflow, and patient safety needs. But hospitals must maintain ultimate control. Clinicians and administrators must not abdicate their responsibility for patient safety. They must maintain vigilance while systems are implemented, evaluated, repaired, and updated.
- HIT system design must incorporate up-to-date standards for user interface design.
- In buying HIT systems, hospitals should focus on basic functionality, flexibility, interoperability, and robust design. The cost of the soft-

ware—which is massive—is only a small fraction of the cost of implementation, integration, training, and use.

- Contracts should be negotiated in a way that maximizes vendor responsiveness to clinical, workflow, user, and safety needs. In particular, they should oblige vendors to address technical problems that lead to patient safety dangers.
- Post-implementation assessments to identify user, environment, policy, workflow and patient issues are critical. User needs that can be evaluated pre-implementation include software interface characteristics, device size, nature and location of information in the HIT software, and methods for data acquisition. These issues must all be considered together and not independently.
- Post-implementation assessments should drive hospital educational efforts, policy, workflow changes, and requests to vendors.
- New workarounds will emerge in response to changes in technology, workflow, and patient types. Evaluation of actual technology use—in the context also of communications, workflow, and teamwork—must be ongoing.

There is a vast gap between the use of HIT and its promised outcomes. The published evidence reports some successes, but fewer than half of medical organizations have installed HIT, and those that have are often disappointed.[40] Even where HIT applications have been implemented, many of the studies report only modest gains. Moreover, at least some of these improved outcomes disappear over time.[41]

Much more focus is needed on how well the design of HIT applications complements health care work and workers. The effect of HIT on nurses, doctors, and other health care workers is the least studied aspect of HIT implementation and is probably one of the most propitious for enhancing HIT's adoption and benefits. Understanding the effects of HIT on, for instance, nurse-doctor or nurse-nurse interactions is essential and essentially unexplored. Similarly, there is little careful study of the effects of HIT on nurses' workloads. Many nurses, for example, find that automated barcoded medication administration systems require *extra* time to use, on top of the additional time needed for scanning each medication.[42] Yet this technology is sold as a time-saver for nurses (in addition to its many other virtues). Nurses also report spending an average of an hour and a half every shift just logging onto computers and smart devices—often fifty times per shift for the same device. In general, despite ubiquitous claims of productivity enhancement, the workplace implications of HIT are too often an afterthought to the technology development. Also, the need to help patients quickly means that clinicians must get the job done either with or in spite of any HIT help. And even if technology developers gave more attention to workplace processes than they currently do, determining what happens when HIT is installed in a health care facility is a difficult task, obscured by workarounds and by small ad hoc repairs that enable work to continue. The press of time—both to keep the system going and to serve the very ill—often means that hospitals are slow to learn from their mistakes. They are patching problems because they are not afforded the time to examine those problems with the consideration they would like to give them. In a coal mine, dying canaries signaled problems. But in a hospital, nonresponsive HIT systems are temporarily resuscitated and everyone goes back to work. Often the abilities of clinicians to solve problems, and the press of urgent work, mean they soldier on—even while systemic HIT faults are sidestepped.

HIT holds extraordinary promise, but its role as a health care panacea is premature. HIT is sold wrapped in an altruistic cloak of patient safety, health care cost reduction, universally available patient information, and the automated creation of research-rich databanks. But that altruistic garb is carefully woven by corporations, their lobbyists, and true believers. There are very real fragments of that cloak that already provide elements of a solution. And an integrated HIT system could provide the threads linking these fragments into a coherent cloth that would benefit patients, health care institutions, and those paying for health care. The elements are in place; the promises are currently unreachable. The irony is that the same market forces that are developing useful software programs (and promoting the industry) are also retarding growth of the technology with proprietary restrictions, software sold before it is ready, compliant evaluation structures, and creation of certification systems that exist to benefit marketers rather than to ensure quality. At this time, the cloak is closer to the emperor's new clothes than to a useful garment. Eventually that cloak will be real. In fact, nothing we say here should retard that progress. On the contrary, we argue that an honest evaluation of HIT will help reach that goal faster than blind faith.

HIT cannot be considered independently of its role within the entire health care system, including the social, physical, and existing technological environments. Use of HIT must include an analysis of the far more complex social, economic, medical, and physical systems into which the technology is incorporated. The effects of IT systems are usually much more nuanced, complex, and dramatic than most health care providers anticipate or are easily able to recognize. Unintended side effects as well as intended effects are discovered slowly, and only with vigilance, thoughtful examination, and an openness to surprises. Policymakers, health care executives, and clinicians should gain a balanced understanding of the powers, problems, and implications of the technology before they continue to devote resources to expensive systems. The often oversold technology—a belief lovingly nurtured by an HIT industry with much to gain—does not negate the significant benefits it can offer. And as HIT evolves, it will be of even greater value to patients, clinicians, and budgets. Ironically, the extravagant hype, the rush to market, and the refusal to address or honestly acknowledge its problems may be more of a danger to its continued growth than are its multifaceted failures. The continuing, and well-orchestrated, chorus of promises may deafen the industry's ability to hear its customers and recognize their needs. Patient safety, which has so much to benefit from good HIT, will suffer until the HIT industry is willing to really listen to the clinicians who use these systems.

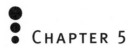

CHAPTER 5

A Day in the Life of a Nurse

Kathleen Burke

As a condition of participation in Medicare, the Centers for Medicare and Medicaid Services (CMS) in its Conditions of Participation Interpretive Guidelines, has made a requirement that scheduled medications be administered within thirty minutes before or after the specified time. To the outside observer, this rule seems quite a reasonable expectation—that a patient would receive a medication close to the time that it was scheduled or ordered. But from the perspective of a bedside nurse, this rule seems to have been devised by people who have little experience with the way nursing work is organized and who have had little direct observation of the work of bedside nurses. I am one of those nurses. I have the practical experience of frontline patient care that seems to have been missing when this rule was devised. So recently, when completing the Institute for Safe Medication Practice (ISMP) survey asking frontline nurses our opinion about this rule, I not only sent in my survey but also wrote the following short essay about what it's actually like to give out meds in a busy teaching hospital.

You asked: How does strict adherence to the thirty-minute rule create an opportunity for error? As a bedside nurse, I can tell you firsthand. But first, let me give you a little peek into what the process of medication administration looks like on my unit.

First, it is important to understand that many patients come into the hospital from home on multiple medications. I may very well be administering

five to ten medications per patient (in addition to administering pain medication, antibiotics, managing IV lines, etc.) during my 0900 medication pass
time. Second, medication administration does not happen in isolation.

Despite trying very hard to minimize interruptions during medication
pass time, I nonetheless have to give out meds while attending to all my
other responsibilities and demands for my attention. On a typical day shift I
have four patients. Many times I must wait in line for access to one of two
automated dispensing cabinets (we are a thirty-six-bed unit), especially during 0900 medication pass times. Then I must safely take out each medication
while double-checking it against the electronic medication administration
record (eMAR) for that patient.

After that, I must find any medication that is not stocked in the automated
dispensing cabinet. These medications may be in any one of four locations:
(1) the patient's individual medication cassette, (2) the refrigerator, (3) the
other automated dispensing cabinet, or (4) the pharmacy (e.g., a missing
medication). I must prepare a paper label for any medications that I need to
draw up into a syringe. For IV piggyback medications, I must first mix them
and then prepare a paper label.

Next, I travel down the hall with my eMAR and all the medications.
Hopefully, when I arrive in the room, the patient is ready for me, water cup
in hand, for his or her medications. I check the eMAR against the patient's
armband and individually open each little packet of unit-dose medication.
I do this while confirming and explaining to the patient the medication,
dosage, purpose, and so on, and responding to any concerns or questions the
patient may have. (I tease my patients that some of those little packets are
"nurse-proof"—they can be so cumbersome to open.)

Hopefully, I make it from the countertop, where I opened all the medications successfully, to the patient without dropping anything or knocking
over the medicine cup. Then I watch as my eighty-three-year-old patient
takes *one* pill at a time ("Honey, I can't take all those pills at once"), while I
cautiously survey her every attempt to reach her mouth, so as to catch any
medications that may fall out of her hand or cup and into the bed sheets or
down her gown. Then I stop and take her blood pressure before she takes her
antihypertensive medications. Finally, I go back to my eMAR and document
with my initials every medication I administered . . . and the *time*.

On to the next patient, right? Not so fast. The patient I have just so
carefully watched as she puts pill after pill in her mouth needs to use the
bathroom. Because she is an elderly postoperative patient with a knee replacement, I need to help her get up to use the bedside commode. This can take
twenty minutes or longer. Of course, assisting my patient out of bed and to

the commode is the perfect opportunity to assess the patient's strength, ability to follow commands, and scan and assess her skin, etc. But it also means that there is no way to get to the next patient within the time allotted.

I hope you are getting the idea that medication passes are time-consuming. Nurses are not administering medications to robots but to human beings. And during a med pass, my patients may express other needs that I cannot ignore at the time. I just gave you one very common scenario. Many more opportunities for distraction and interruptions to workflow occur that cause medication administration times to be delayed.

So where's the opportunity for error? There are many. One of the most prevalent is the time crunch and the level of frustration with the whole process of medication administration. This frustration causes distraction—one of the most frequent contributors to medication administration errors. The push to administer medications within the thirty-minute rule causes nurses to find workarounds . . . like pilfering another patient's cassette for a missing medication, documenting that the nurse gave a medication at 0900 (to keep in compliance and not get "caught" on audit) when it was really given at 1005, or withdrawing and preparing two different patients' medications at the same time to save time. Here's an example: Both patients are in a semi-private room. Why walk down the hall, back and forth, twice? Just bring Ms. Smith's meds and Ms. Rogers's meds to the same room at the same time! These are just some examples of a nurse's effort to "be in compliance" rather than do what is in the best interest of safety for the patient.

Giving nurses more flexibility for some medications and administration times, and educating us as to how and why these workarounds put our patients and our practice at risk, is the answer. And, wait, it might just be a good idea to talk to nurses before promulgating rules that make our jobs harder, more frustrating. and thus less safe for patients.

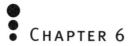

CHAPTER 6

Excluded Actors in Patient Safety

Peter Lazes, Suzanne Gordon, and Sameh Samy

Diane Sommers is an ICU (intensive care unit) nurse at a major East Coast teaching hospital.[1] Over the past few years her hospital has launched a number of pioneering safety initiatives: operating room and ICU checklists, efforts to reduce falls and infections, as well as safety meetings on individual patient care units. On the unit, a specific time is set aside each week so that staff can meet and learn about new safety methods, as well as discuss their concerns and insights. For Sommers, this has been a promising development. The problem, however, is that she and her colleagues have such a heavy workload caring for two intensely ill patients that they cannot regularly attend these patient safety meetings. Increasingly skeptical about her hospital's commitment to the kind of ongoing staff input that is critical to improving patient safety, Sommers wonders: Why doesn't hospital management adjust the nursing workload—just for an hour a week—so RNs like herself can contribute more effectively to patient safety efforts?

Beth Jones is an intravenous (IV) nurse at a Massachusetts teaching hospital. Although her hospital has implemented efforts to reduce central venous line infections, Jones is quite frustrated because these activities have not included the frontline staff responsible for placement of IVs. "We've had a really serious problem with central venous catheter [CVC] line infections. We have an awful lot of problems with PICC [peripherally inserted central catheter] lines. Management got together some nurses, infectious disease people, and doctors but left out the IV nurses, who are responsible for maintaining these lines and who'd complained about this problem for years. After all, we're the ones who take care of the central lines. I don't know why they left us out. I can't really figure it out. It's like they don't seem to think practitioners have valuable knowledge."[2]

Rick Brooks is the executive director of Rhode Island United Nurses and Allied Professionals (UNAP), a union that represents nurses at Rhode Island Hospital and other institutions connected to Lifespan, the largest hospital network in the state. Lifespan is another hospital network that has signed on to various patient safety initiatives. For example, one of Lifespan's physicians has partnered with an airline pilot to train staff in the kinds of teamwork lessons that have been essential to promoting safety in commercial aviation. Although the union is an influential "stakeholder" in hospital culture, Lifespan administrators have never asked UNAP to encourage its members to attend such seminars. In fact, the first Brooks heard of these meetings was when one of the authors asked him about them. Brooks acknowledges that he and fellow union activists could be more proactive when it comes to patient safety, but adds that members tend to be quite cynical about hospital safety initiatives. He explains, "Whenever union members identify workplace issues—mandatory overtime, unsafe staffing, failure to utilize lift equipment when moving heavy patients or failure to empower staff to challenge surgeons who refuse to use operating room checklists—the hospital ignores their concerns." When worker safety and patient safety intersect, says Brooks, "the hospital seems uninterested in pursuing either."[3]

Pamela Brier is the CEO of Maimonides Medical Center in Brooklyn. Over the past several years, her institution has also initiated a variety of patient safety initiatives. One concerned hospital cleanliness; others focused on patient falls and medication errors. Another was triggered by problems in the cardiology program. Although initiatives that are taking place at Maimonides seem similar to those going on in other hospitals, there is a significant difference. Unlike top-down management- or physician-led patient safety initiatives in many other U.S. institutions, those at Maimonides have been developed, implemented, evaluated, and refined in partnership with the hospital's three unions and led by frontline staff—not only RNs but also nursing aides, lab techs, and even cleaning staff. Brier feels that the inclusion of frontline staff and unions has transformed stalled efforts to make Maimonides a safer hospital, and she and her colleagues in the executive suite are committed to pursuing a bottom-up approach to patient safety.

These four anecdotes highlight one of the most significant issues related to the realization of the patient safety agenda in hospitals today. In the contemporary American hospital, when patient safety initiatives are planned and designed, this work is almost always done at the top. Physician leaders, safety champions, "green belts," safety researchers, nurse managers, hospital administrators, outside consultants, patient safety advocacy groups, or hospital regulators identify problems, craft solutions, design and plan initiatives, and/or issue mandates requiring their implementation. As initiatives move from top to bottom, managers are generally enlisted to encourage worker compliance. The evaluation and refinement of safety efforts also takes place with little input from the front lines of care—nursing, nursing assistants, cleaning, food services, and other hospital occupations. In a similar vein, in many hospitals in which unions represent a significant segment of the workforce, union leaders and activists are rarely enlisted as allies and may not even be notified about patient safety projects or plans.

Furthermore, when workers identify patient safety problems that target workload, equipment, supplies, or fatigue and worker safety and health—anything that involves the allocation of significant financial resources or involves significant changes in work organization—hospitals often turn a deaf ear to their concerns. When workers, particularly unionized workers, propose legislative, regulatory, or contractual remedies that could improve patient safety, hospitals generally fight to defeat these efforts. Indeed, rather than allying with workers who have identified significant safety problems, administrators often perceive workers as adversaries rather than allies. When it comes to patient safety, there is also a disconnect between initiatives designed to make patients safer and those that also target the health and well-being of the hospital workforce. Although the two are intimately connected, in the modern patient safety movement and hospitals' responses to it, worker safety lies on one side of a very wide chasm that separates the health of hospital workers from that of the patients for whom they care.

In this chapter we explore this blind spot in the effort to make hospitals safer, providing an argument for the inclusion of frontline workers and unions, analyzing some of the reasons for their exclusion from safety efforts, and suggesting a different model that would help strengthen safety activities.

Why Frontline Workers and Unions Matter

Including frontline workers in the full spectrum of patient safety initiatives is important for several reasons. While high-level buy-in is critical to patient safety, hospital culture is changed not only through dictates elaborated in the C suite (the hospital department where we find the offices of the chief executive and operations, finance, and nursing officers), or by experts and researchers at a patient safety conference, or on grand rounds, but also at the grass-roots level, where care is delivered and where the environment in which it is delivered is shaped: in the patient's room, hospital corridor, nurses' station, on-call room, laboratory, X-ray suite, or housekeepers' locker room. The people who must carefully manipulate IV lines, administer medications, wash their hands before and after touching a patient, read tests correctly, keep hospital corridors and patients' rooms clean, or make sure that a patient doesn't die while being transported to or waiting for an X ray are also the people who can best help identify the problems they have doing these things safely and effectively. They are also the people who must help craft workable solutions as well as workable ways to implement and evaluate them. These staff have the implicit knowledge of what works and what doesn't. If hospitals are to learn from their mistakes and thus produce and sustain institution-wide learning, the process of institutional transformation must be circular, not linear—from bottom to top and top to bottom in a continuous manner.[4]

Let's look first at how patient safety problems are identified. Many researchers, policy experts, administrators, and managers have very accurate and innovative ideas about what is wrong in health care institutions and how to fix it. Safety initiatives must be supported by the top of the health care hierarchy and be implemented by—and overcome the resistance of—traditional medical elites. Higher-level administrators and middle managers have control over the resources that make change possible.[5] They also have a lot of good ideas about what needs changing and how to change it. Nevertheless, many of the things that jeopardize patients are invisible to top management because they occur in what the great sociologist Erving Goffman called "backstage spaces" and involve backstage and often invisible health care workers. These are spaces that upper-level executives or managers (and sometimes even middle-level managers or physician leaders) rarely have access to because they spend very little time actually delivering patient care at the sites where care is delivered, or communicating directly with backstage workers. As the ones who deliver care or tend to the environment in which care is delivered, frontline workers are far more familiar with processes of care delivery and infrastructural maintenance and can thus far more effectively identify aspects of patient care delivery that are unsafe. As Amy Edmondson has put it, "In hospitals senior managers often do not know which group has which culture, making it difficult to ascertain whether and when they are getting the true data on errors."[6]

According to Carol Porter, director of nursing at Mount Sinai Hospital in New York City, "to create an effective patient safety process, frontline staff need to be involved, not just to assure compliance with major initiatives once they have been designed but to assure that the choice of initiatives, the strategies pursued, and plan for implementation and monitoring of activities include [them]."[7] Porter found "it was impossible to improve patient safety in our hospital without the full involvement of frontline staff and the support of their unions. Past management refused to see these groups as allies and instead spent time fighting their involvement."[8]

The renowned business professor Michael Porter (no relation to Carol) pointed out in an interview that institutions that have succeeded in creating a culture of safety have found ways to encourage and include frontline staff in the identification of safety problems without fear of reprisal. They not only involve staff in the design and implementation of appropriate and practical solutions but also, like other high-reliability industries (the aviation and chemical industries, for example), provide staff with the necessary time and resources to create, learn, and master new procedures and processes. Finally, they encourage staff to identify new problems that arise as solutions are rolled out. And, as Edmondson adds, they create an environment of psychological safety so workers can identify problems without risk and suggest if and when safety efforts are not succeeding.[9]

Because "solutions" always create unintended problems, these industries involve frontline staff and management. These two groups are central to any effort to illuminate clearly the dynamic interaction between work organization and the allocation of financial resources to patient care and safety. Clarity around this issue is absolutely critical. When it comes to patient safety, the devil that can undermine the best of patient safety activities often lies in the details of work organization. Consider, for example, the effort to reduce the spread of hospital-acquired infections. When a hospitalized patient acquires an infection, it is important for all staff and visitors to put on a gown and gloves before entering the patient's room. They must also discard them before exiting the room. To make sure that these procedures are followed consistently, not only RNs but also hospital cleaning, dietary, and any other staff who enter and exit a patient's room must be carefully and recurrently trained in the proper infection control technique.

In one hospital we visited (a Magnet hospital that had won many other prestigious awards), one of us (Suzanne Gordon) watched closely as nurses gowned and gloved appropriately before entering a room and discarded their protective gear before exiting. A few minutes later, after the RN had left the room, a hospital cleaner entered, similarly gowned and gloved, and proceeded to clean the patient's room. She, however, exited the room without discarding her gown and gloves inside and then, in the hospital corridor, took them off and threw them into a garbage receptacle. As she was walking by just by chance, an RN chastised the aide for failing to execute patient safety precautions correctly. The aide had not done this correctly because cleaners had been left out of the patient safety information loop and were not sufficiently educated about the entire infection control procedure.

In another hospital, Gordon and Ross Koppel observed a similar problem. Workers, if consulted early and often, can identify problems and obstacles in the way their work is structured, information communicated, and care planned. The following example illustrates this often ignored fact.

We know that one of the most effective infection control measures is also one of the most simple: hand washing before entering and after exiting a patient's room. Yet we also know that many hospital workers don't wash their hands appropriately. As a recent article in the *Lancet* documented, it is not simply ignorance or laziness that keeps workers from using the soap and water or hand-sanitizing gel available in hospitals—when, that is, it is made available. The lapse also has to do with work organization. The article reported that understaffing and too much emphasis on patient throughput supersede hand washing even when indicators point to the acute need for more of it. Frontline staff are not ignorant of this problem. They know what discourages them from appropriately following hospital policies. As one RN commented tersely, "Don't tell me about hand washing. I know all about universal precautions. My hands are so cracked they are painful because I have them in soap and water all the time."

This RN works on a medical surgical unit where the average patient load is between seven and eight patients. This may help explain why her hands are so cracked and painful. Increasing a physician's, nurse's, or nurses' aide's patient load significantly increases the number of patient encounters he or she has per day, which in turn increases the number of times he or she must clean his or her hands. To wash hands correctly would eat up a significant amount of time. Clearly if, because of heavy workloads, hospital staff lack the time to wash their hands and perform assigned patient care duties and/ or find it too painful, they won't wash their hands.

Frontline workers may also be the only ones who can identify how institutional financial priorities are impacting the success of patient safety initiatives. Once again the issue of hospital cleanliness comes to mind. Cleanliness doesn't involve only washing one's hands or discarding gowns and gloves in the proper place. It involves the basic cleaning activities that Florence Nightingale identified over 150 years ago at the military hospitals in Scutari during the Crimean War. What is usually considered to be the prototypical example of "mindless" work can have lethal consequences if not done properly. Yet a number of studies have highlighted the fact that devaluation and outsourcing of this kind of work have increased hospital-acquired infections, not to mention worker injuries and illness.[10]

The sociologist Dan Zuberi, for example, has analyzed the impact of a trend that began in the United States and has swept hospital systems all across the globe. The job of cleaning the hospital is no longer performed only by staff employed, trained, and controlled by the hospital but has been outsourced to private for-profit contractors. These contractors often try to save money and increase profit by skimping on the number of workers they hire, failing to train workers adequately to do their work safely, and even failing to provide them with adequate cleaning supplies. Zuberi states: "In an era in which about one in ten patients will suffer from a hospital-acquired infection, it is more important than ever that hospitals invest in the training of adequate numbers of cleaning staff. In fact, by disinvesting in cleaning through outsourcing, hospitals are doing the opposite."[11] In his research Zuberi has found that managers frequently lose control over every step of the process. In many hospitals they can no longer choose whom to hire, what kind of training staff get, the number of staff assigned, or the kinds of chemicals used.

Zuberi explains that infection control nurses, who used to meet and work regularly with housekeeping staff to provide them with training and supervision or to address critical issues, are no longer able to work directly with housekeepers because they are no longer working directly for the hospital. "When cleaning workers work for outside contractors whose main mission is to maximize profit, patients suffer,"[12] Zuberi says. Using contract employees often leads to reduced communication with nursing and clinical staff, since they are accountable not to the hospital but instead to their contract supervisor. As an article in the *Journal of the Royal Society of Medicine* describes the situation in Great Britain "'outsourcing' of services such as hospital cleaning has produced a demoralized, exploited workforce and a management that has lost touch with what the job entails."[13]

Loss of control over the process of keeping hospitals clean can compromise any and every patient safety initiative that is proposed and implemented. Indeed, this loss of control jeopardizes the very mission of the hospital as well as the fundamental ethical promise of physicians and nurses to "first do no harm." Problems are also caused by the lack of clear, appropriate procedures for these staff, on the assumption that "everyone knows how to clean a room." Making sure that these phenomena do not jeopardize the nonnegotiable aspects of patient care will require discussing workload and working conditions with workers who often fail to capture the attention and imagination of elite experts.

These and other workers can also help us understand the roles that time, energy, and burnout play in the implementation of patient safety. Over the past decade or more, health care has seen a flood of patient safety dictates not only from regulators or accreditors but also from outside consultants coming into the workplace to reorganize, restructure, or reengineer work processes. In one large Manhattan teaching hospital, the chief nursing officer recalled that over a period of ten years, almost the same number of consultants made their way into and out of the hospital, each with a contradictory way of organizing care, creating teams, or structuring work processes. These consultants entered hospitals in a whirlwind of promises and activity but rarely stayed around long enough to implement changes or evaluate what had happened to patient care and the hospital workforce as a result.

Patient safety has also become part of this flavor-of-the-month consultant trend. One week some staff may be asked to attend trainings in Crucial Conversations led by Vital Smarts, teamwork trainings given by NDelta, or Top Gun (founded by former airline pilots), or Six Sigma or Toyota Lean Production, delivered by yet another cohort of consultants. Hospitals are the site of initiatives pioneered by the Institute for Healthcare Improvement, one of the leaders in the patient safety movement. Over the past several years the IHI has launched the 5 Million Lives campaign, which began as the 100,000 Lives campaign. Its website lists programs like the State Action on Avoidable Rehospitalization (STAAR), or WHO Surgical Safety Checklists,[14] with new initiatives announced sometimes on a weekly basis. In nursing there is the Robert Wood Johnson Foundation's Transforming Care at the Bedside, and the American Nurses Credentialing Center's Magnet hospital movement, as well as the American Association of Critical Care Nurses' Healthy Workplace Initiative. Every one of these initiatives demands time and energy from frontline staff. The crucial questions here are: Are units allocated enough staff, and are staff given enough time to absorb and master these new activities—activities that are too often an add-on to an unadjusted workload? How can these activities be financially sound investments for hospitals? How can they be seen as important critical investments that will reduce outcomes such as medical errors, lawsuits, and length of stay for patients?

The time and energy required by the introduction of new technologies that are discussed in chapters by Koppel and his colleagues also complicate the patient safety picture. Depending on an individual's age and computer literacy, mastering these technological changes takes a great deal of time and effort. Often, staff need to manage both the old system and the new system while technological bugs are ironed out. Again the question arises: Are staff given enough time, and is their workload adjusted so they can master these technologies? If not, the sheer number of initiatives that workers are asked to implement and absorb can result in the kind of "consultant fatigue" that may, in turn, lead to cynicism.

Frontline workers can be very helpful in identifying how much time it will really take to deal with new initiatives and their accompanying technological demands, as well as in suggesting how staffing levels and workload need to be adjusted so that workers can change practice. Frontline staff, Edmondson writes, must also have the time to do second-order problem solving, not just first-order "workarounds,"[15] whereby a problem is not effectively resolved but instead a temporary solution is implemented in order to resolve the immediate issue. Unfortunately, current staffing patterns leave workers little time to do more than the latter—engaging in time-consuming workarounds. This failure to consider long-term solutions is not merely rewarded on hospital units; it is embedded in medical and nursing education.

"The topic of improving patient safety and problem solving in terms of organizational and system issues are rarely taught in nursing and medical [schools]," commented Dr. George Thibault, president of the Josiah Macy Jr. Foundation, which supports the development of a clinical education–reform curriculum in medical and nursing schools.[16] When programs for health care administrators and middle managers tackle the issue of patient safety, they tend to focus on problem-solving tools but not the processes and skills needed to engage the workforce in activities to identify critical problems and to assist in implementing changes. When hospital staff are promoted out of the ranks of frontline workers and into the ranks of management—when RNs become nurse managers, for example—the hospital generally fails to teach them the kind of coaching and team-building skills that are key to patient safety. As one nurse manager expresses it, "If we were able to figure out how to involve frontline staff sooner, we would be able to improve our performance—not just improve our performance, but improve performance faster."[17] Furthermore, they are certainly not part of the training of workers on the lower rungs of the health care ladder—workers who, because of class, race, and ethnicity, are unlikely to be asked to participate in problem-solving and decision-making activities when it comes to patient safety. This is ironic, since these workers tend to be long-term employees who know firsthand about systems that work and those that don't.

Frontline staff must also be involved in patient safety initiatives because they are the ones who directly experience the unintended consequences or glitches of safety initiatives. We know that unintended consequences are common outcomes of well-intentioned projects. High-risk, high-reliability industries that have successfully changed their cultures have long recognized that safety requires a lot of trial and a lot of error. You can't work out the glitches, however, if the people who can best identify them are not encouraged to speak up and/or aren't heard when they do.

Citing just one of these glitches, Krishna Collie, a consultant who works with the National Institutes of Health (NIH) in Washington, D.C., comments: "A common breakdown is that computer systems for outpatient, inpatient, and specialist and primary care doctors using EMRs [electronic medical records] don't talk with each other. Many of these problems could be controlled if not eliminated if [hospital] staffs had been included in the selection of vendors and the actual software that is used."[18] Many physicians and nurses report that they are evaluated on their display of enthusiasm for newly installed health information technology (HIT). Koppel elaborates:

> Even though they experience significant problems with HIT that has profound negative patient safety implications, many doctors and nurses say that they are discouraged from reporting these problems. If they fail to show enthusiastic support for HIT or report problems, they risk being labeled "technophobes" or "troublemakers." Rather than acknowledging that the technology has problems that require remedy, doctors and nurses are accused of being dumb, technophobic, or incompetent. In this way dangers to patient safety are allowed to propagate, workers become increasingly frustrated, and the software is not improved.[19]

Failing to include frontline workers in hospital initiatives is clearly documented in an influential article by Harvard Business School professors Anita Tucker and Amy Edmondson, "Why Hospitals Don't Learn from Failures." They write, "Front-line employees in service organizations are well positioned in these efforts to help their organizations learn, that is, to improve organizational outcomes by suggesting changes in processes and activities based on their knowledge of what is and is not working."[20] Or as John le Carré expressed in a more literary vein in his novel *Absolute Friends*, "in a mammoth bureaucracy obsessed with its own secrecy, the fault lines are best observed by those who, instead of peering down from the top, stand at the bottom and look up."[21]

Backstage Attitude Change

The most promising patient safety initiative involves more than a technical fix or a brilliant campaign slogan. Patient safety, like any other cultural transformation, involves changing attitudes and not just changing behavior.

Changing attitudes, however, is not simply a matter of individuals acquiring the right information and then applying it under the watchful eyes of an alert expert or manager. Changes in attitudes and beliefs occur in the web of social relationships in which individuals reside. As David Dickinson has pointed out in his excellent book on HIV/AIDS prevention, *Changing the Course of AIDS: Peer Education in South Africa and Its Lessons for the Global Crisis,* changing behavior involves a complex interplay between the front stage, backstage, and private spaces.[22] These terms are taken from Erving Goffman, who, in *The Presentation of Self in Everyday Life* (1959), described human interaction as a performance that is executed in a variety of spaces—front stage, backstage, and private.[23] Elite actors, the proverbial experts, generally occupy the front stage spaces, where they give performances and hand down information, advice, and recommendations. They expect their audience of less elite players to accept this information and adjust their behavior accordingly. Actors who are barely recognized by experts as "players"—or, in the new health care jargon, as "stakeholders"—occupy backstage and private spaces. In front stage spaces the powerless or lower-level player may often seem to assent to or comply with the powerful. In private or backstage spaces, to which the powerful do not have access, the less powerful say what they really think and act upon their true beliefs and feelings.

In the hospital or patient safety movement, front stage spaces would involve conferences like those conducted by the IHI, or seminars given inside or outside the hospital by prominent patient safety experts or hospital higher-ups. Backstage spaces would include the hospital ward and even the patient's room, which managers will try to penetrate through a variety of championship efforts or management by walking around. Private spaces include the nurses' station, lunchroom, staffroom, hospital corridor, locker room, and so forth. These are the "cultures" that Porter and Edmondson refer to in quotations cited earlier.

What one learns in the culture of backstage and private spaces is key to both attitude and behavioral change, for example, the role played by demoralization and burnout in workers' responses to patient safety initiatives. As we said earlier, over at least the past decade and a half, hospital management has hired a raft of consultants to help cut costs and reengineer hospitals. These cost-cutting efforts have largely targeted frontline staff such as nurses, as well as cleaners and other nonclinical workers. During this period, hospital workers have also fought for a clear and structured process to work jointly with management on patient safety activities, bans on mandatory overtime for RN staff, safe nurse-to-patient staffing ratios, safe needle technology to prevent the spread of HIV/AIDS and other blood-borne pathogens, safe lifting technology, the reduction of medical errors, the use of appropriate checklists for critical procedures, and the creation of increased teamwork among doctors and nurses, among other goals. With few exceptions, hospital management has resisted these efforts.

Many hospital staff members are thus deeply suspicious of what they perceive to be hospitals' sudden embrace of "safety," when, in their view, they have been pleading with hospitals to attend to the safety of both their patients and their workers for years. In the private spaces of our interviews, one health care union leader put it this way: "Our attitude is, really, you care about safety? Where were you when we were trying to get safe needle technology to protect patients and us? Now you blame staff for not caring enough about patient safety. Is something wrong with this picture?" Or as Diane Sommers, whom we met at the beginning of this chapter, explains: "We can't even get off the wards to attend safety rounds. Our hospital will just not allocate the financial resources to things like staff that help make patient safety a reality. So when I hear about a new patient safety initiative, I just sigh and roll my eyes."[24]

The same is true of the outsourced hospital cleaner or food service worker. According to Polly Toynbee, author of *Hard Work: Life in Low-Pay Britain*, "when you combine low pay, low regard and high turn-over what you get is a hospital industry in which there is no loyalty to its outsourced employees and no loyalty of outsourced employees to the institution in which they work. This can be a toxic brew when it comes to patient care and safety."[25]

In backstage and private spaces, workers also express their concerns about the impact of patient safety initiatives on their perceived status and authority. Just as airline pilots at the beginning of the airline safety movement in the 1980s believed that cockpit (later crew) resource management programs were an industry effort to erode their authority,[26] many frontline staff are concerned that patient safety initiatives are really wolves in sheep's clothing. One nurse who was highly critical of the impact of patient restructuring voiced concern about efforts to utilize the SBAR *(situation, background, assessment, and recommendation)* technique to enhance communication between doctors and nurses. "This is just a way to deprofessionalize nursing," she insisted.[27] Other nurses have objected on similar grounds to, for example, asking two nurses to check IV medication administration. Many nurses are concerned about the computerization of bedside nursing and the introduction of medication administration records and PDAs (personal digital assistants). As Koppel and his colleagues highlight in chapter 4, their concerns are warranted. If there is no institutional vehicle—no attempt to create the psychological sense of safety that is a prerequisite for institutional learning—through which staff are made to feel comfortable about voicing their concerns and working to make technology and other safety initiatives not only helpful to patients but also worker friendly, staff may continue to resist such initiatives.

Under these circumstances, resistance, which is all too often viewed as an irrational fear of change, may in fact be a rational response to a poorly planned and executed patient safety agenda. If hospital executives and patient safety advocates are to succeed in transforming institutional culture, they will have to understand the limitations of top-down approaches and the importance of working in backstage and private spaces. New knowledge obtained through frontline staff involvement is also critical to arriving at appropriate and sustainable solutions.[28] Organizations able to encourage and capture this knowledge can go on to achieve breakthrough changes and thus effectively improve the quality of the services they provide.

In addition to their generating new knowledge, co-workers are the only ones who can navigate backstage and private spaces by lowering resistance to any ill-conceived and autocratic dicta from above. When one co-worker leads another because that co-worker has been involved in the planning of initiatives, he or she can recognize what a peer understands, what information peers need, what beliefs have to be challenged, what hostilities or resentments need to addressed and overcome, and how best to negotiate them.

Why Unions Must Be Involved

Many hospital administrators and patient safety advocates are well aware of the successes of the safety movement in aviation and frequently cite the literature of crew resource management (CRM) in discussions of patient safety.[29] Yet there is one aspect of CRM that is consistently downplayed: union involvement in the creation of an aviation safety culture was central to its success.

At United Airlines, the first major commercial airline company to initiate CRM training, top-level management began its change initiative with the full participation of the Air Line Pilots Association (ALPA). When cockpit resource management morphed into crew resource management, the Association of Flight Attendants (AFA) participated in trainings and their implementation. "The industry has learned that we are integral to a successful safety process. They would never contemplate going back to the old way,"[30] says Keith Hagy, a safety officer for ALPA. ALPA continues to work with management to design and conduct the training for all flight crews. It is also responsible for helping to monitor safety problems of the airline industry. "The involvement of ALPA has been critical to the success of our safety program," Hagy continues. "The unions have helped to make sure the approach we used was practical and relevant, and they helped to create a process that their members would trust since they were critical players in the process. If they were not involved, there would still be issues of whether or not employees would trust this process."[31] Just as it was critical to the creation of a safety culture in the aviation industry, the involvement of union leadership and activists is similarly critical to changing culture in health care. In many areas of the United States, aides, janitors, unit clerks, and a variety of other health care workers are represented by trade unions. Almost 20 percent of hospital RNs are in unions, as are many licensed practical nurses (LPNs) and nurses' aides. In some locales, even medical residents are unionized.[32]

In a workplace that is unionized, engaging union leaders is one of the most viable routes to mobilizing the support and input of frontline staff. In hospitals that are unionized, many frontline staff—particularly those who are the most vocal, active, and motivated to help with change activities (precisely the kind to be the "black belts" or "champions" of change)—may feel greater loyalty to their union than they do to hospital management. As we said earlier, since the endless cutbacks and restructuring that began in the 1990s, many workers are deeply suspicious of hospital management. They believe that the C suite does not represent their interests or the interests of patients. Involving union leaders and activists can help overcome the belief that projects pitched as efforts to increase patient safety are in reality ploys to increase productivity from the health care workforce.

Another reason why union participation is critical is that unions can protect workers from either actual reprisals or the fear of reprisals. If reporting problems is the key to addressing them, then protecting those who report problems is essential. In the aviation industry, protecting workers who report safety concerns has been critical to enhancing safety for both passengers and crew.[33] Many lower-level workers, however, are very concerned that their reward for identifying patient safety problems will be disciplinary procedures or even being fired.

In unionized settings, frontline staff, which at times can include supervisors, are protected from reprisals as a result of collective bargaining agreements with management. (For instance, workers cannot be fired without just cause, such as documentation of clear violation of safety procedures.) Unions can protect members from the all too common dangers facing frontline workers who champion safety in nonunion hospitals. To cite just one example, a veteran nurse at Huntington Memorial, a nonunion hospital in Pasadena, California, was recently fired when she tried to challenge an intern's order to ventilate a patient on a busy medical unit. Not only did she lose her job, but also she was disciplined by the State Board of Nursing. An even more recent case is the trial in 2010 of nurses in Texas who reported a physician to the medical board and were brought up on felony charges as a result.[34] Incidents like these do not help to assuage workers' fears, and prevent them from becoming fearless patient safety champions.

Soliciting the input of unionized frontline workers is particularly important since they may be the only ones who are able to discuss candidly the unintended consequences of patient safety initiatives. Ironically, managers who are responsible for implementing patient safety initiatives may not be comfortable identifying significant and troublesome problems for fear of being reprimanded or even fired. "Many times management sees critical patient safety problems but fear that their job is at risk if they identify a specific problems that upper management would prefer to ignore," says a vice president for human resources at a hospital in the Northeast. "I had this happen to me. I am now more reluctant to share significant patient safety problems with upper management for fear of losing my job."[35] This is why managers must also be protected if patient safety is to become a reality.

The fact is that hospital administrators who have put their reputations on the line by spending millions on hiring consultants and/or purchasing new technologies may not want to hear that these are not working as well as expected. Under current conditions, where nonunionized workers, both staff and managers, are employees "at will" (meaning they can be fired without just cause) and there are no guaranteed protections for speaking up and identifying specific problems in the workplace, the sad truth is that many workers and managers are fired if they voice concerns about significant patient safety problems which management is unwilling to address.

Another way in which unions can be extremely helpful is their ability to create education and funds for hospitals to train frontline staff and managers in effective methods to improve patient safety. Often it is difficult to create needed training and education just for one hospital. But if multiple hospitals can be persuaded to contribute to a common fund, important training and education activities are possible. Two significant examples of this arrangement are the 1199/SEIU and League of Voluntary Hospitals Training and Upgrading Fund in New York City, and the Worker Education and Resource Center in Los Angeles established by SEIU local 721. Both of these educational centers were created by unions to provide hospitals with educators and trainers to assist in the development of patient safety programs. These educational centers have provided hospitals in New York City and Los Angeles with thousands of dollars in training funds. Unions can also be helpful in working with management to obtain local, federal, and private foundation funds for patient safety projects, since hospital reimbursements will increasingly be based on higher levels of quality of care and patient safety, and it is clear to many of these funders that training and education activities for frontline staff and supervisors are needed to improve patient safety outcomes. Lobbying for training, education, and pilot projects is another positive way for unions to work with hospitals. Through these activities, health care unions can help expand access to politicians, state and federal agencies, and foundation staff to which management alone does not have access. This is because health care unions represent a large numbers of workers from multiple worksites and thus have larger constituencies than management commonly has.

Finally, given the fact that so many of us resist change no matter where it begins or ends, enlisting every single ally in the cause seems not just simple common sense but something one would avoid at one's—and at patients'—peril. In workplaces where union members are active, they can become significant advocates for making the change to a safety culture. Given their insistence on recruiting stakeholders and on the power of informal leaders, one wonders, therefore, why managers and safety advocates do not spend more time and energy recruiting union leaders and activists in their efforts for cultural change.

Why Frontline Workers and Unions Are Not Sufficiently Involved in Patient Safety

In a study conducted by Peter Lazes and other researchers at Cornell University and the University of North Carolina School of Nursing at Chapel Hill, hospital staff in charge of quality and/or performance improvement at thirty-one U.S. hospitals were interviewed. The researchers wanted to ascertain if—as well as how—frontline staff were involved in patient safety and quality-of-care activities. All of these hospitals had received some sort of publicity, accreditation, or award which suggested that hospital management was deeply committed to engaging frontline staff in quality and safety activities within the hospital. The researchers asked four primary questions: To what extent is your hospital involving frontline staff in improvement activities? How are they involved in these activities? What have been the outcomes? And what role have unions had in these improvement activities?

In spite of their reputations and awards, there seems to be a disconnect between the public stance and reality at these hospitals. Many of those interviewed indicated that frontline staff were only marginally involved in problem solving and had almost no role in identifying problems in the first place.[36]

If, for example, a hospital was trying to reduce central line infections, the researchers asked about the extent to which frontline staff were involved with devising solutions to the problem. Moreover, and perhaps more disturbingly, frontline staff had almost no role in implementing safety efforts like these. Only 17 percent of hospitals engaged frontline staff in both problem identification and implementation activities. For the most part, only nurses were engaged in such activities. When hospital workers were represented by unions, they were active partners in only some cases and were often not included in monitoring and seeking ways to improve the impact of safety and improvement processes. Indeed, all too often they were sidelined. The researchers were concerned with improving the accuracy of information about frontline staff engagement. Although interviews were conducted with only one staff person involved with the hospital's quality or safety activities, it was nonetheless clear that the level of frontline staff involvement in these cases of excellence was limited. Perhaps the most significant thing researchers uncovered was the fact that management rarely consulted frontline staff about daily patient care issues, concerns, or problems, nor did they ask staff for suggestions for improvement. Even in the few cases where frontline staff were involved in identifying problems, they were not involved in implementing solutions.[37]

The exclusion of frontline workers is often the result of managerial and professional attitudes. Hospitals are not only some of the most complex but also some of the most hierarchical institutions in industrialized society. Organized into rigid, stratified groups, hospital professionals and workers are divided by both financial and professional status. These sharp divisions are reflected in traditional hospital language. Doctors are called "chief medical officer" or "house officer," and they issue "orders" to other hospital employees as well as patients. Lower-level workers, such as nurses, are termed "physician extenders." Physicians and managers consider themselves to be the designated problem identifiers and solvers. They are the mindful leaders who deliver dictates to workers who do what has often been characterized as "mindless" work.[38]

Trained and referred to in their higher-level role in the health care hierarchy, many managers and physician leaders do not believe that workers have anything to add to their own knowledge of the big picture. "I don't see a need to involve frontline staff. They don't know enough about the real problems," is a familiar "leadership" refrain. Kamilla Kohn Roadberg, an international management consultant who works for Odhe and Company in Gothenburg, Sweden, notes that it is the job of management "to create needed procedures to improve patient safety and by so doing reduce the variances in how actual work gets done. This approach is at the core of [the] lean manufacturing process, which has not proven to be an effective process of improving health care delivery problems by itself."[39]

Instead of exploring ways to engage frontline staff in the initial stages of planning and development of patient safety processes, the most common approach in hospital management today is the recruitment of management staff who are assigned to find solutions to specific patient safety problems. Referred to as "champions," "black belts," "ambassadors," and "internal consultants," they are picked by upper-level management and assigned the mission of creating appropriate solutions to a variety of problems—solutions that line management are then required to implement.

This top-down approach is promoted by the many consultants who offer their services to hospital administrators. One has only to Google any one of these terms—"champions," "internal consultants," "black belts"—to unleash an avalanche of advertisements posted on consultants' websites that will tell you where, and how much you have to pay, to get patient safety advice, information, and training. The American Academy of Management, the American Hospital Association, and the Institute for Healthcare Improvement all encourage an approach that concentrates on creating more and more champions, black belts, quality fellows—the list seems endless. The price of their services, seminars, and conferences makes it clear that the audience most consultants target is composed of physician leaders, upper-level, and sometimes middle-level management. Rarely are frontline staff and unions involved.

This top-down approach often produces dismay and resentment in many staff. One nurse at a northeastern teaching hospital described upper-level management's efforts to encourage hand washing in her institution. A hand washing initiative was designed and implemented at the top, and then a managerial hand washing "champion" walked around the units rewarding staff members with a box of Skittles if he saw them comply with hand washing policies. "It was like we were a bunch of children whom they could pacify by giving out a box of cheap candy," an RN commented.[40] Not only did frontline staff resent the fact that they weren't involved in the design and implementation phase, but also they were deeply offended at being treated like children rather than adult professionals. These resentments were never directly made known to managers but were heartily expressed in private spaces.

From our observations, top-level leaders may at times solicit ideas from staff. One common practice is to conduct interviews, create a team, and survey staff about initiatives that have already been decided. Frontline workers, however, are rarely included in the overall design of patient safety processes. Once initiatives are designed, workers are then cajoled or exhorted to comply with new practices or activities. Like the patient who either acquiesces or refuses to do what the doctor orders, workers become either "compliant," and thus good, or "noncompliant," and thus difficult, and are blamed or disciplined for their failure to obey.

Even when frontline staff are recruited to join patient safety initiatives, the choice of staff tends to be limited to RNs. Patient safety, however, "is not simply nursing's work, it is the work of the whole organization," says a CEO in a study of frontline staff involvement.[41] Depending on the specific nature of a particular problem, other clinical staff, physicians and house staff, respiratory therapists, social workers, pharmacists, lab techs, and non-clinical staff such as housekeeping and food services need to be engaged. As another chief nursing officer (CNO) at a hospital steeped in patient safety activities comments, "I wish we could have done more in a multi-disciplinary fashion. We tend to hand off pieces to each other and work in silos. Nurses themselves are very involved, but a lot [of] what happens is beyond just the nurse."[42]

If the positive potential of frontline staff is too often ignored, the potential of unions as allies in the patient safety project is ignored even more so. In Europe, unions are viewed as critical "stakeholders" in any workplace activity. Important social partners, they help ensure that the voice of workers is part of public discourse, and they play a central role in lobbying for funding of hospitals and other health facilities. Reflecting traditional American management's hostility to unions, many health care employers view unions as hostile at worst and obstructive at best. "The feeling is that unions add to the complexity of an already complex job," observed a chief nurse executive of a major hospital.[43] As Gordon has written in an article analyzing nurse managers' attitudes toward unions, nursing executives and even nursing academics often socialize nurses and managers to view union leaders and activists as spiders catching flies or manipulative militants trying to dupe goodhearted but ultimately mindless prey. At best unions are considered a necessary evil, at worst the devil incarnate.[44]

"They [unions] have no awareness of management's difficulties. They just cause us problems," echoes a middle manager at a hospital in the Northeast.[45] "We actively keep them out of our hospitals, and if they were present, we would keep them out of any organized patient safety process," adds an officer of a northeastern hospital association. "They can only cause problems for us."[46] Other administrators think that including unions in planning and implementing needed changes takes too much time. "We need to make important changes now and cannot wait for everyone to be consulted," remarked one administrator.[47]

In our work and discussions with managers and union staff, these sentiments were repeated over and over again. One physician at a major teaching hospital in Boston, which has been an exemplar of patient safety activity, remarked: "I have been very surprised about their [patient safety leaders'] attitude toward bringing the union on board when it comes to patient safety initiatives. People will sit around and talk about something and then someone will say, 'Oh, the union won't like that.' And I say, 'Well, did anyone ask the union?' 'No.' 'Is anyone going to?' 'No.'"[48] In the United States there tends to be an untested assumption that unions will invariably be an obstacle rather than an ally in any positive transformation.

It is not surprising, then, that union leaders say they are often excluded from the planning, implementation, and evaluation of safety initiatives. One RN union representative at a Massachusetts teaching hospital described her frustration at the failure of management to consult the union about safety initiatives: "They seem to consider us to be an obstacle. We are not advised about safety initiatives before they happen. When, after the fact, we come into the process, it's often in a backdoor way to put out fires or fix problems that didn't have to happen in the first place." This nurse gave the following example. To make sure that RNs practice safely, her hospital decided that they would have to be tested to prove their competence. To do this, the nurses were given a test on medication administration. Seventeen percent of the nurses flunked the test. Why? According to this union representative, it was because the test asked them questions about areas and medications with which they had no familiarity. "Psych nurses were asked about cardiac meds," she recounted.

> They don't give cardiac meds. I was given the test, and I haven't passed meds in ten years. The nurses were told that if they flunked the test three times, they would be fired. But they weren't given any review or teaching. We [the union] suggested that they get some classes going to help our nurses get more familiar with medications that are needed for cardiac patients. Some nurses haven't taken a test since they passed their boards twenty years ago.

Finally, management agreed to these classes after a whole day of bargaining to arrive at this solution. "Without the union rep, many would have continued to flunk the test. Did the hospital consider that it would then lose hundreds of nurses? We had to play catch-up and then try to fix the problem. When we were bargaining we asked management, 'Did you ever think that you could have a floor where five nurses flunked the test and only one nurse passed? Who's going to be giving the medication?'"[49]

Cathy Stoddart, vice president of health care for the Pennsylvania chapter of SEIU, summed up: "It is quite frustrating. We see problems affecting patient care on a daily basis . . . but rarely have a chance to help management solve them."[50] Stoddart decided to move beyond her frustration and started a quality improvement process at Allegheny Medical Center, where she works. She got several managers to join her and other union leaders to establish patient care committees in all of the hospital's medical-surgical units. But most frontline staff don't have Stoddart's confidence and may not feel comfortable trying to push management to listen to their ideas and suggestions.

Far too many unions, as we stated earlier in this chapter, are not invited to participate in patient safety programs. "Many times managers keep us at a distance; they don't value our input," comments David Schildmeier of the Massachusetts Nurses Association.[51] "We have participated on various quality and safety committees, but our suggested solutions don't get implemented. When we have gotten involved, many times members' ideas often get voted down without attempts at genuinely analyzing their merits. This is not only discouraging members from participating in these activities, but puts union leaders at risk for suggesting that it is important to work with management on such issues," says Schildmeier.[52] "Why should we put out when they won't accept our advice? I have better things to do with my time,"[53] says Michael Chacon, organizer for the New York State Nurses Association (NYSNA), expressing a common frustration. "In our hospital, management has established a parallel performance improvement and professional development process to our partnership structure. This parallel process reduces our ability to help improve the safety of patients and leaves our members questioning the value of our activities with management," says Janet McCarthy, staff nurse and negotiating team member at Allegheny Medical Center.[54]

To be fair, unions have not always been proactive enough about involving themselves in certain patient safety agendas and initiatives. While it is true that some nursing unions have fought for transformations in work organization and working conditions that would definitely improve patient care—bans on mandatory overtime, safe staffing, safe needle technology and lifts—union involvement in patient safety issues more generally may be too limited.[55] "We need to be part of the process to improve patient care," comments Mary Lehman McDonald, director of the American Federation of Teachers' (AFT) health care division.

Most of our members don't have grievances or labor relations issues [traditional areas for the union], but instead they want a voice in what goes on with patients. We as union leaders need to help use our influence to improve their ability to have input in activities to improve patient care. It is no longer just management's responsibility to be concerned with patient care and safety and costs. We have always been concerned about these issues but most of our work was focused on the traditional work of the union [such as handling grievances, negotiating contracts, and organizing new members]. There now needs to be a much broader balancing of these activities; we too need to expand our areas of work.[56]

Rick Brooks, executive director of UNAP, the Rhode Island nurses' union, acknowledges:

Frankly at times, we have not pushed our way into patient safety improvement work. We know that there are quality and safety committees organized in many of the hospitals where we have members, but we have been reluctant to get involved; we decided to stay on the sidelines. We have resisted getting involved in these activities. To some extent this has been caused by being comfortable in just doing our traditional union work. And to some extent we have been hesitant to learn new skills. Why change? Things are pretty good for now. Also, it is discouraging for us to have to fight our way to be heard by management and then get ignored. Many of our members feel that improving patient safety is a critical part of our responsibility as health care workers but many times question the value of needing to spend hours convincing management to listen to us.[57]

Nursing unions, as is pointed out in chapter 9 by Alison Trinkoff and Jeanne Geiger-Brown, have also taken some contradictory positions on patient safety. Unionized nurses have fought for bans against mandatory overtime on the grounds that it is not safe for nurses to work more than one shift, but have defended nurses' right to work as many shifts in a row and as many hours as they want, as long as working more than eight hours is voluntary, not mandatory. When advised that the safety literature documents that errors increase after eight hours on the job and escalate dramatically after twelve, the union response tends to be that "nurses like twelve-hour shifts." Obviously unions and their members can't have it both ways. If it's unsafe to work more than twelve hours when they are mandated to do so, it's also unsafe for them to work more than twelve hours voluntarily.[58]

How Involving Frontline Staff—and Their Unions—Makes a Difference

In this chapter we argue that it is necessary to create a fundamentally different patient safety template. Creating that template can produce impressive results. Maimonides Medical Center in Brooklyn has been successful at creating a safer hospital environment because it has involved both unions and frontline workers.

Maimonides Medical Center has seven hundred in-patient beds and employs over six thousand workers, who are represented by three unions: 1199/SEIU, which represents non-nursing staff; New York State Nurses Association (NYSNA), which represents registered nurses; and the Committee of Interns and Residents (CIR). The hospital, like most others in the country, has had its share of patient safety problems. A cardiology patient had died because staff "did not seem to respond to monitors and alarms in a timely manner." The hospital was not consistently kept clean. Hospital administrators and staff were also concerned about patient falls, among other medical errors and injuries.

CEO Pamela Brier, cited earlier in this chapter, comments that the hospital attempted to deal with a variety of safety issues in the past, but with limited success. In 1997 the hospital finally took a different approach. Rather than initiate safety efforts from above, it formed a labor-management joint process with the three unions and established what became known as a "Strategic Alliance." The purpose of the alliance was to ensure that labor and management worked together to improve patient care and to increase employees' input in decision making. This would, the hospital hoped, have a positive impact on employee recruitment and retention.

The alliance established a hospital-wide Labor-Management Council as well as Departmental Labor-Management Committees (DLMCs). To deal with the problems that were occurring on all of the cardiology units, the alliance went into action. Before the union, management, and frontline workers began to meet, management had contemplated disciplining nursing staff "because they were not responding to monitors and alarms in a timely fashion." Instead, the cardiology DLMC began to investigate why staff—particularly nursing staff—response time to monitors and alarms fluctuated between two and a half and eight minutes rather than the minute or less required to rescue patients successfully.

To understand this discrepancy fully, the twenty-member DLMC decided to do an in-depth analysis of what was going wrong on its units. For five months, registered nurses, patient care technicians, information specialists, physician assistants, nurse practitioners, nurse managers, physicians, nurse educators, performance improvement specialists, and a resident met weekly. Staff from departments such as Patient Transport, Radiology Health Information Technology (HIT), and Materials Information Systems (MIS) also attended when needed.

The DLMC group began by tracking patients' trajectory into and out of the hospital. This detailed analysis illuminated a number of serious problems. Acuity (severity of illness) measure of patients was not uniformly established or adequately understood. Thus, the proper numbers of RNs and nursing assistants were not assigned to care for patients. Patients were transferred to other departments—say, X ray—without a knowledgeable licensed staff member accompanying them. If a patient's condition deteriorated off-unit, people there were not always equipped to help. At change of shift, information about patient acuity was not conveyed to the next cohort of caregivers, precluding effective coordination of care. Finally, the DLMC discovered that staff did not know how to make simple adjustments to medical equipment, which meant that minor problems would often sideline a piece of equipment.

Because frontline employees from all shifts participated—including attending physicians and nurse practitioners—workers felt far more comfortable expressing their real concerns and making suggestions. The group was therefore able to get an accurate picture of the problem and propose solutions that had been designed with the involvement of these different groups. The solutions—to which all disciplines and occupational groups agreed—included:

- Establishing new clinical protocols to define patient acuity correctly.
- Making sure all patient acuity is assessed on a daily basis.
- Communicating acuity assessments in daily rounds with all staff, including physicians, to ensure accurate staffing levels.
- Including information on acuity in shift-to-shift reports on patients and making sure that acuity information is in the patient's chart.
- Establishing a new procedure to ensure that patients would be accompanied by a licensed practitioner when they leave the unit for tests, and involving patient transport in the implementation of the procedure.
- Creating the same standard for individualized alarm settings, checking the settings at the start of a new shift, and using the same standards on all four cardiology units.
- Providing more training on equipment to make sure it operates properly.

- Retraining nurses in how to set alarms and suspend a monitor without disabling others.
- Creating a logging system for tracking equipment failure and repairs, as well as tracking when patients left and returned to their floor.

Once these solutions were agreed on, DLMC members and nurse educators trained all staff, including physicians, on new procedures and protocols, and the group designated an RN and a nursing assistant to monitor the implementation of all changes to make sure all solutions were implemented and sustained. As one nurse involved in the effort remarked: "What was the tipping point for us was when we realized that blame for these problems was no longer automatically assigned to nurses, that other disciplines were ready to accept accountability for problems and help solve them. That made all the difference."[59]

Because the group understood that patient safety depends on sustaining solutions over the long term, it continues to meet, collects data about response time and new procedures each month, and reviews reports from each unit to determine whether or not gains have been maintained. If the data show that staff are having problems continuing to follow the procedures just listed or response times to alarms exceed one minute, the DLMC analyzes the particular situation and makes recommendations for needed changes. As a result of the multidisciplinary, all-encompassing work of the cardiac staff, the response time to monitors fell to less than one minute on all four cardiology units and has remained at this level.

At Maimonides, frontline staff were also involved in improving hospital cleanliness. When Pamela Brier was a patient in her own hospital, she discovered that the hospital simply wasn't clean enough. To deal with this problem, five staff members (four cleaners and one supervisor) were relieved of their regular duties and assigned to work as a Study Action Team. For four months their full-time job was to interview staff, analyze work processes on all three shifts, and visit other hospitals to check on their procedures and equipment. They also engaged nursing staff, physicians, unit coordinators, and various administrators throughout the hospital to gather their ideas and concerns about unit and hospital-wide cleanliness.

Again, the fact that the group was made up of cleaners, not just managers, allowed members to enter backstage and private spaces and to understand the actual work processes and concerns of those whose job it is to keep the hospital clean. What the Study Action Team discovered when it looked at the problems of the environmental services departments was that staff lacked the requisite equipment and supplies because the inventory system that should have made sufficient supplies available didn't function effectively. For example, all supplies were rarely available at the beginning of shifts for employees. There also wasn't enough cleaning staff, particularly on the graveyard shift, which in turn created problems for workers on day and afternoon shifts. As a result, morning or afternoon staff would come into a room or corridor and discover that garbage hadn't been removed, as it should have been on a previous shift. The group also identified another important issue. Even though many workers had been employed as hospital cleaners for a number of years, some weren't adequately trained in how to keep the hospital clean. As a result, cleaning staff weren't really sure if a room was clean and couldn't turn rooms around quickly enough for new patients. Moreover, housekeeping and nursing staff didn't communicate well with each other. Thus housekeepers often didn't know which rooms needed to be cleaned urgently and which less so.

Rather than rely solely on standard hospital satisfaction surveys, such as Press-Ganey scores, to help address these problems, the Study Action Team developed its own survey instrument to determine whether patients' rooms as well as all public areas and nursing stations were cleaned in a timely fashion. Members of the Study Action Team were responsible for making sure that staff had the appropriate training not only in housekeeping skills but also in infection control and dealing with bodily fluids and chemical hazards. The team was also responsible for helping to establish a new process for purchasing cleaning equipment and supplies. In addition, it took responsibility for negotiating with management, particularly around issues of staffing on the graveyard shift. The team also worked on developing more effective communication between nursing and housekeeping staff.

As a result of these activities, Maimonides is now a cleaner and safer hospital. Moreover, these joint efforts did not end with cleanliness and changes on the cardiology units, but continues to target a variety of patient safety problems. The decision to involve frontline staff and unions on an ongoing basis produced not only a genuine group of allies but also an ability to strategize continuously about crucial patient safety and worker safety issues. It uncovered not only problems and solutions but also aspects of work organization that needed to be changed to sustain safety over the long term.

Another important example of a major patient safety initiative that involved frontline staff took place throughout the Veterans Affairs health care system. Beginning in October 2007, acute care hospitals in the VA system addressed one of the most vexing hospital-acquired infections—methicillin-resistant *Staphylococcus aureus* (MRSA). Efforts to reduce incidence of the infection had stalled at the VA, and researchers and clinicians recognized the need to act more assertively and effectively to decrease MRSA infections. The VA thus implemented what it called a "MRSA" bundle," which included a number of different activities: "universal surveillance, contact precautions, hand hygiene, and institutional culture change was associated with a decrease in health care–associated transmissions of and infections with MRSA in a large health care system."[60]

During the study period, all patients admitted to a VA acute care hospital had their nose swabbed to test for the presence of the MRSA organism. If a patient tested positive, that patient was then isolated. Hand hygiene—critical to the spread of infection but sometimes not sufficiently practiced—was emphasized in each facility, but it was done in a way that encouraged culture change by making "infection control the responsibility of everyone who had contact with the patient." The results of the study were dramatic. Between October 2007 and June 2010, rates of health care–associated MRSA infections in ICUs decreased by 62 percent and in non-ICUs by 45 percent.

According to Dr. Rajiv Jain, principal investigator on the study, the early and consistent engagement of frontline staff to ensure prevention of the spread of infection was key to the success of this effort. Jain commented: "In our view, frontline staff are the experts. On in-patient units, they provide care everyday 24/7. You can have all the policies and procedures you want on the books, but the practice staff follow in delivering care is what makes the difference between safe and unsafe care."

To make sure that staff followed hand hygiene policies and procedures, it was critical to talk with staff to understand why some people use the proper hygiene and some don't. "Complexity science," Jain explains, "teaches us that knowledge does not equal practice because there are lots of filters that impact whether knowledge becomes practice." As Jain points out, it is hard to find anyone who works in health care who does not know that hand hygiene is the single most important mechanism to fight the spread of infection in hospitals. That said, not everyone who "knows" follows policy when it comes to hand hygiene. Why not? "By engaging frontline staff," says Jain, "we began to understand the barriers to practice and to understand how some people overcome those barriers."

Next Jain and his colleagues held focus groups with staff. Unlike typical focus groups, these were not led by an outside consultant or by a physician or other institutional leader. "The staff who do it correctly were the ones who led the discussion," Jain says. "They explained to their co-workers and colleagues how they overcome the barriers they experienced. That was what led to positive behavior change."

Another aspect of their project that reinforced this kind of positive change was universal testing. Some experts claim that testing everyone who comes into a hospital is too expensive and unnecessary. Jain and his colleagues disagree. They believe that universal testing has both a clinical and a behavioral rationale. From the clinical point of view, testing anyone who is going to be admitted helps the hospital discover who does and who does not carry the MRSA organism. Jain says:

> Obviously there is a scientific reason to test people. That is to find out whether the patient has the organism. This allows you to make clinical decisions, like whether to place them in isolation. But there is another reason to test patients. When, in the process of admitting a patient, the staff are doing the swab test, this becomes a reminder that they need to do all the things they need to do to prevent the spread of the organism.

Testing serves as a reminder, and reminders, Jain notes, are very important in real life. "I think of testing like I think of signs that remind us of the speed limit that's posted on a highway. When we see the sign we remember that maybe we ought to slow down. Without that reminder we might continue speeding and eventually hurt someone." Although Jain and his colleagues did not scientifically test this particular hypothesis—that universal testing acts as a reminder that in turn leads to improvements in practice—they firmly believe that is the case.

As Robert Reich, secretary of labor in the Clinton administration, has argued, in the new global economy, the workers whom policymakers focus on today are the symbolic analysts, the so-called knowledge workers, who have captured the biggest share of global wealth.[61] Gone are the manufacturing jobs and blue-collar workers of old. In the contemporary universe, the ones who matter are the professionals with minds that can manipulate facts, data, and the latest management theory. Our society, as Mike Rose has pointed out in his excellent book *The Mind at Work,* is now strictly divided into mindful and mindless work. In a twenty-first-century version of early-twentieth-century Taylorism, the frontline worker in an office, hospital, or nursing home is often viewed as a mindless worker who is managed by those who have the minds and the knowledge to do so.

Although health care is a shining temple of twenty-first-century technology, much of the realpolitik of health care management and policy is grounded in classic Taylorist perceptions of the division of labor, updated superficially to address pressures for return on investment, profit maximization, and production speed-ups. Just as the early-twentieth-century factory owner would not have consulted his workers about better automobile design, few contemporary hospital administrators (rhetoric about teams and inclusion notwithstanding) consult their nurses or other workers about how to provide more effective and safer patient care.

It is thus hardly surprising that some in the modern patient safety movement reproduce and reinforce this paradigm. As we have argued, workers at the bottom of the totem pole are not viewed as having the kind of knowledge that is truly valued. Although there is a great deal of rhetoric about the need to involve frontline staff, the definition of involvement is all too often limited to bringing staff on board solely to ensure compliance with programs that have been designed without their input. Managerial and professional attitudes toward frontline staff can, in fact, create a self-fulfilling prophecy. If higher- level professionals such as physicians or top-level managers see themselves as "the designated problem solvers" for departmental and interdepartmental problems, they won't consult frontline staff. If frontline staff are never consulted, they can never develop the kind of confidence needed to address controversial issues. If and when they are asked to offer their ideas or suggestions, they may be so intimidated by the education and "expertise" of those above them that they hesitate to contribute. If they are suddenly given leadership roles, without any prior training in how to fulfill those roles, they may fail. If they are reluctant to contribute good ideas, are silent when finally asked to sit at the table, or fail to act in a leader-like manner, physicians or managers may consider them to be useless time wasters. "Why are they here at all," one physician asked in frustration after a meeting in which RNs sat silently around a table. The RNs spoke to us about some excellent ideas after the meeting was over, but they were hesitant to share their knowledge openly in a very physician-dominated hospital. Rather than delve into the reasons for the nurses' silence, the elite simply decided to exclude them from future meetings. This in turn convinced nurses that doctors never listen to them and are not interested in their concerns and insights, which simply reinforced the cycle of reluctance and resistance.

Similar resistance is created when managers, administrators, and safety researchers and advocates neglect the safety problems identified by frontline staff (safe lifting, needle-stick injuries, work overload, long hours and lack of sleep, access to medical records and lab results, coordination with other departments, and so on). In a similar vein, managers often focus on regulations and scores—patient satisfaction scores, Medicare payments for hospital-acquired problems, and Joint Commission requirements—and ignore worker concerns. All of the problems that managers and workers identify are important. They are not, however, given equal weight on the patient safety agenda and in the priorities of hospital administration. Nor are they always integrated into the agenda of unions as representatives of frontline workers.

We are arguing here for a fundamentally different paradigm—one that recognizes that frontline workers and the unions that represent them can have a positive role to play in resolving patient safety problems as well as in contributing to a comprehensive patient safety program. It is not only their compliance that matters but also their insights, their knowledge, and yes, their mindfulness. Recognition of their mindfulness when it comes to patient safety must begin at the beginning, in the identification of patient safety problems, and continue in the design of methods to resolve them; the implementation of those programs and processes; the follow-up; and recurrent training, evaluation, and constant refinement of these programs and processes. Education and training not of but *with* frontline workers, managers, and other hospital players is crucial. So is the kind of recurrent training in safety methodology and practice that has made the airline industry safety movement so successful.

Culture changes not through episodic intervention but through constant repetition and reiteration. Safety training sessions, safety conferences, seminars, and webinars should, therefore, target not only physicians, nurses, and administrative leaders but also other frontline workers, who should not merely attend such conferences but actually present at them. Imagine the message that would be delivered to frontline staff (not just RNs) if they were asked to speak at such events and were offered educational materials and discounts to attend such conferences and seminars. Making such participation possible by including their comments in programs and making participation affordable is critical for those whose jobs are located at the point where the rubber of patient safety meets the road of patient care practice.

Currently our country is involved in various activities to make needed reforms of our health care system. No matter where this discussion leads, health care cannot be reformed without a fundamental reconsideration of the way frontline workers influence the fate of people once they enter the health care system and become patients within it. Nor is reform possible unless the health and safety of frontline staff is considered to be part of, not apart from, the patient safety agenda.

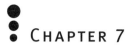

CHAPTER 7

Nursing as Patient Safety Net

Systems Issues and Future Directions

Sean Clarke

In most industrialized countries, nurses are the largest group of health care providers working directly with patients. They are responsible for implementing much hands-on patient care, particularly in acute care hospitals, monitoring patients for complications of illnesses and untoward reactions to treatment as well as protecting them from the "hazards" of medical care.[1]

Recent years have been marked by unprecedented attention to patient safety and quality of care issues and the introduction of many programs and initiatives intended to reduce hazards and improve consistency of services in health care institutions around the world. In their frontline roles in clinical practice, nurses directly experience the impacts—both negative and positive—of changes in operating practices and systems. They are often charged not only with complying with a dizzying array of changes but also with monitoring other workers' adherence to guidelines and practices.

While many safety-related reforms are well intentioned, sometimes both the nature of the interventions themselves and the schemes used to implement them clash with the realities of daily operations in health care facilities. Incomplete understanding of the processes clinicians and other workers use to provide care can doom efforts to improve safety. Furthermore, safety initiatives are often designed without much attention to the realities of group functioning. For instance, the impact of local history and professional and institutional culture on behavior is often underestimated, the complexity of communication and coordination that can be consistently achieved in busy settings overestimated, and little attention given to addressing the factors required to produce and sustain change. As Peter Lazes, Suzanne Gordon, and Sameh Samy point out elsewhere in this book, conflicts between intentions and realities are not only true on an initiative-by-initiative basis but also are reflected in the sheer volume of changes many facilities attempt to implement at once. To many nurses it seems that new guidelines and quality-monitoring programs appear with dizzying frequency, each demanding almost instant implementation.

To complicate things further, the safety movement is evolving at the same time that health care systems, the health professions and occupations, and health care practice worldwide are undergoing profound changes. One such change involves the health care labor supply. Decades of a revolving door of entry and exit in nursing have contributed to a steady aging of professional workforces. Despite high numbers of new graduates in the recent past, nurse supply is projected to shrink with an onslaught of retirements expected shortly. This, along with rapidly expanding clienteles for health services in most Western societies, is expected to create severe imbalances between the supply of and the demand for health care providers in the coming years.[2]

This means that a diminishing number of nurses are being asked to deliver an expanding volume of services to—at least in the West—an aging population. These nurses are also asked to implement a dazzling array of safety initiatives that are often necessary to deliver safer and more effective care. What is missing, however, is attention to whether nurses can effectively manage their current roles alongside added tasks or changes owing to patient safety technologies and practices. Nor is much discussion occurring around which changes in practice will produce the biggest improvements in outcomes or how nurses can be assisted in integrating the most relevant changes into their work.

Contexts of Struggles to Improve Safety in Nursing Practice

Nursing practice is affected by a great number of external forces and priorities. As a result, as safety initiatives have multiplied, it is not surprising that nurses have been responding to directives to change health care delivery rather than participating in the construction of the reforms. Why is it so difficult for nurses and their leaders to shape nursing practice in a manner that achieves improvements in a systematic and efficient manner? Why are isolated aspects of care so often addressed at the expense of broader aspects of work environments?

One major reason relates to blurriness in the nature of nursing practice. Nurses have difficulty explaining the cognitive and relational (as opposed to technical or task-based) aspects of their work to those outside the profession. This has devastating consequences because judgment and relationship building (within health care teams and with patients) are extremely sensitive to the contexts of practice, especially the presence or absence of critical masses of competent professionals and skillful managers. A second reason that helps explain the difficulty of securing outside support for investments in or protection of nurses' work environments is the tendency to think about safety and error in individual versus systems terms, that is, in a manner that frames quality problems as the fault of poorly prepared, insensitive, or disorganized professionals rather than poor working conditions.

Understanding Error: An Individual or Systems Phenomenon?

Historically, institutional responses to error focused on the worker or workers who were the "last pairs of hands" to touch the patient before an incident. Responses to errors causing serious harm were often swift and severe.[3] Conscientious, talented clinicians and health care workers having a bad day or in the midst of an unfortunate set of circumstances could watch their self-confidence and even their careers evaporate in the space of a few hours. Not surprisingly, clinicians and managers tended to hide errors or attempted to shift blame to others. Secrecy was probably the more common of the two responses. Sadly, hiding errors can compound patient injuries by delaying definitive treatment to correct reversible problems. Moreover, secrecy erects a wall between patients and their providers that can cause great psychological damage on both sides. But most important, secrecy all but eliminates the potential for errors to be used to as learning opportunities to improve care in the future.

Many commentators now recognize that most patient safety problems are, at their root, systems problems and are therefore best handled as such at the levels of both prevention and response. Indeed, an emphasis on systems of care, work system design, and organizational factors has been one of the hallmarks of the present era of safety research and attempts to reengineer care.[4] Nevertheless, there is still a great deal of emphasis in actual practice settings on the immediate circumstances around errors as well as the actions and judgments of the individuals involved. When we consider the actions that institutions take to deal with error, it is apparent that errors are still viewed primarily as issues of ignorance or carelessness requiring direct instruction and, potentially, disciplinary intervention. As a result, one of the most popular tools in the arsenal of quality and safety work in health care facilities has always been education aimed at improving individual (rather than team) practice.

For very understandable reasons, many institutional administrators and managers, as well as professionals and the public, tend to believe that impressing the importance of doing things "right" upon individual workers is the best defense against error. Safety experts stress that well-designed systems are probably one of the best defenses against human fallibility, and researchers have demonstrated that organizational conditions have important connections to quality of care. Nevertheless, there is still a lingering fear that focusing on circumstances or conditions surrounding errors and adverse events will limit health professionals' accountability for their behavior and wind up endangering patients.

Thus, in the end, many safety interventions, even ones touted as systems redesign initiatives, admonish individual providers to change narrow aspects of their behavior at work. Nurses and others are taught specific ways to carry out tasks either in groups or in one-on-one counseling sessions, and their compliance is monitored. Some changes in work practices include banning certain types of equipment or supplies and replacing them with others that are presumably safer or less error-prone, developing checklists and timeouts before procedures, and adding steps to procedures.

A number of relatively narrow changes in practice have been achieved fairly easily. For instance, at one time vials of concentrated electrolytes such as potassium for intravenous administration could be routinely found across all patient care areas in hospitals around the world. Because of their medical condition or the treatments they undergo, and often as a result of both, many hospitalized patients need some sort of replacement of low levels of essential minerals delivered as electrolytes. Nurses were made aware of the risks of overly rapid infusions of these solutions—including the possibility of sudden patient death. Over time, in many countries, staff across many areas of hospitals routinely prepared diluted solutions of electrolytes. Strong concentrations of electrolytes were administered only in settings where patients could be monitored closely. These were very common practices that few questioned until it was found that the concentrates were sometimes inadvertently administered—often when vials were confused—leading to serious complications and even death for thousands of patients worldwide every year. Lengthy discussions ensued around whether or not patients' interests were served by allowing the situation to continue for the sake of tradition and, perhaps, the wishes of prescribers, who wanted to have the freedom to prescribe unusual concentrations and mixes of electrolytes at any time and in any setting. Regulators in North America were ultimately successful in banning concentrates from all but a handful of clinical areas within hospitals and in shifting the handling of concentrates from direct care units to hospital pharmacies. Deaths from electrolyte overdoses dropped precipitously.

Other top-down modifications in local practices, such as requiring double-checks and timeouts to limit wrong-patient and wrong-side/wrong-site surgeries and procedures, have not been as easy to implement, especially because they require extra steps or work or create inconveniences. But particularly over the longer term, even if the events being prevented are rare, many of these changes are seen to produce returns on the considerable investments of time and energy required at the local level because the risks to patients are so serious. The successes of the Institute for Healthcare Improvement's multiple campaigns to engage American hospitals in evidence-based practice change provide some good examples.[5]

Change initiatives, however—even well-designed ones, based on sound rationales and implemented with skill—can produce unintended consequences such as "workarounds" or "overrides," and result in outcomes that were never intended because the so-called solutions generated new problems. Furthermore, no one questions the time and energy savings that might have been realized in addressing common underlying causes rather than specific aspects of narrow problems in the delivery of clinical care.

What, specifically, might a "systems focus" really mean in the context of organizing nursing practice? It would begin with a consideration of the web of organizational features affecting nurses' work. Leaders applying a systems focus would integrate overarching factors such as staffing levels and staff development (to ensure that there were enough workers with the right knowledge, skills, and attitudes), hours at work, communication within and across occupational groups and disciplines, and broader cultural issues into their overall strategy for ensuring safety in their health care facilities.

Leaders and clinicians adopting a systems focus recognize that safety issues often have common underlying causes and therefore try to strike some type of balance between error-specific solutions and broader system improvements—but not necessarily an equal one. High-volume, high-cost, or high-risk aspects of practice are certainly worthwhile targets for focused intervention, especially errors and omissions that risk patients' lives or create the potential for permanent patient disabilities. Lethal medication errors, avoidable pressure ulcers (bedsores), and complications from intravenous (IV) lines that are ubiquitous in acute care today are good examples of issues meriting targeted tracking, dedicated staff education, and practice improvement projects.

Not every narrow aspect of practice, however, can be directly monitored and managed. There are simply too many. Nor can the importance a particular advocacy group accords an issue always be used as a guide to the urgency of implementing a potential solution. Systems-oriented leadership questions the scale of the problem to be solved in relation to the costs of the proposed solution and carefully examines the potential impacts of any corrective interventions before implementing them. For instance, a systems-oriented leader might pause and ensure that a safety or quality issue is really worth pursuing before rallying resources for a new initiative and verify that simpler solutions have been explored, sources of resistance to change have been thought through and understood, and the change process has been designed with overcoming barriers to change in mind. All of this is often easier said than done.

Challenges for Managers in Systems-Level Thinking

There are considerable pressures on managers that lead them away from systems-based approaches and toward narrow foci: these include an emphasis on measurement and measurable indicators, fears that systems approaches provide a blanket excuse for inattention to detail by clinicians, and difficulties in arguing for systems-level resources with their superiors.

Managers and executives in health care are increasingly being held accountable in the court of public opinion for the safety and quality of the care their institutions provide, not only by politicians, journalists, and others, but also by funding and reimbursement schemes. In the United States, the national Medicare program requires hospitals seeking full reimbursement to collect quality data for posting on publicly available websites, and is moving toward rewarding hospitals and providers that are "best in class" on specific measures and withholding payment for costs of care related to complications believed to be due to poor practices.[6] This feeds into a command-and-control view of management and a marked preference for measurable inputs and outputs that many health care administrators hold. The problem, though, is that because of rapid growth in the complexity and volume of health care services without a parallel evolution of information systems, what is immediately measurable can often be a considerable distance from what is truly important in terms of the outcomes of patient care or the factors that are most proximately connected to it.

Managers and executives may or may not have a theoretical and/or practical understanding of quality and change management that is consistent with a systems approach. They may or may not have embraced approaches to management and leadership that emphasize teamwork and participation of workers in decision making. Yet even among health care leaders who accept systems thinking, there is a fear, as mentioned earlier, that it could be dangerous to provide health care workers with a pat excuse for poor performance. ("It wasn't me, it was the *system*.") A good illustration is an article describing medication errors as "more basic than a system issue" and fundamentally about poor mathematical skills.[7]

There are many reasons why issue-specific as opposed to systems-level safety interventions are preferred by many. Frontline and middle-level managers in health care are held accountable for holding the line on operating costs. Systems-level resources—particularly additional staff, better-prepared staff, and staff development or team development programs—tend to be expensive. Not surprisingly, managers are often reluctant to ask for more staff or more qualified staff (or more training for existing staff), even though such strategies might provide better prospects for improving quality than some of the narrow safety measures they are asked to implement. Managers will not suggest increasing staff unless they are in an environment where investment of additional resources is possible and are reporting to executives who share their perspectives and invite this type of input. Furthermore, managers can be so bound by competing demands from their superiors regarding smaller performance issues that they are unable to address higher-level, "softer" issues, such as staff development and enhancing safety climate and culture. Finally, initiating systems-level change is likely to be difficult, outside their span of control and scope of resources, and time-consuming, and may well fail to lead to the types of measurable short-term results for which they will be held responsible. In the end, regardless of what managers and executives may espouse publicly about the need for evidence-based staffing and improved patient safety climate, they may not perceive any rewards for working on these issues in the clinical areas they manage.

Despite much research and discussion to the contrary, many health care managers proceed as if it were possible to provide safe, high-quality care in work environments where systems factors are unmonitored and unmanaged. Clearly, managers and executives need development and support to recognize broader and deeper systems causes of problems in patient care quality and safety. They need to argue effectively for investments in staffing and practice environments in addition to changes in equipment or other narrowly focused quality efforts.

Financial and Other Incentives in the Safety "Industry"

The safety movement has generated an extensive number of public and private initiatives that have engaged both the for-profit and not-for-profit sectors. Not surprisingly, a formidable safety "industry" consisting of vendors of safety-related equipment and consulting services has developed. Governments and their departments and agencies, as well as professional and trade associations, want to be seen as vigorous and effective advocates for the public. They want to demonstrate that they are making relevant investments and sending appropriate signals to health care facilities and workers. They certainly do not want to be seen as uninterested in or "soft" on questions of patient safety. While all movement toward safer health care is to be applauded, it sometimes appears as if the motivations behind the statements and imperatives, as well as the soundness of initiatives being proposed, are beyond question.

The various commercial or industry providers of products that are involved in the high-volume and/or high-risk aspects of care include pharmaceutical companies, medical equipment and supply manufacturers (for example, of intravenous medication delivery systems, ventilators, and monitors), and developers and manufacturers of various types of information technology products. In competing for the attention and dollars of health care managers and executives making decisions under time and budget constraints, companies propose "niche" solutions to very focused problems, and frequently sell equipment and systems that are not compatible with other systems. These approaches protect their market share and build in a near-guarantee of obsolescence of the products down the line which ensures long-term sales as well. Many companies feed on a sense of urgency about particular issues (for instance, concerns about errors in the administration of intravenous medications or the perceived need for barcoded medication delivery systems). They play on institutions' wishes to portray what appears to be a forward-looking and vigorous approach toward patient safety improvement among institutional leaders.

Unfortunately, as Ross Koppel and his colleagues also discuss in another chapter, sales pitches for new equipment and information systems rarely include much discussion about impacts on the work of caregivers or larger impacts on systems of care. Equipment manufacturers promote the distinctness of their products, even though this distinctness commonly builds in incompatibility with other systems and even with earlier versions of the same systems. Extraordinary similarities in health care delivery in hospitals and clinics across countries and regions and around the world would suggest that standardized design of equipment, work systems, and supplies might lead to considerable improvements in care. Manufacturers, however, often offer opportunities for hospitals and units to tailor systems extensively, especially in the case of provider order entry and electronic patient care records, to deal with a puzzling culture in health care, in which encouraging extensive input into seemingly minor design features (for instance, screen layout) is equated with offering high-quality and user-friendly products. Because companies need to sell individual products, they seldom seek to promote comprehensive or integrated patient safety solutions, unless, of course, those solutions involve adopting many or all of their own products. Distributed or decentralized decision making across clinical areas and departments multiplies the potential for incompatibilities between systems. Using multiple models of the same devices across various settings within a facility (for instance, monitors, ventilators, or intravenous infusion pumps), can create safety issues. This can become particularly risky when staff move from setting to setting even within the same facility (for instance, when they are "floating" to cover staffing shortfalls) and find themselves operating unfamiliar equipment.

Overall, the involvement of both for-profit and not-for-profit entities has injected energy and money—and perhaps stimulated innovation—in the safety movement. Nonetheless, it has spawned technologies with a strong potential to generate unintended consequences (for systematic discussions, see Michael Harrison's and Ross Koppel's work) and initiative overload.[8]

Technophilia and Program/Project Mania

Nurses in many organizations quickly absorb technologies and special projects and programs because these solutions seem to offer satisfying "fixes" for patient safety problems. Nurses tend to be deeply invested in their patients' well-being and sometimes unquestioningly accept arguments that specific practices will improve outcomes. Even if they have doubts about the usefulness and the sustainability of the interventions, there are many motivations for health care workers and managers to remain silent. Sometimes nurses lack the energy or interest to argue against poorly thought-out initiatives. In other cases, they may lack the knowledge or skills to articulate their concerns or unease. They may also fear that speaking up will brand them as being "against" patient safety, which is tantamount to being a "bad nurse." Sometimes they lack the institutional power to oppose problematic initiatives. Not only are there many disincentives to speak up, but they have a vested interest in going along as well: often those involved in implementing technologies or practices receive real or imagined credit and reward capital in their facilities and sometimes even beyond the walls of their facilities.

Certainly the search for the "new" is not unique to health care but can also be found in the social service and education sectors. For instance, in American elementary and secondary public education, an accountability movement intended to improve student achievement (often known colloquially by the name of the federal legislation penalizing low-performing schools, "No Child Left Behind") has had widespread impacts on teachers' work. Specific curricular packages (textbooks, exercise books, tests, and teachers' manuals) purchased from publishers come and go on a regular basis as schools and school districts attempt to find the "magic bullet" to increase student achievement, or at the very least scores on statewide tests.[9] Teachers, like nurses, face intense scrutiny of their work, while relatively little attention is paid to variations in the environmental conditions that affect the outcomes of their "clients" (patients in the case of nurses, students in the case of teachers). A market for consultation services to increase scores by managing teachers' (and health care workers') behavior on the job is flourishing. Interestingly, consultants rarely suggest increasing staffing levels, changing management style, or engaging in broad-based staff development. They most often recommend micromanagement, not higher-level organizational change.

Many U.S. public school teachers are now "teaching to the test"— tailoring the content of their interactions with students to mirror questions that appear on tests with the intent of increasing scores—and are either ignoring or being forced to ignore broader issues in curricula and the organization of their schools and communities. So, too, nurses are encouraged to do the same in the care of their patients, the organization of their work, and the management of their hospitals. There is much incentive to adopt narrow programs that promise to improve high-stakes, publicly released performance measures.

Consequences of Failure to Adopt a Systems Stance

What are the consequences of not attending to systems issues? As mentioned earlier in the chapter, an obvious consequence is that when errors and accidents occur, the individual workers involved may well receive intense and unfair scrutiny, an approach commonly referred to as "shaming and blaming." These approaches demoralize staff and can encourage the hiding of errors. Performance cannot improve when individuals on the front lines are held accountable for the failings of entire systems.[10] Sadly, blaming individuals may indirectly contribute to the shortage of nurses by compounding public perceptions of the work as stressful and risky, reducing people's willingness to go into and remain in frontline nursing care. Within institutions or units, instead of ensuring the safe passage of patients, the focus becomes achieving narrow goals with as little friction in the short term as possible, regardless of the larger consequences for particular patients or for quality of care. Just as serious is the tendency in the absence of a systems approach for nurse managers and executives to be forever managing crises and running from fire to fire without longer-term and higher-level foci.

Without an approach to quality management grounded in an awareness of and attention to systems factors, the proliferation of externally imposed guidelines and dictates can create significant problems. Agencies and expert panels tend to give little thought to the additional labor created by the introduction of new guidelines, programs, or technologies or to the tradeoffs in staff time or money that are necessary to implement new safety recommendations or safety- and/or quality-tracking guidelines. New or lengthened forms, checklists, and methods of assessment or documentation are commonly created by these mandates. In some instances, additional screening or procedures become mandated across facilities regardless of whether or not they are relevant for all patients. For instance, the rate of falls or pressure ulcers may be extraordinarily low among laboring obstetrical patients, but regulations and policies may require that baseline assessments be completed for all hospitalized patients, thus creating what is arguably pointless documentation work for nurses on labor and delivery floors.

Because budgets are finite and staff have limited time, targeted actions will often displace other work and activities, because individuals and organizations naturally direct their energies toward avoiding punishments and receiving rewards. Evidence suggests that an emphasis on one set of initiatives typically leads to neglect of other interventions, as illustrated by the findings of a 2007 paper about standards in geriatric primary care. Under a provider education and reward program, the specific screening and treatment recommendations targeted by the scheme increased, while other evidence-based practices decreased, and patient outcomes overall were not improved.[11] In 2008, Diana Mason commented on the rise in pressure ulcers in some critical care units as a result, directly or indirectly, of an emphasis on keeping the heads of patients elevated in bed and other interventions to prevent ventilator-associated pneumonias over other hygiene, comfort, and position-ing interventions.[12] She provides further examples of the neglect of basic nursing care that has sometimes accompanied focused attention on specific measures and/or evidence-based practices. Specifically, she cites getting patients out of bed to prevent complications of immobility, feeding, and patient teaching as areas that have been dropped under pressure of time and resources. All of these developments are, of course, variations on the simi-lar concern that public school teachers are forced to "teach to the test"—to omit from their work with students important concepts and skills not addressed by the tests.

Without a systems focus, the relationship of parts to the whole (in this case patient safety and positive health outcomes) is lost. When regulators and/or payers demand that hospitals and other agencies track too many different safety or quality measures at once, each according to very particular guide-lines, the information tends to degrade. Worse still, resources are diverted from care to documentation of care beyond what is necessary to promote patient safety and continuity of care.

Furthermore, when too many modifications of too many different aspects of care delivery are attempted at the same time, they can rarely be sustained for long. Scattered efforts create confused and anxious staff. Managers, who are also vulnerable to overload, can easily become confused and anxious, too.

When performance stagnates on one or more measures, it can be tempting to revert to targeting isolated behaviors in individual providers in a manner that negatively affects performance. Pressure to comply with very narrow aspects of protocols can send contradictory messages to staff about thinking "critically," deepening the problems created by overload and micromanage-ment. Stakeholders who are not on the front lines of care may be tempted to blame recalcitrant staff or poor leadership for indicators that fail to improve. Fortunately, there is a distinct (and growing) voice within the health care community that recognizes a need to stem initiative overload, especially in agencies facing major workforce challenges.[13]

In practical terms, managers and quality personnel must spend at least part of their time addressing higher-order aspects of nursing work and the systems factors that influence performance because they cannot possibly oversee all minutiae of practice. While there are repetitive aspects to nursing work, and some of the individual tasks nurses perform may not appear particularly challenging or dangerous, the overall flow of the work is remarkably varied in focus and tempo and cannot be managed the same way as, for instance, repetitive factory work. On a daily basis, nurses make dozens, if not hundreds, of potentially critical decisions that have impacts on patient safety. While no one is proposing or advocating the mechanization of nursing work or the work of health care providers, neither has anyone proposed workable solutions for the flurry of standards and data elements for which providers are held responsible.

This is not to say that attention should not be paid to high-frequency, high-risk aspects of clinical practice or that clinicians and leaders shouldn't be made aware of problematic procedures, medication errors, or unsafe conditions revealed by analyzing trends in incidents and incident reports. And it certainly is not meant to imply that individual practitioners and their agencies shouldn't be held accountable for remaining alert to recognized, well-documented hazards in care and ensuring that dangers to patients are minimized. Nevertheless, the number of simultaneous demands on clinicians and their leaders is reaching a critical point. And so, when a particular unit or institution is not willing to jump at every new initiative suggested, this may not always represent resistance to progress but could reflect the wise exercise of leadership under conditions of limited resources. Resistance is not an easy thing, especially when an initiative gains a critical mass of popularity; the popularity of an intervention, however, is rarely a guarantee of its effectiveness, as we will see in the case of rapid response teams.

Limitations of the Quick Fix: Failure to Rescue and the Organizational Intervention of Rapid Response Teams

Apart from massive overdoses of chemotherapy and other dangerous drugs, wrong-side surgery, and wrong procedures, perhaps few patient safety incidents in hospitals are met with as much sorrow and anger as situations in which patients have clearly deteriorated past the point of no return because health care workers have failed to monitor them or have been unable to treat their complications in a timely manner. The notion behind "failure to rescue" (the term that has been applied to the concept in the clinical and research literature) is that late and/or ineffective treatment of complications leads to needless death and disability.[14] One of the most highly publicized—and frequently adopted—solutions to this problem is known as the "rapid response team" (RRT, also known as the medical emergency team). The RRT is the equivalent of the 911 call in the community. When a patient becomes medically unstable, a call to an RRT is often (but not always) launched by a frontline nurse, who summons a multidisciplinary team to the patient's side. The RRT, which has been promoted by the prestigious Institute for Healthcare Improvement and has been widely adopted in hospitals in Australia and

New Zealand, North America, and Europe, provides an interesting context for discussing some of the challenges in reengineering health care settings and achieving enduring improvements in safety.

RRTs always include nurses and often involve physicians as well as health professionals from other disciplines. While historically, under certain circumstances, cardiac arrest or "code" teams in many facilities have been called in when patients are becoming compromised but have not necessarily gone into cardiac arrest, the RRT is officially charged with troubleshooting the patient's situation and preventing a cardiac arrest before it happens. In its assessment and management, the team aims to reverse the underlying problem or prevent further deterioration by arranging for timely transfer of the patient to a higher level of care, often the intensive care unit (ICU).[15] Since most areas of hospitals outside critical care have less than ideal layouts, staffing, and equipment for executing intensive life-saving interventions, even when deterioration cannot be halted, timely transfers can avoid the panic of a disorganized resuscitation effort and post-resuscitation stabilization outside the ICU. Consequently, a number of leaders have described a "code outside the unit" (that is, a resuscitation effort outside a critical care area) as a de facto failure of the clinicians and/or the system in place to deal with emergencies.

Part of the intent behind RRTs has been to overcome the delays in initiating definitive treatment of deteriorating patients under the "chain of command" model of medical care in hospitals. Under this system, the most junior medical clinicians are often called upon to deal with unfolding clinical crises, then call in more senior clinicians for help as needed. In principle this approach of scaling up the intensity of medical attention as necessary meets the dual goals of offering learning opportunities for junior staff and sparing the time and energy of the most experienced physicians for activities requiring a high level of training and expertise. Unfortunately, this model has sometimes led to considerable delays in initiating treatments—and patients have been seriously harmed.[16] RRTs have been designed to overcome nurses' hesitancy and fears around calling and disturbing physicians, and ensure that those responding to emergencies are fully equipped to handle them so that patients are not jeopardized by the delays in treatment that can be created by a need to "go up the chain" when initial efforts are inadequate.

When hospitals adopt the RRT, they commonly provide caregivers, including nurses, with a list of assessment parameters (vital signs suggestive of physiological compromise, for instance) that would normally be triggers for calling in the team. Clinical leaders, however, often emphasize that nurses should feel free to alert the team when they have even a vague sense that something isn't "right" and that the team will take things from there.

The hope is that the RRT will not only respond to specific events but also educate staff and improve practice both during and after the event takes place. Non-ICU nurses have reported feeling more secure with such teams in place. Research indicates that teams are called in for a wide range of reasons, and that some care processes appear to improve overall as a result.[17]

While the basic idea appears sound, it's interesting to consider why this patient safety fix has been proposed and implemented at this particular historical juncture and why it may not necessarily work in all situations or in all facilities. Intervening to treat patients whose condition is deteriorating before it reaches a point of no return is obviously important. But is the RRT necessary because delayed or ineffective treatments are an inevitable byproduct of a complex high-tech medical system? Are most direct care staff not competent or experienced enough to detect problems? Or is another phenomenon at work here: Could delayed or ineffective "saves" be more common when nurses—and physicians—lack adequate resources? Are they paying close enough attention to identify emerging clinical problems and function effectively in a crisis? Why are nurses fearful of calling physicians? The intensity of care delivered to patients in acute care hospitals has increased because thresholds for admission have risen, and patients are discharged back to the community earlier and earlier. The numbers of nursing staff per patient-day may have increased, but probably not in proportion to the work that needs to be done to care for these patients and the risks the average patient runs for complications.[18] And the issue of hierarchy in nurse-physician and other relationships, as we see in other chapters in this book, has been poorly addressed.

Certainly, very different organizational interventions are called for depending on whether patients are not being observed closely enough, they are not being observed astutely (that is, the right observations are not being made or interpreted correctly), or patients identified as being in trouble are not being treated effectively. If staffing levels are insufficient to allow nurses to watch over patients frequently enough to "catch" complications in time to allow correction, without better staffing that enables nurses to sound the alarm quickly, even the best-functioning RRTs will fail to rescue at least some of the patients who might otherwise be salvaged. For instance, Daniel Allen presents the case of a patient in the UK who died of complications from massive postoperative bleeding following a hysterectomy. The registered nurse–to–patient ratio on the surgical unit where this woman was transferred was apparently one to thirty, and by all outward appearances, thin nurse staffing seems to have been to blame.[19] Indeed, research on the predictors of failure to rescue at the hospital has found that registered nurse staffing is among the most consistent predictors in studies to date.[20]

Non–critical care hospital units do not have the same numbers of nurses and physicians present on nights, weekends, and holidays as on weekdays, and this may compromise the recognition of patient problems and the effectiveness of rescue efforts. Analyses of multiple years of data from over five hundred hospitals suggest that patients experiencing cardiac arrest on weekends or at night are likely to face delays before resuscitation efforts are begun and less likely to be successfully resuscitated.[21]

Yet sufficient staff presence may not necessarily be a guarantee of timely identification of complications. Linda Aiken and I reviewed several cases in which surveillance was insufficient under relatively favorable staffing conditions.[22] One involved delayed detection of postoperative bleeding in an abdominal surgical patient, and a second concerned a failure to recognize well-known early signs of drug toxicity before an overdose proved fatal. A similar case was reported in Scotland, where a fifty-year-old woman hemorrhaged to death after breast cancer surgery, and poor staff training rather than low staffing was pinpointed as the underlying cause.[23] If bedside staff are unable to recognize early signs of complications or communicate their observations and concerns to other clinicians in order to mount a response, improving staff development (rather than increasing staffing levels) is the logical solution.

The developers and popularizers of the rapid response team concept have indeed begun to address some systems issues in rescue. For instance, they have suggested that difficulties in communication among providers may impair a timely response to patient crises. Experience suggests that the presentation of data in calls to providers can be disorganized, and this may force health care workers and providers to second-guess one another. Experts have proposed staff education in structured communication to help frontline staff structure their calls to physicians and other providers, since concise, focused calls will increase the likelihood of rapid, appropriate action. The SBAR mnemonic (situation, background, assessment, recommendation), which is being taught to staff in many hospitals, guides nurses and others to present, in order, the patient's situation, the background leading up to the event, the bedside nurses' assessment of the situation, and finally their recommendation or desired response.[24] Nevertheless the explicit omission of a number of other systems factors from consideration—particularly the workloads and practice of staff nurses, as well as their education and clinical proficiency as individual practitioners and as a group—may be undermining the success of RRTs.

Indeed the many unanswered questions about RRTs and their effectiveness are indicative of a broader problem in the patient safety movement, which is that a number of initiatives seem to become popular in spite of questions about their ultimate utility. The RRT may well offer a significant advantage in situations in which attending physicians are not on-site and limited or no house staff is available to cover emergency situations, or physician-nurse communication is poor. In some institutions, however, RRTs may be addressing a non-problem if the numbers of nursing staff are sufficient to provide adequate oversight to prevent the kinds of incidents RRTs are designed to address. The clinical acumen of these nurses might be sound; a sufficient number of house staff clinicians (such as nurse practitioners, physicians in postgraduate training, or physician's assistants) and attending clinicians may be available to deal with emergencies quickly; and nurses may feel comfortable co-managing patients with the clinician or team treating the patient. In such cases, a rapid response team may not be necessary. Interestingly enough, the majority of both the anecdotal reports and research on RRTs originate in facilities whose leaders would likely describe them as having all of these elements (staffing, well-trained providers, and so forth) in place. Whether they actually are well equipped in these respects according to any objective criteria is open to debate, of course. Research suggests that significant problems of staff workload and competency are found even in hospitals with RRTs (see, for instance, the work of Annie Chellel and her colleagues).[25] It is also possible that the support provided by RRTs is helpful regardless of the composition and structure of the nursing and medical staffs as a "backup" or "safety valve" for the increased workload created by rapidly evolving patient situations, but that is not yet clear.

The potential problem with the RRT is that health care facilities are arriving at a solution to a serious problem by jumping to the end of the process (the rescue portion) rather than undertaking a full analysis of the issue. Why are there failures to rescue in the first place? The part of the process that is likely to be the culprit in many if not all facilities—insufficient numbers of adequately trained nursing staff to oversee patients and interpret clinical observations accurately—is all but ignored. Could it be that the drama of rescue which the RRT represents is so seductive that it has eclipsed other considerations and more nuanced alternatives? Or is the appeal of RRTs that they appear to represent a cheaper alternative than hiring sufficient numbers of nurses to staff hospitals and educating them to handle their patients' needs?

The better organized and more effective the response to emergencies and the better able health care teams are to handle near-emergencies before they become full-blown disasters, the better off patients, as well as health care workers, will be. No one wants to be involved in a doomed or failed rescue effort, least of all the patient. Nevertheless, offering a solution to a significant problem doesn't rule out the possibility that the solution is not the right one or could create unintended consequences. An important potential consequence of shifting the involvement in emergencies from floor nurses to nurses on RRTs is that these teams concentrate the expertise in managing emergencies in the hands of a relatively small number of staff and therefore deskill other staff. Not so, say some. The expertise found on many RRTs is well beyond that commonly found outside ICU settings. In at least one vision of the RRT, the staff nurse assigned to care for the patient remains at the bedside to participate in the rescue and to learn by watching the team assess and intervene. Some have expressed hope that over the long term, RRT clinicians will share their expertise and thus increase the competence of all involved in rescuing patients.

In the real world of busy units, however, anecdotal evidence suggests that when the RRT arrives, staff nurses quickly hand over their patient to the RRT and move on to their other patients. That's because, given today's heavy patient assignments, a nurse caring for a patient whose condition has deteriorated knows all too well that her or his workday has unraveled. Once someone else is available to cope with the crisis, overburdened nurses will tend to gravitate to their other patients—all of whom have their own urgent needs and potential near-emergencies. If staff nurses are to stay with a patient in order to learn from an RRT call, not only must RRT members encourage them to do so, but also the structure and culture of the hospital unit must allow for coverage of all their other patients while this is going on. This can happen only if there is enough staff on a unit to permit mutual support. Without both encouragement from RRT members and the right workloads, nurses who consistently hand over emergencies to others risk losing their self-confidence and competence in handling emergencies. This raises some very real concerns about the potential for unintended consequences for patients if RRTs (or qualified team members) cannot function effectively at all times, or if the RRTs should ever need to be disbanded because of cost.

All in all, it is not yet clear whether the goal of RRTs—to improve short-term patient survival—is actually being met in some or most, let alone all, settings where they are being introduced. In terms of rigorous empirical support, the jury is still out on their effectiveness in improving rates of survival to discharge,[26] although one meta-analysis suggests they may be effective in addressing the problem referred to at the beginning of this discussion: cardiac arrests occurring outside critical care units.[27] The mixed results of RRT evaluations may be due to the limited understanding of the underlying problems this intervention is intended to address. What we need to know is: Where is the problem? To what extent does it lie with identifying patients in need of rescue and to what extent does it lie with action? And is a specialized team that handles the "rescue" portion of the process the right approach to work redesign?

Finally, the leadership role on RRTs and the enthusiasm of critical care nurses for these teams also deserves probing and discussion. Experienced ICU nurses tend to have a wealth of hands-on experience in the management of emergencies. They become accustomed to making a variety of judgments but may not always be able to function autonomously or claim credit for them. Not surprisingly, many ICU nurses have been particularly excited about playing an expanded role outside critical care units. Many have joined these teams, and some have even spearheaded RRT initiatives without thinking more deeply about the systems issues that may underlie failures to rescue patients in their facilities. These ICU nurses do not usually reflect on the impacts in terms of developing knowledge and maintaining competency for nurses on non–critical care units of transferring away from floor staff the responsibility for troubleshooting situations and handling emergencies. Is it time to build a broad base of skills across clinical staff in addition to creating an elite "SWAT team" of providers to deal with emergencies?

RRTs are discussed here because they are emblematic of a number of organizational interventions whose outcomes can at times fall well short of what is intended. The overall approach has been accepted uncritically. In the case of RRTs, no doubt some hospitals experienced an increase in successful patient "saves," or at the very least saw declines in staff anxiety and improvements in staff satisfaction after implementing these teams because they appeared to address recognized issues in patient care. Indeed research, product development, and on-the-ground safety work relating to specific safety issues (such as medication errors), as well as the causes of a broad array of other problems (including late and ineffective rescue efforts) are and always will be needed. Nonetheless, critically examining safety interventions can help us understand what may happen when safety problems are caused by underlying systems issues that no one is able (or willing) to discuss.

When hospital leaders decide whether to introduce RRTs, new equipment, or intervention bundles to reduce complications or participate in quality-monitoring efforts at a state or national level, the question that should arise is which initiatives make the best uses of limited resources. The important questions to ask are:

- How many narrowly targeted efforts can be implemented at once?
- Are we choosing the initiatives we pursue wisely?
- Are we critically examining the outcomes of our choices?

Without sound answers to these questions, at best we are guilty of negligent stewardship of scarce resources, and at worst of endangering our patients' well-being in the interests of short-term professional and financial rewards.

Where Next?

Some of the first and most systematic and cogent analyses of the problems facing health care systems worldwide have been commissioned by the U.S. Institute of Medicine (IOM).[28] Not surprisingly, many of the observations have special relevance to nurses and nursing care. Health care systems and providers are reported to be distressingly unaccountable for safety and other areas of their performance and are too slow to change.[29] An IOM report that focused on nursing urged careful attention to human resources and systems issues in care, but it has been cited principally by nurses and rarely beyond the profession.[30] Implementation of many of its recommendations is proving to be slow and difficult. The strategies being suggested, however, are likely the types of interventions addressing the "root causes" of quality problems that will be necessary to create lasting improvements in quality. Here I review several recurring and vital systems elements discussed in the IOM reports and elsewhere, including staffing reforms, work design, and attention to safety culture and climate.

Staffing Levels

An obvious systems-level feature of hospital care, and of the role of nursing in it, which many institutions are examining more closely in light of a burgeoning research literature, is staffing levels. Hospitals clearly need to have enough personnel with appropriate credentials (and in the right proportions relative to lesser-trained or untrained assistants) to provide safe care. A critical mass of research, particularly in acute care hospitals, has found that negative patient outcomes (including complications of care and unexpected patient mortality) are more common in settings with lower staffing levels.[31] Having enough properly trained nursing staff physically present to provide the required patient care and surveillance is unquestionably a necessary, but not a sufficient, condition for achieving high-quality or even merely safe care in hospitals. In other words, meeting or exceeding certain thresholds of staffing levels may not guarantee that the "right" things will be done for patients, although falling below them surely makes safe care difficult, if not impossible.

Policy approaches by governments and regulatory or accreditation authorities for ensuring consistently safe staffing levels are quite controversial. Examples include requirements that institutions report staffing schemes for state inspection, and requirements for the use of formal systems to estimate patient needs and to adjust staffing accordingly. For some time the Joint Commission (formerly the Joint Commission on Accreditation of Healthcare Organizations) in the United States has asked accredited facilities to track variations in staffing and verify whether safety-related events (and human resource indicators) seem to vary with them.[32] Among the strictest approaches are minimum mandatory nursing staff–to–patient ratios enforced by governments.

The unfolding story of mandated ratios in California and the Australian state of Victoria,[33] and the arguments of both critics and advocates of ratios, bear careful reading in the context of the ideas raised in this chapter. The importance of adequate staffing levels as the basis for safe care must be balanced against an awareness that staffing levels alone can never provide a guarantee. Many fear that a single-minded focus on staffing levels could divert attention and resources from other important aspects of safety and environments for safe care. The tensions between the two stances (pro-ratio versus anti-ratio) are considerable and are often played out in debates that oversimplify the very complex issues involved, with ratio advocates ignoring the subtleties in staffing that go well beyond nurse-to-patient ratios, and opponents sidestepping the tremendous variations in staffing approaches within and across hospitals, which surely cannot always be in patients' best interests.

One of the most important elements of context in the connections between staffing and safety, and one that needs urgent attention, is the workforce crisis affecting most, if not all, health care systems worldwide. Fortunately, there is a growing viewpoint within the health care community that human resource stability and safety are linked issues.[34] Keeping turnover to a minimum, encouraging new entrants to the field, and attracting critical masses of both recent graduates and experienced nurses are becoming priorities for nursing and health care executives. Some institutions and regions are destined to hold their own, while others may experience a profoundly different workforce from the one they are accustomed to. Analysis of the forces drawing nurses in and out of work in health care, and in specific regions and at specific facilities, is desperately needed. Currently, staffing is often thought of as a parameter that can be adjusted upward or downward at the discretion of managers and executives (depending mostly on cost considerations). This is destined to change—and soon. The availability of qualified nurses will soon be the major constraint on staffing levels in hospitals in most communities, and if predictions are correct, safety issues related to nursing are destined to become much worse.

Broad Workflow Issues

The wise use of the personnel who are actually on hand to provide care is another critical issue that has not received much discussion. A recurring problem in nursing has to do with a lack of clarity around—or at least an unwillingness to confront—the essence of nursing care.[35] It has been said that academic nursing is charged with developing the full menu or repertoire of what professional nurses can offer patients and with teaching these approaches to new generations, and that societal and health systems forces (particularly economic ones) influence which portions of these services are ultimately delivered to patients.[36] It is probably time to tackle this dichotomy head-on.

Disconnects between available resources and the expectations of patients, facilities, and the health care system for the types and quality of care to be provided must be addressed. There has been little discussion, let alone research, about the physical and practical limits of what can be expected of nursing staff. How many patients of high acuity, how much surveillance, and how many procedures represent too heavy a workload to carry out well? How many tasks, responsibilities, and initiatives constitute an untenable workload? Is it possible that quality of care or its cost-effectiveness could be improved by adding assistive personnel to the mix of nurses and judiciously delegating some aspects of care? What about the issue of downtime in nurses' workdays? What are the costs and benefits of building in "slack" (a certain proportion of "extra" time beyond what is necessary to perform minimal care in order to cope with the unexpected or to allow reflection and system improvement)? Given shorter lengths of stay, very high patient acuity, and a steep decrease in the number of stable patients occupying beds only because they are awaiting services provided on day shifts from Monday to Friday, is it time to revisit the question of staffing needs at night and on weekends? Are today's patients any less sick and their needs for nursing care dramatically slimmer in the "off hours," as staffing levels at night and on weekends would suggest?

Discussion is probably also overdue with respect to simplifying and streamlining the work nurses do, finding higher-order principles to guide practice instead of ever-lengthening checklists of tasks, and coaching staff in setting and resetting priorities in relation to the activities that have the most influence on patients' outcomes. Is continuous monitoring on multiple parameters, particularly with high-technology devices, equally helpful for all patients? Is "more" of some types of care always "better," or could fewer nursing treatments of certain types offer patients parallel or even superior benefits?

Perhaps there are concerns about slippery slopes and how little staff would do if told there were limits in terms of what can and should be provided. Precautions should be taken to avoid a race to the bottom in terms of care for some or all patients in hospitals, but perhaps the time has come to think of the nurse shortage many countries are facing as a shortage not just of bodies but of nursing time and nursing attention. If we do not, then safety problems, particularly in hospitals unable to recruit and retain experienced staff and to maintain minimal staffing levels, might become especially severe sooner rather than later.

Hospitals are plagued by unquestionably inefficient and ineffective work systems. Securing materials and supplies and communicating with other departments and professionals is notoriously inefficient and frustrating, and can lead to distractions that jeopardize patient safety, for instance, in calculating drug dosages or preparing medications. The breakdowns and detours in obtaining basic tools and in the exchange of critical information, as well as constant interruptions, are routine elements of nursing work.[37] Given the central place of nurses in delivering care to hospitalized patients, the problem of interruptions may be quite difficult to remedy and may require deeper redesign of their work, including rethinking communication systems and physical layouts of units.

Similarly problematic are the antiquated systems for handling the large quantities of information that nurses deal with. Information is managed in nursing practice in more or less the same way it has been since the origins of the profession—with narrative notes, flow sheets (notably, graphic vital signs forms), and a panoply of forms, and of course the near-ubiquitous scraps of paper that nurses use to track minute-to-minute developments. Forms are used in idiosyncratic combinations from hospital to hospital and even across units within the same hospital. Entries of questionable relevance and duplicative recording of some kinds of information (such as certain types of medications) are very common, along with huge gaps in the documentation of important clinical observations. Access to nurses' observations and records to enhance the provision of care and drive quality improvement remains very difficult. Systematic computerized recordkeeping is the obvious solution.

Most involved in health care, including information technology companies, admit that IT has not yet fulfilled its potential to help clinicians deal with the cognitive demands of caring for many patients with complex needs all at once. Care is still organized in most settings in a manner that relies on humans' notoriously fallible short-term and long-term memory to provide complex services, share information among clinicians, and follow an evergrowing array of best practices and safety considerations. Information technology may not provide a complete answer for all of these problems, but it can be a start, even though experience suggests that at least in the short term it may add to clinical workloads.[38]

The use of technologies, from handheld input devices, touch screens, and various computer formats to processing functions, has been limited, and heavy financial investments have often created much labor with limited proof of return on investment. What is needed is a thorough examination of the potential applications of IT in nursing practice and a shift from niche applications to integrated IT solutions across care settings which mirror and smooth workflow. Practical considerations in nursing work are too often considered an "extra" layer of complexity to be addressed at the end of the health IT design process. Without thoughtful analysis and a willingness to make considerable investments in design, equipment, software, and training, IT—including its absence from many settings where nursing care is delivered—will continue to be a drain on nurses' time and energy rather than the force for improving the safety and quality of care that it could become.

Safety Culture and Climate

Creating a culture of safety is another system element that can decrease, if not always eliminate, the need for intensive management of many narrow aspects of practice. Safety cultures are grounded in shared understandings among health care workers of best practices and quality-improvement principles. Safety cultures—enduring patterns of thinking and behaving among members of an organization—influence what is known as safety climates, which are the impressions and perceptions about safety conditions over shorter time periods experienced and described by workers.

Safety cultures can either facilitate or pose barriers to sound practice, good communication, and process analysis and change. Culture is built over time, as expectations are created and upheld concerning the costs and rewards of reporting errors and near-misses, managers' and leaders' true values around honesty and openness, and the size and scope of investments in benchmarking performance, educating staff, and analyzing safety and quality issues. The existence of a safety culture within an institution or facility can be charted on a continuum. At one end is profound dysfunction: unhealthy communication across groups of clinicians and between managers and clinicians, active hiding of errors, and the unwillingness to confront any safety problems.[39] At the other extreme are organizational cultures in which continuous attention to safety issues not only includes but also goes beyond being proactive about risks and having a constant awareness of and focus on safety. By analyzing systems of care and drawing from discussions of problems that have occurred elsewhere, workers in organizations with cultures of safety attend to issues or conditions that may not yet have resulted in an error or accident.[40] Safety climate, the more "local," personal, and time-limited form of safety-related organizational environments, and safety culture, like minimal staffing levels, are likely to be necessary but not sufficient ingredients for maintaining high-quality care in complex systems. Obviously, achieving the high end is not easy, and a number of interventions that have been put forward to improve safety—such as having clinician and non-clinician executives walk around facilities, observe conditions, and exchange perceptions, experiences, and information with one another—have been somewhat narrow. More research and discussion of the practical aspects of producing change in safety culture and climate are clearly needed.

A Leadership Focus on Higher-Level Organizational Forces and a Commitment to the Systems Approach

Today's health care leaders are inundated with an array of patient safety strategies. They are asked to allocate time, money, and energy to improve many aspects of care delivered by clinicians. There is a tremendous temptation to deal with safety problems on a piecemeal basis. Wanting to show that one is "doing something to enhance patient safety" can blind leaders to the patchwork of initiatives that results. The acceptance of a systems approach, not just in theory but in practice, is essential. Recognizing and modifying obvious safety hazards is important, but so is understanding and remedying problems with health care organization structure and functioning that undermine safe practice. Caution must be exercised to avoid devoting all, or nearly all, available resources for safety and quality improvement to equipment, education, and monitoring focused on very specific and narrow aspects of care or unit performance. In the end, institutional leaders, managers, executives, and senior clinicians need to take control of their institutions' destinies. They also need to provide practical assistance for other clinicians as they try to sift through multiple priorities and imperatives. They must think beyond the immediate and the narrow and look to longer-term and higher-order features of their institutions' practice environments.

Every system has capacity limits, and a change in one part of a system affects aspects or areas of others. So while they must listen carefully to regulators, payers, and other stakeholders, leaders need to give feedback and unite to speak with one voice when initiatives are excessively burdensome and/or unlikely to achieve their intended ends. Somehow, in the face of staff shortages and understandable demands for accountability, they must find ways to create conditions under which staff can hold more on their plates, perhaps by optimizing staffing and workflow.

In order to resist the temptation or pressure to sign on to all initiatives that come along, health care leaders must be supported by their peers. They need to speak out against bandwagonism and speak up for those who challenge orthodoxy in safety work. Voices in nursing and the other health disciplines, in management, and in national and international safety circles need to confront the uncontrolled proliferation of demands for reporting indicators, as well as information and initiative overload in the safety field. Health care leaders must listen without prejudice when their staff raise concerns about having to handle too many practice changes and demands at once and not leap to accuse direct care providers of being afraid of change. Enduring improvements in safety and the avoidance of unexpected negative consequences of safety initiatives will depend on it.

While it's difficult to know whether health care is any safer or more dangerous than it has ever been, the risks inherent in high-intensity health care treatments have certainly never been greater. This is true of patients receiving concurrent medical therapy for multiple chronic conditions in the community and in long-term care settings, for patients receiving curative treatment in acute care facilities, and for many other clinical populations. The supply of a critical mass of qualified nurses and other health personnel has never been as much in peril as now, nor have so many forces within health care systems been as determined to control costs and improve quality in so many ways at once, seemingly at any price. Without careful reflection and strong leadership, well-meaning but poorly planned and executed safety initiatives could needlessly divert nurses from keeping patients safe in the face of a severe and deepening nurse shortage.

Ensuring the safety and quality of nursing work requires a deep commitment to patients and their well-being as well as compassion for providers who want to do the right thing but may not always find it easy to prioritize or to see the larger picture. Leaders and authorities must exercise intellectual curiosity, carefully scrutinize safety issues, be willing to rethink many operating practices, and look before leaping into the latest safety or quality initiatives. They must consider the involvement of nursing staff in the delivery of care, not only by involving nurses in the design of programs and initiatives, but also by ensuring that the impacts of these initiatives on the actual delivery of care are thought through. Managers have a duty to understand and respect the limitations of systems that place caps on what can be accomplished, and to communicate about safety issues, organizational performance, and patient outcomes to those they supervise in a way that allows health care workers to retain their dignity, self-esteem, and passion for their work. This is true not just for nurses, of course, but for all health care workers. The extensive scope of nurses' involvement in delivering care, the historical neglect of many aspects of nursing work and the adequacy of the nursing workforce, as well as the potentially devastating magnitude of the coming shortage of professional nurses worldwide all make critical examination of systems issues in the delivery of nursing care particularly important—and urgent.

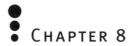

CHAPTER 8

Physicians, Sleep Deprivation, and Safety

Christopher P. Landrigan

In the mid-1990s, when I was an intern in pediatrics, here is what one of my typical days "on call" looked like. I dragged myself out of bed at about 5:30 AM (an hour and a half later than my friends who went into surgical residencies, but similar to most other interns), showered, threw on some scrubs, and ran out the door. After grabbing a cup of coffee and a doughnut, I hopped on the T—the public transportation system in Boston—and headed in to work. Arriving at about 6:30, I scurried around to the rooms of the four or five patients still on my census from the last time I was on call three nights previously, gathering data that would be needed during rounds. From 7:00 to 9:30 I rounded with the attending physician, the unit charge nurse, my three fellow interns, and several medical students, discussing each patient on the service in detail, and seeing the sickest as the attending made teaching points for the trainees regarding sickle cell disease, perhaps, or the optimal management of pneumonia in adolescents. Afterwards, the attending physician headed out for the day, and my fellow residents, the medical students, and I were left to care for the twenty-five patients on our service in the hospital. Over the course of the next eight hours, with perhaps a one-hour break at noon to take in a lecture on a medical topic of interest, I was busy examining my patients, writing notes, ordering medications, answering pages, ordering tests and labs, doing minor procedures such as placing intravenous lines and performing lumbar punctures, speaking with consultants, and arranging the follow-up plans for those heading home. Over the course of the afternoon, things typically intensified as I gradually assumed the care of all of the other interns' patients, as first the "post-call" intern (at the tail end of a thirty- to thirty-six-hour shift) and later the "swing interns" (those on a relatively short ten-hour workday) signed out their patients to me and went home. By 6 PM I was fielding pages and heading to patients' bedsides to deal with everything from minor concerns to major crises that arose. To complicate things further, at roughly the same time, about three to ten admissions per night from the emergency room would start to roll in. I would see each new child admitted, speak with his or her parents, take a detailed history, do a full physical exam, review and attempt to interpret his or her laboratory studies, electrocardiograms, and X rays, and write admission orders, general care plans, plans for diagnostic testing, and perhaps two to twenty new medication orders per patient, depending on the complexity of the problem. After midnight I was sheltered from further new admissions by activation of a "night float," a resident who came in to help with late-night admissions, but any patients called up before midnight—who often did not arrive from the ER until after 2 AM—were my responsibility. By the time these patients had been worked up and I had completed all of my work, it was usually about 3 AM, at which point I was able to sleep for perhaps two to four hours, a sleep most often interrupted by between one and five hazily recalled pages from nurses. After struggling to awaken, I would pre-round, round with the team, and take care of the next day's work for my new patients. Sometime in the afternoon I would depart bleary-eyed and feeling oddly euphoric (a known consequence of sleep deprivation) after signing out to the intern taking the next night's call . . . around thirty to thirty-six hours after I had first arrived in the hospital.

When I was on call at night, some help was certainly available—the senior resident discussed each case with me, at least briefly—and in the case of an emergency, backup teams of physicians could be called, but for the most part I acted alone, seeing patients, writing orders, interpreting tests, and performing procedures without any direct supervision, inexperienced and exhausted. I cannot count the number of times that an error I made in ordering a medication was intercepted by an alert nurse or pharmacist. How many more mistakes made their way through these defenses to the patients I will never know.

At the time, few hospitals were attuned to patient safety. Within a few years, however, with the publication of the Institute of Medicine's 1999 report *To Err Is Human,* the landscape began to change, at least in some respects.[1] Computerized order entry systems were put in place to intercept medication errors in many hospitals. In other hospitals, clinical pharmacists were hired to oversee interns' and residents' orders. Efforts to eradicate hospital-acquired infections increased. Yet at a deeper level, our system of care remains fundamentally unchanged from what it was when I was an intern.

Academic medical centers continue to run on an engine that is continuously in overdrive, where junior doctors fresh out of medical school provide most direct patient care with minimal supervision in a state of near-complete exhaustion. Inexperienced resident physicians are still on call every three to four nights in most hospitals. Senior residents and attending physicians are now more often physically present somewhere in the hospital to provide backup in emergencies, but interns and junior residents continue to write most orders and provide most medical care without any direct, minute-to-minute oversight. Despite the introduction of token work hour limits for doctors in training in 2003 (eighty-hour-per-week and thirty-hour-per-shift maximums), actual work hours have changed only minimally,[2] and as the condition of hospitalized patients has become more acute, there are some data showing that the amount of sleep interns are obtaining on call has actually dropped. A series of studies has emerged unequivocally demonstrating the hazards of interns' and residents' long work hours,[3] but this issue remains largely unaddressed by hospitals, physicians, professional societies, and policymakers.

Even the patient safety movement itself has seemed reluctant to tackle the issue of physician sleep deprivation. While it is clear that traditional resident work schedules built on frequent shifts of twenty-four to thirty consecutive hours increase the frequency with which errors occur,[4] efforts in the United States to address this hazard have been weak and ineffective. The 2003 ACGME (Accreditation Council for Graduate Medical Education) work hour limits for residents permit hours far in excess of those proved safe, and even at these permissive levels are inadequately enforced.[5] A more stringent sixteen-hour-shift limit for first-year residents (interns) was implemented in July 2011, but second-year and higher residents continue to be permitted to work for up to twenty-eight hours in a row. No limits of any kind have been established for senior physicians. By contrast, the United Kingdom and some other European nations have taken strong action to limit work hours for both physicians in training and senior physicians.[6]

This chapter provides an introduction to the nature of medical error, the neurophysiology of human alertness and performance, and the manner in which sleep deprivation and circadian misalignment conspire to induce error in medical settings. It reviews recent studies investigating this issue and current efforts to translate sleep and circadian science into public policy. It concludes with a call for more effective action. If the patient safety movement is to achieve its promise of optimizing the safety of American health care, physician sleep must be an integral part of the agenda.

Human Fallibility

Psychologists and human factors engineers have long known that even the smartest and most conscientious individuals make mistakes, and make them frequently. While humans can process and retain enormous amounts of information, and are capable of innovation and intuitive leaps of understanding, we are also prone to certain predictable cognitive failings. An awareness of our capacities and constraints provides some insight into the genesis of error.

Rasmussen and Jensen have categorized human thought processes into "automatic" and "active" modes of processing as a means of explaining human performance and error.[7] The automatic mode is used in the completion of routine, day-to-day tasks such as driving a car or, in a doctor's case, carrying out a familiar procedure. An experienced driver does not need to think about inserting her key in the car door, turning it to open the door, sitting down, pulling on her seatbelt and inserting it in the buckle, inserting her key in the ignition, turning it, stepping on the brake, shifting the transmission from park to reverse, and so on. These steps happen smoothly and effortlessly. Likewise, an ICU doctor rapidly learns the proper way to place a supraclavicular venous line, and once experienced, can relatively effortlessly set up a central line kit, gown and glove herself, sterilize the skin, access the vessel, thread in the line, and secure it in place. The ability to conduct complex, routine tasks with this low-effort mode of cognition affords us efficiencies, as it allows us to focus our minds on other tasks while we accomplish the mundane routines of daily activity. During an emergency, however, or when an unusual situation occurs, a need arises to take more "active" control of this automatic process. Failing or forgetting to do so at the right moment leads to a "slip" or a "lapse," and can have consequences from the simple (driving past the intended exit on the highway or missing an attempt to place the central line) to the profound (crashing the car, or inadvertently puncturing the pleural space).

When faced with a novel or difficult problem, we employ the active mode of thinking. This mode is slow, labor-intensive, and prone to its own set of well-characterized mistakes. An example of a specific type of common failing is "confirmation bias." That is, if a physician, for example, prematurely jumps to the conclusion that a patient presenting with abdominal pain has gastroenteritis, there is a natural human tendency to accept confirmatory data and to ignore or downplay data that refute this preliminary diagnosis. A substantial effort is required to take a step back and carefully confront one's conclusions, to recognize that this particular patient has a little more right-lower-quadrant pain than is typical, and perhaps a hint of rebound tenderness suggestive of appendicitis. Interruptions, time pressures, sleep deprivation, or other factors can prevent us from taking this step back, potentially leading to error.

Physicians in training in their first year (interns) work an average of sixty-seven hours per week, with 40 percent of all workweeks exceeding eighty hours, 24 percent exceeding ninety hours, and 11 percent of all workweeks exceeding one hundred hours. Overnight shifts last an average of thirty hours, with an average of 2.6 hours of sleep obtained during these overnight shifts.[8] On many nights no sleep is obtained at all. Under these circumstances, cognition, vigilance, and performance are greatly impaired, as described in detail later in this chapter.

Health System Design

In addition to individual human fallibilities, the design and complexity of the health care system play a role in error. Human cognition, and thus the propensity for error, is not constant under all circumstances but varies with changes in working conditions. Moreover, work environment and systemic design determine in part whether an error will be intercepted or will go on to cause harm. A well-designed work environment can reduce both the risk of an individual's making an error and the risk of that error's causing harm, just as a poorly designed environment can increase the risk for each.

Human factors engineering is a discipline focused on the mental and physical parameters of human functioning and the interface between individuals and their work environments. *To Err Is Human* described the nature of error in complex systems. Based on the work of James Reason and others, it concluded that complex systems fail because of the combination of multiple small failures, each of which is individually insufficient to cause an accident. These failures are latent and their patterns change constantly.[9] When an error occurs in health care (as in other complex systems), there are typically multiple opportunities to correct it that could potentially prevent harm. The "safety nets" that exist are usually dependent on human action, however, and are therefore imperfect; from time to time an error slips through all safety nets and causes harm.[10]

An example in health care of the "multiple small failures" paradigm is the manner in which a medication ordering error causes harm. If an intern inadvertently makes a decimal point error in calculating the dose of morphine to administer to a patient, it is not the case that such an error immediately results in harm. Rather, in order for harm to occur, many secondary failures must occur as well. First, the intern herself must fail to notice that she has made a calculation error when placing the order. At a minimum, the order must then make it past the nurse or pharmacist who transcribes the error, the pharmacy technician who fills the order in the pharmacy, the nurse who receives the medication from the pharmacy and administers it, and the patient himself. Each of these individuals has an opportunity to catch the error; it is only through a failure at each stage in the process that the medication overdose reaches the patient. The probability that each of these individuals will catch or fail to catch such an error is, like the commission of the initial error, a function of both that individual's cognitive processes and the system in which he or she is working. He or she must be awake, alert, and vigilant to serve as an effective safety net.

Unfortunately, as Alison Trinkoff and Jeanne Geiger-Brown point out in chapter 9, there is increasing evidence that nurses as well as doctors are feeling the effects of sleep deprivation and long hours. Nurses now routinely work twelve-hour shifts, many of which extend out in practice to thirteen hours or more.[11] With longer shifts, nurses appear to be less effective safety agents, both making more errors themselves and likely catching fewer errors made by doctors and others.[12]

Sleep Deprivation and Human Performance

Like distractions, excessive workload, and other environmental factors that degrade individual performance, provider sleep deprivation exerts its influence by increasing the risk of slips, lapses, and mistakes in judgment. Patients are dependent on providers' judgment and performance in their completion of both routine and complex tasks. Sleep deprivation increases the chances that providers will fail to recognize an evolving problem or will make a mistake in the writing of a prescription or the performance of a procedure. Given the medical fragility of many hospitalized patients, even minor lapses of attention or calculation errors can have serious consequences. In health care, where physicians and other providers are routinely scheduled for long work hours, sleep deprivation can have very substantial system-wide consequences.

Human alertness and neurobehavioral performance are codetermined principally by two neurobiologic systems: the sleep homeostat and the circadian system. The homeostatic system mediates time spent awake and asleep, and has a direct effect on performance across a range of cognitive and motor tasks. The circadian system superimposes a nearly twenty-four-hour cycle of performance over these homeostatic effects, with the minimum performance normally occurring a few hours prior to waking. Under normal sleep-wake conditions, the homeostatic and circadian systems work together to maintain alertness and performance throughout the waking day. Under rotating and shifting schedules, however, the two systems can interact in a manner that causes performance deficits greater than would be observed during a normal waking day. Chronic sleep loss and sleep inertia (described later in this chapter) can lead to further deterioration in performance. Particularly during the early morning hours, if one has been awake continuously for a protracted period of time, the combined effect of the sleep homeostat and circadian pressure can create a critical zone of vulnerability in which decreased performance on the job may occur, increasing the risk of fall-asleep incidents, errors, and accidents.

Circadian Misalignment

Laboratory studies and studies in the field have shown that during extended wakefulness, alertness and performance exhibit daily variation with a near-twenty-four-hour period.[13] This circadian pattern of alertness and performance is superimposed on the steady deterioration induced by sleep loss, discussed later in this chapter.[14] Human circadian rhythms are driven by an endogenous circadian pacemaker located in the suprachiasmatic nucleus of the hypothalamus,[15] which drives the rhythms of core body temperature, cortisol, and melatonin, as well as neurobehavioral functioning. In laboratory studies in which subjects are made to live on a sleep-wake schedule outside their norm, in a protected environment absent any information about what time of day it is,[16] their circadian pacemakers continue to oscillate at their intrinsic periods (24.2 hours on average), so that they must sleep and wake up at many different circadian phases.[17] In these circumstances it has been found that the largest number of neurobehavioral performance problems are seen near the minimum of the endogenous core body temperature rhythm, which occurs approximately one to three hours before habitual wake time in most individuals.[18] In addition, these experiments have revealed that the ability to sleep varies with circadian phase;[19] circadian misalignment impairs not only one's neurobehavioral performance when awake but the quality and duration of sleep as well. This effect is common among night workers— including medical residents and other physicians working at night—who frequently have difficulty sleeping during daytime hours.[20] Since alertness and performance depend heavily on sleep quality and duration,[21] circadian misalignment therefore causes neurobehavioral function to decline indirectly, via its effects on sleep, as well as directly.

Acute Sleep Deprivation, the Sleep Homeostat, and Performance

Independent of the circadian system, acute sleep deprivation has been systematically documented to cause reduction in human alertness and performance.[22] Every hour of wakefulness increases the homeostatic drive to sleep, which results in deteriorating performance. In industrial settings this is illustrated by the increased risk of fatigue-related fatal truck crashes with increased hours of driving.[23] Compared with the first hour, there is a more than fifteen-fold increase in the risk of a fatigue-related fatal crash after thirteen hours of driving. Federal regulations strictly limit the number of consecutive hours that truck drivers can drive and that pilots can fly, but residents are permitted to work as many as eighty hours per week. Senior physicians' work hours are not limited at all.

Chronic Partial Sleep Deprivation

The history of nightly sleep duration over the preceding days to weeks has also been demonstrated to affect performance. Sleep loss on a nightly basis, also known as chronic partial sleep deprivation, results in a "sleep debt."[24] Loss of two hours of sleep for five to seven consecutive nights impairs performance to a similar degree as twenty-four hours of continuous sleep deprivation. After twelve to fourteen consecutive nights of sleep restriction, lapses of attention on the psychomotor vigilance task (PVT) can increase to the level seen after forty-eight hours of total sleep deprivation.[25]

Sleep Inertia

Alertness and performance are also impaired immediately after waking,[26] even in subjects who are not sleep-deprived;[27] this phenomenon is called sleep inertia.[28] Sleep inertia then gradually dissipates over time, with residual effects lasting up to around two hours.[29] A study of U.S. Air Force flight accidents due to pilot error found that pilots were much more likely to make errors shortly after awakening than later.[30] In hospitals, sleep inertia may be extremely important, as physicians awakened from their brief nightly sleep regularly make decisions and perform interventions within minutes of waking. A physician woken up urgently who must immediately perform a resuscitation on a patient in cardiac arrest is far more likely to make a mistake than if he or she had been awake for a few hours; indeed the propensity to err in the first few minutes after awakening may exceed even that which is induced by twenty-four hours of total sleep deprivation.[31]

Sleep and Occupational Safety

Night work and sleep deprivation have been identified as root causes of accidents and adverse events across high-risk industries, including nuclear power and transportation.[32] The Three Mile Island and Chernobyl nuclear power incidents, as well as the grounding of the oil tanker *Exxon Valdez,* were caused in part by operator fatigue. Gas meter readers and train drivers make more errors during the night shift, and commercial pilots suffer increased sleepiness, microsleeps, and performance lapses during the night.[33]

Night workers are prone to increased errors for several reasons. First, their endogenous circadian rhythms and the imposed sleep-work schedule are typically out of phase. For the night worker, the timing of meals, work, and sleep remains permanently out of phase with the timing of environmental light, the most powerful synchronizer of the human circadian pacemaker.[34] As a result, most permanent night workers fail to fully adapt physiologically to their work schedules.[35] Second, as alluded to earlier, circadian misalignment leads to a substantial loss of sleep efficiency during daytime sleep.[36] Third, night shift workers often begin their workday eight to ten hours after awakening,[37] which leaves them with more accumulated homeostatic pressure to sleep at the beginning of their shift compared with day workers. For residents and other physicians working shifts of twenty-four to thirty hours or longer, this accumulated homeostatic pressure is inevitable.

Motor Vehicle Crashes

Motor vehicle crashes are an especially common and hazardous consequence of sleep deprivation, especially among night workers. In approximately 56,000 motor vehicle crashes (MVCs) and 1,550 fatalities per year in the United States, fatigue is cited by police officers as the cause of the crash, but these statistics likely underestimate the problem.[38] Data on sleep are not routinely gathered in many states, and drowsiness is typically deemed the cause of a crash only when all other possible causes have been excluded. The 100-Car Naturalistic Driving Study, in which one hundred vehicles were equipped for a year with sophisticated sensors, found drowsiness to be a cause of 22 percent of all MVCs and 16 percent of all near-crashes.[39] Making a very rough extrapolation from this figure to the annual number of MVC fatalities, we find that as many as eight thousand fatal crashes each year in the United States could be due to drowsy driving.

The risk of fatigue-related crashes is especially high in certain occupational groups. A report from the National Transportation Safety Board Studies found fatigue to be the most frequently cited probable cause of all heavy truck crashes that are fatal to the driver (31 percent), exceeding alcohol and other drug use combined (29 percent).[40] As described later in this chapter, resident physicians have likewise been found to be at high risk of fatigue-related motor vehicle crashes.[41]

Health

In addition to its effects on alertness and performance, chronic, recurrent sleep deprivation is associated with significant health problems. Sleep deprivation and working in an adverse circadian phase have been linked with an increased risk of obesity due both to changes in leptin and ghrelin activity in the body and to altered eating behaviors.[42] Gastrointestinal disease, particularly peptic ulcer disease, is common in shift workers.[43] The risks of high blood pressure, myocardial infarctions, and cardiovascular disease are elevated as well.[44] In addition, regular night shift workers have been found to have an increased risk of breast and prostate cancer, as well as other cancers,[45] leading the World Health Organization in 2007 to declare shift work a probable carcinogen.[46] Since the schedules of resident physicians in particular, as well as those of senior physicians in some specialties, are among the most extreme of any profession, they may convey even greater risks of long-term health problems than typical shift workers experience.

Mood and Mental Health

While these long-term health risks are an obvious concern, shift work and sleep deprivation have more immediate effects on mental health. Sleep deprivation due to extreme work hours is well documented to affect mood adversely. In residents in particular, the frequency of nights on call is associated with marital discord and failure to meet social commitments.[47] Sleep-deprived interns report more sadness and lack of self-worth, as well as depression, irritability, depersonalization, inappropriate affect, and memory deficits.[48] A small study conducted in 1984 found that approximately one in seven residents reported having experienced a major depression, and almost half reported having experienced a less severe depressive episode.[49] More recently, a series of studies administering standardized depression and burn-out screening tools to residents found that three in four residents are burned out, and fully 20 percent score at high risk of major depression.[50] Residents report significantly elevated rates of anger, tension, confusion, depression, and fatigue after six months of residency.[51] Depression has been shown directly to increase the risk of medical errors.[52] This is likely a consequence of decreased vigilance on the job, as well as the adverse effects of poor mood, decreased empathy, depression, and burnout on team performance and communication. As each of these is induced by sleep deprivation resulting from extreme work schedules in residency, reducing resident work hours may have a significant beneficial effect on teamwork and communication as well as resident mental health and cognitive performance.

Resident Physicians, Sleep, and Performance: Laboratory and Simulator Studies

Many studies have attempted to assess the effects of sleep deprivation on resident physicians' performance. These studies have measured reaction time, memory, and manual dexterity, and the performance of clinical skills in laboratory or simulated clinical environments. Though a few have not found performance to degrade as a consequence of sleep deprivation,[53] the overwhelming majority have identified significant deteriorations in performance.[54]

In the 1970s, Friedman and colleagues had interns read electrocardiograms to detect arrhythmias when they were sleep-deprived and again when rested.[55] Sleep-deprived interns made nearly twice as many errors, a finding substantiated by more recent studies using similar methods.[56] In surgical simulator studies, surgical residents who are sleep-deprived have been found to perform less efficiently[57] and to make more overt errors in the completion of manual tasks.[58] More recently, Arnedt and colleagues demonstrated in 2005 that working a traditional schedule with shifts of twenty-four hours or more every four to five nights impaired residents' neurobehavioral and driving performance to the same degree as a blood alcohol level of 0.04–0.05 percent, despite the fact that the residents obtained an average of three hours' sleep while working overnight shifts in the hospital.[59] Philibert found in a meta-analysis of sixty studies that residents' mean performance on clinical tasks after twenty-four hours of sleep deprivation dropped nearly two standard deviations, to the seventh percentile of the level at which they performed when rested.[60] The findings included failures in the performance of routine tasks such as conducting an adequate physical examination or taking a thorough patient history, as well as failures in the performance of procedures and interpretation of diagnostic tests.

Resident Physicians, Sleep, and Performance:
Harvard Work Hours, Health, and Safety Studies

In light of concerns derived from laboratory and simulator data that physicians' traditional work hours might be exposing them and their patients to excessive risk, as well as concerns that current physician work hour standards might be inadequate to address this risk effectively, colleagues and I in the Harvard Work Hours, Health, and Safety (HWHHS) Group began conducting a series of studies several years ago. These are described in detail in this section.

Harvard Work Hours, Health, and Safety Study I: A Nationwide Study of Interns' Sleep and Safety

Barger and colleagues conducted a nationwide prospective cohort study of 2,737 first-year medical residents (interns) in their first year after graduating from medical school. On a monthly basis, detailed data were collected on work hours, extended-duration work shifts, motor vehicle crashes, near-miss accidents, self-reported medical errors, needle-stick and other occupational injuries, and fall-asleep incidents. Motor vehicle crash risk during the commute home from work was found to be more than doubled over baseline risk, and near-miss motor vehicle crash risk was increased sixfold after extended-duration shifts compared to non-extended-duration shifts.[61] In addition, Ayas and colleagues found that interns working for longer than twenty consecutive hours had 61 percent increased odds of suffering a needle-stick or scalpel injury on the morning after working all night, compared with the risk of such an injury on other mornings.[62] In a third related study, Barger and colleagues found that those interns working more than five extended shifts of twenty-four hours or longer in a month were seven times as likely as those who worked fewer hours to report a fatigue-related medical error that injured a patient, and four times as likely to report a fatigue-related medical error that led to a patient's death,[63] including a delayed diagnosis of a ruptured aneurysm leading to a patient's death and a delay in initiation of antibiotics leading to overwhelming sepsis and death.

The Intern Sleep and Patient Safety Study

Concurrently we conducted an intensive randomized controlled study of the effect on intern sleep and patient safety of an intervention schedule that limited interns' work to under sixteen consecutive hours. Interns working in the coronary care unit and medical intensive care unit at Brigham and Women's Hospital in Boston were studied. Sleep and work hours were documented through the use of daily logs validated by electroencephalography (EEG) and third-party confirmation. We systematically monitored the units for errors, using a four-pronged data collection methodology that included hiring a team of trained physician-observers to monitor the performance of the interns continuously around the clock, as well as daily medical record review. All suspected errors were subsequently classified by two independent investigators blinded as to study conditions. The intervention schedule reduced weekly work hours from eighty-five to sixty-five per week. Interns on the traditional schedule were found to obtain approximately one less hour of sleep per night than those on our intervention schedule and had twice as many objectively documented attentional failures during night work hours. In addition, interns on the traditional schedule made 35.9 percent more serious medical errors and 5.6 times as many serious diagnostic errors on the traditional schedule as compared to the intervention schedule.[64] Examples of serious errors from that study include:

- Patient with history of flash pulmonary edema admitted for congestive heart failure. Several days into the hospitalization, intern reported that patient was clinically stable, having miscalculated that 24 hour input and output volumes were well matched (20cc positive). Nurse was concerned that patient seemed fluid overloaded and in mild respiratory distress, and requested a re-evaluation. A re-calculation by the senior resident revealed a 100-fold error in calculation: the patient was in fact 2000cc positive for the prior 24 hours. Furosemide was promptly administered and patient's symptoms improved.
- Patient with implanted defibrillator on left side urgently needed central access for inotropic support. Intern inserted a central venous catheter in the left subclavian vein. The intern did not recognize that the vein was occupied with the wire from the defibrillator, and was having repeated difficulty advancing the introducer. In the middle of the placement, the cardiology fellow entered and asked the intern to abort the procedure immediately. The catheter was removed before it interfered with or dislodged the defibrillator wire.
- Patient developed a right-sided tension pneumothorax, after a technical error during placement of a subclavian venous catheter led to pleural space puncture.[65]

Physician Work-Hour Policy in the United States and Abroad

Given the considerable data on sleep deprivation and performance, as well as public concerns about resident physician work hours, the Accreditation Council for Graduate Medical Education—the professional body that regulates residency programs in the United States—implemented nationwide work hour limits for residents for the first time in 2003. These standards limited shifts to no longer than thirty hours in a row, with a maximum of eighty weekly work hours, averaged over a four-week period. These limits, however, are not commensurate with work hour limits in other safety-sensitive industries in the United States or with limits for physicians in other industrialized countries, and address only work hours for physicians in training. Senior physicians' work hours are not limited in any way, and in some intensive specialties (such as surgery, obstetrics, cardiology, and intensive care), senior physicians routinely work for more than twenty-four hours without sleep.

While some studies have found small drops in mortality for certain hospital subpopulations following implementation of the ACGME standards,[66] the largest study conducted as of this writing has found that the standards had no effect on patient mortality.[67] This is likely due to the fact that (1) the standards reduced nationwide work hours by only 5.8 percent and increased sleep by only 6.1 percent, which was likely insufficient to yield a substantial reduction in fatigue-related errors; and (2) compliance with these standards has been extremely poor.[68] As part of the HWHHS nationwide prospective study of interns, we evaluated compliance with the ACGME standards and found that 84 percent of interns violated the standards during at least one month in the year after their release, and in any given month 61.5 percent of interns working in hospital settings were in violation. Interestingly, the rates of noncompliance we detected were far higher than those detected by the ACGME itself, most likely because of systematic underreporting to the ACGME; interns (and residency programs) have a disincentive to report violations to the ACGME, as such reports can in theory result in a program's being suspended or shut down altogether.

Perhaps even more important than compliance, however, is whether the number of hours U.S. resident physicians are allowed to work (twenty-eight hours in a row for most residents, eighty hours per week) is appropriate. Having years ago recognized the risks of sleep deprivation, regulatory bodies in other high-risk U.S. industries established consecutive work limits of eight to twelve hours.[69] The United Kingdom and continental Europe, recognizing the strength of the data on sleep deprivation, have passed laws limiting all workers, including physicians and nurses, to thirteen consecutive hours and forty-eight hours per week. While considerable controversy has surrounded this change in the United Kingdom as in other countries that have implemented work hour limits, preliminary data suggest that a forty-eight-hour workweek may be even safer than the fifty-six-hour limit that existed in the United Kingdom until the summer of 2009,[70] never mind the eighty-hour workweek that is common in the United States. New Zealand has had a sixteen-consecutive-hour work limit for physicians in training in place for over twenty years, and while few high-quality data exist comparing safety and quality between nations, those data that do exist suggest that New Zealand's health care system is at least as safe as that in the United States, and possibly safer.[71]

Although several hospitals around the United States, including Children's Hospital and Brigham and Women's, both in Boston, have been taking major steps to reduce consecutive work hours much more substantially than is required by the ACGME, such efforts have occurred in only a handful of institutions. Indeed, in the national push to implement safer care, the issue of provider fatigue has received remarkably little attention, despite the fact that the evidence base supporting its importance is far more robust than that underlying many other common interventions. Ironically, failing to take human fatigue into account may erode the effectiveness of other interventions, such as efforts to reduce nosocomial infections or improve medication safety, since exhausted providers may have difficulty implementing new safety protocols just as they have difficulty providing direct clinical care.

Moving Forward: From Sleep Science to Safer Schedules to Safety Improvement

Given the slow pace of progress in improving scheduling safety, as well as in implementing other patient safety initiatives in the United States and abroad, concerns have begun to surface that rates of medical errors might not be improving, despite over ten years of federal investment in patient safety.[72] It is becoming increasingly apparent that the research and improvement funding devoted to patient safety has not been as effective as hoped, most likely because of the failure to address certain key root hazards in the system, as well as the difficulty of disseminating proven interventions.

The perpetuation of the traditional twenty-four- to thirty-hour marathon "on-call" work shifts of physicians in training (residents) is a quintessential example of the disconnection between state-of-the-art safety science, the allocation of funds to improve safety, and current practice. As described earlier in this chapter, shifts exceeding twenty-four hours have repeatedly been proven to pose very substantial safety hazards to both residents themselves and their patients. Extrapolating from the HWHHS data to the full national cohort of 100,000 physicians in training, we find that there are apparently thousands of fatal yet preventable fatigue-related medical errors made by residents each year, and thousands of fatigue-related motor vehicle crashes. Neither this series of studies nor congruent research by other investigators,[73] however, has led to evidence-based reductions in most residents' work hours, even as considerable resources have been poured into addressing other safety hazards. ACGME has continued to endorse twenty-eight-hour shifts and eighty-hour workweeks for second-year (PGY2) and higher residents—who represent about 80 percent of all residents nationwide—despite more substantive steps to limit consecutive work hours for first-year residents (to a sixteen-hour maximum) as of July 2011.

Reduction of work hours has proven difficult for many reasons. First, while recognition of the risks of extreme work hours has increased, it is not universal.[74] Many physicians remain deeply committed to traditional on-call schedules despite data about their risks, and others believe that implementation of the ACGME duty hour standards has effectively addressed the problem, despite data to the contrary. Concern about discontinuity of care,[75] particularly in hospitals where supervision and sign-out systems have been inadequate,[76] has slowed reduction of work hours. Concerns also exist about how to reschedule residents effectively, how to train and hire more providers, and what effects these new personnel might have on the physician workforce. In the United Kingdom, active efforts have been under way for years to train more physicians and bolster the resident workforce through the opening of new medical schools, among other initiatives. In the United States, no parallel efforts have occurred. Inadequate resources have been invested in hiring needed personnel and establishing safe systems to allow for shorter hours. In addition, medical educators have expressed concern about how reduced residency hours might affect education, although conversely, data have emerged demonstrating that sleep deprivation impairs consolidation of memory and learning as well as safety.[77]

In 2008 the Institute of Medicine (IOM) convened a panel to review the data on resident work hours systematically and make new recommendations.[78] On the basis of the data accumulated, the IOM concluded that working for more than sixteen hours without sleep is unsafe. The report recommended that residents work no longer than sixteen hours unless a fully protected period of five hours of continuous sleep is provided during a traditional extended shift. Alternatively, the IOM recommended that consecutive work hours could be limited to a sixteen-hour maximum. It suggested improvements in resident supervision and handoff procedures to facilitate these changes and further improve overall safety.

The ACGME chose to accept the IOM's recommendation to limit intern shifts to sixteen hours but, as mentioned earlier, continued to allow second-year and higher residents to work up to twenty-eight hours in a row. As new policies are developed, attention will have to be paid to the work hours of attending physicians as well. While data on senior physicians are largely lacking to date, and while senior physicians fall outside the jurisdiction of the ACGME, some preliminary data suggest that senior physicians, like residents, may be prone to err when sleep-deprived. In a ten-year retrospective study at Brigham and Women's Hospital, we found that surgeons who were working overnight and had less than a six-hour-long opportunity to sleep had nearly a threefold increase in complication rates compared with those who had more sleep opportunity.[79] Further studies of senior physicians will be needed, as will appropriate strategies to mitigate identified risks.

Ultimately, only with implementation of evidence-based work hour limits will significant reductions occur in physicians' fatigue-related errors and occupational injuries in health care. Initial efforts to implement solutions in individual centers are under way, but wider-scale implementation and testing of solutions will be needed to ensure that these efforts lead to substantive improvements in safety at a national level, and that improvement occurs continuously. Efforts will also be needed to ensure that any limits implemented are enforced effectively, and testing of the relative effectiveness of alternative scheduling solutions will be required to identify which solutions are most effective.

Moving the Patient Safety Movement

While the recommendation of the Institute of Medicine to eliminate shifts in excess of sixteen hours without sleep may seem extreme to many physicians accustomed to traditional residency schedules, the need for such a change has been apparent to patients for years. In a 2002 National Sleep Foundation poll, 70 percent of respondents believed that physicians' work should be limited to no more than ten consecutive hours; 86 percent reported that they would be very anxious if they learned their surgeon had been awake for twenty-four hours, and 70 percent reported that they would ask for a different surgeon if they learned their surgeon had been awake for twenty-four hours.[80] In a national survey of the U.S. public in which respondents were asked to identify important causes of medical errors, "overwork, stress, or fatigue on the part of health professionals" was the highest ranked of nine possible causes, with 74 percent of respondents believing it to be a very important cause;[81] in a second survey it ranked second of eleven possible causes at 70 percent.[82] In both surveys, 66 percent of the public believed that "reducing the work hours of doctors in training to avoid fatigue" would be "very effective" in reducing preventable medical errors; by contrast, only 33 percent of physicians thought that reducing resident work hours would be very effective.[83]

From this contrast, and in light of the objective data that have emerged on the hazards of sleep deprivation, it appears that the public may well have insights into the risks of sleep deprivation that health care providers themselves cannot see. It is not clear if physicians' lack of recognition of this problem stems from professional enculturation—acceptance of a cultural norm that values self-sacrifice for the benefit of the patient, taken to an unhealthy extreme whereby this self-sacrifice ends up harming the provider and patient alike—or is the product of sleep deprivation itself, which may impair the ability to perceive impairment.[84] Regardless, it is likely that physicians' indifference to sleep deprivation has bled over into the patient safety movement itself, which has not prioritized this issue to the degree that the public's concerns or the data would suggest is necessary.

Altogether, a wealth of data unequivocally demonstrates that sleep deprivation impairs physicians' performance. The extreme work hours of physicians in training (and most likely senior physicians as well) put them and their patients at risk. While implementation studies are needed to measure the relative effectiveness of diverse approaches to solving this problem, there is no longer any credible scientific doubt that the problem exists. Nevertheless, the patient safety movement has been hesitant to address physician sleep deprivation systematically, and meaningful policy change has been extraordinarily slow. In the interim, patients continue to be exposed to a very significant, avoidable risk. To solve the problem, policymakers and physicians must begin listening to both the data and patients, who appear to be far more attuned to this issue than are physicians themselves. There is an urgent need to begin translating the existing science on physician sleep deprivation and safety into daily practice if we wish to see the promise of the patient safety movement come to fruition.

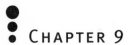

CHAPTER 9

Sleep-deprived Nurses

Sleep and Schedule Challenges in Nursing

Alison M. Trinkoff and Jeanne Geiger-Brown

U.S. hospitals and patients are increasingly relying on nurses who are working rotating shifts that, in many cases, involve longer and longer hours. Current work patterns can and do adversely affect sleep. In turn, inadequate sleep increases the risk that nurses may make more errors and sustain more injuries. When nurses do not sleep enough for several days each week over the course of several years, they also increase their risks for obesity or diabetes and cardiovascular diseases along with other health problems. Sleep deprivation also negatively affects their interpersonal interactions with patients and colleagues, as well as with family and friends.[1]

Despite studies demonstrating that nurses suffer from poor sleep, health care administrators have been slow to adjust schedules, improve working conditions, or increase staffing levels so as to reduce nurses' work-related sleep disturbances or promote their alertness. This is a missing element in the robust debate about patient safety, which focuses on improving processes of care (for example, handoffs, rapid response systems, teamwork training) and the use of technology to prevent errors (barcoding, electronic reminders). Nurses are critical to the implementation of many of these important initiatives, and these initiatives will not succeed if nurses are exhausted when on the job.

Given its importance to patient safety, why has nurses' sleep not been framed as a component of the patient safety agenda? One reason is that sleep occurs away from the workplace and is often considered a private matter. Sleep problems may be unacknowledged because fatigue can go undetected by others until nurses (or other professionals) become severely impaired. In addition, hospital administrators and other employers worry that their costs would increase if nurse workloads and shifts were adjusted to provide adequate opportunity for sleep and a reasonable amount of time away from work. It is therefore not surprising that hospitals and other employers have not put sleep deprivation "on the radar" as the modifiable risk factor it actually is.

Evidence of Nurses' Sleep Problems

Sleep deprivation for interns and residents, as Dr. Christopher Landrigan points out in chapter 8, has received some limited attention, and as a result of public outcry, there has been some reduction in their work hours. Nurses' sleep needs have not, however, been addressed. This lack of attention persists despite several studies documenting unhealthy sleep patterns for nurses. The first major descriptive study of nurses' sleep was published in 1992. K. A. Lee studied 760 nurses working a variety of shift patterns in use at the time and found that a high proportion of nurses experienced poor sleep quality and inadequate sleep.[2] These sleep disturbances varied according to the shift patterns the nurses were obliged to work, with 43 percent of night nurses, 28 percent of rotating-shift nurses, and 30 percent of day shift nurses complaining of inadequate sleep. Ten years later Ulla Edéll-Gustaffson and colleagues studied a group of Swedish nurses and found that about 40 percent of them reported insufficient sleep.[3] In this study, the link between somatic illnesses—gastrointestinal symptoms, palpitations, muscular and joint pain—unpleasant mood, and inadequate sleep was also strong. A 2003 study by J. S. Ruggiero of U.S. critical care nurses found that 68 percent met the criteria for "poor sleeper"; she detected a strong correlation between poor sleep and increased fatigue, depression, and anxiety.[4]

Poor sleep was also evident in a population-based survey of more than 2,200 nurses, in which Jeanne Geiger-Brown, Alison Trinkoff, and V. E. Rogers found that 29 percent reported restless sleep and 44 percent reported inadequate sleep on three or more days in the past week. The same study found that those who worked mandatory overtime or were on call more than once a month had increased odds of getting inadequate sleep (Odds Ratio = 1.4, 95 percent CI: 1.0–1.9).[5] The evidence that nurses have occupationally based impaired sleep is compelling.

Nurses face two major challenges related to sleep: getting sufficient sleep because of long work hours that reduce their sleep opportunity; and getting adequate-quality sleep due to circadian rhythm disruption from working during the night.

Long Work Hours

Since the 1980s, fewer nurses have been working the traditional eight-hour shift. Twelve-hour shifts are now common in hospital nursing, and these shifts have also spread to other nursing settings such as nursing homes. Unfortunately, a twelve-hour duty rotation often runs thirteen hours or longer, because additional job demands (for example, giving intershift reports, completing unfinished patient care and paperwork) can increase the duration of the workday.[6] Broken down by subgroups of nurses, the proportion of nurses working thirteen-plus hours was even more of a concern. Sixteen percent of the nurses who were single parents, 23 percent of hospital nurses, and 16 percent of nurses reported holding two jobs.[7] In addition to long work shifts, these patterns are often compressed (with several twelve-hour workdays followed by several days off), making it difficult for nurses to establish a consistent sleep schedule and obtain adequate sleep.

There are other ways that schedules create extended hours for nurses. Hospitals may ask—or require—that nurses work overtime to cover for absent nurses or on shifts that need additional staff. Some positions require nurses to be "on call" when they are at home. They must keep their phones on and may have to return to work if needed. In the study by Trinkoff and colleagues, 39 percent of staff nurses had call requirements. Of those nurses, 33 percent were called in monthly, 11 percent weekly, and 7 percent more than once a week.[8]

Because nurses' wages were stagnating in the mid-1990s, many nurses also began working voluntary overtime to make additional money. The shortage of nurses and the accompanying staffing policies provided many opportunities for nurses to work extra hours when they wished. Currently there is no way to control moonlighting (working additional jobs), as there is no regulation that limits the number of hours a nurse may work. A 2004 study found that nearly 14 percent of nurses working a full-time job in nursing also worked a second nursing job, further limiting the number of hours available for sleep.[9]

Long hours Decrease Sleep Opportunity

Working extended hours, such as twelve-hour shifts and beyond, clearly reduces sleep opportunity. If nurses work in excess of twelve hours, they have less time to do chores or attend to family duties and to socialize outside of work. Even when they are tired, they may forgo sleep to maintain a social life away from the workplace. When work and commuting hours are added to the time needed to fulfill home and family responsibilities, little time is left for sleep. In a diary study of nurses working twelve-hour shifts, Geiger-Brown and colleagues found that 58 percent had fewer than ten hours at home between shifts, and 13 percent had fewer than nine hours at home. In this study, nurses averaged only 5.5 hours of sleep between shifts.[10]

Shift work reduces Sleep Quality and Quantity

In addition to a lack of sleep opportunity because of inadequate time at home, sleep quality may be affected by the nature of nursing work during the shift. We know that nurses' work is very physically and emotionally demanding, and that nurses take very few breaks during their work shift.[11] Highly demanding work can reduce sleep by making it difficult to unwind after too many hours in a stressful work environment.[12] Earlier research found that as physical demands on the job increased for nurses, the likelihood of inadequate sleep also significantly increased.[13]

Because of the circadian rhythm that creates pressure to sleep at night, nurses who work the night shift face additional challenges to getting sufficient sleep between twelve-hour shifts. At 7:30 AM, the time when most night nurses are leaving for home, the circadian pressure on the body to wake begins to increase. Despite their being fatigued and sleepy, and readily able to fall asleep after getting home, these nurses' sleep will be short, because circadian pressures for wakefulness will increase further by the afternoon. For example, a nurse who completes her shift at 7:45 AM may make the forty-five-minute drive home, shower, have a snack, and go to bed at 9 AM. By about 2 PM, however, the body's circadian pressure to be awake is quite strong. The nurse will thus wake up spontaneously after only five hours in bed. So even though he or she desires more sleep, the nurse will be unable to get back to sleep. This pattern is hormonally driven and is due to the combination of the circadian drive to alertness with the waning of the body's drive to sleep. Because of these hormonal drives, nurses who work night shifts often get far less sleep than those working equivalent shift lengths during daylight hours.[14]

Although some nurses can acclimate somewhat to working at night, others have strong physiological preferences for "morningness" (that is, they are "larks"). To make matters worse, some nurses with morningness tendencies are forced to rotate to the night shift, even though they are physiologically unable to sleep during the daytime. In the previously mentioned study by

Geiger-Brown, Trinkoff, and Rogers, such nurses had more than twice the odds of inadequate sleep as nurses without the "lark" tendency who worked the night shift.[15] Because this preference for morningness or eveningness is genetically determined, no amount of acclimatization can reverse this inability to sleep during the day. Yet work on the night shift is unavoidable for many nurses in settings that have a need for 24/7 nursing care. Not surprisingly, shift work sleep disorder is common among rotating shift workers.

Sleep Deprivation increases Risk of Unintentional Injury

The kind of sleep deprivation nurses experience not only is unpleasant but also has been shown to cause injury. Some of the most serious sleep-related injuries involve motor vehicle crashes. While the precise number of crashes that are attributable to sleep deprivation will never be known, current estimates suggest that sleep deprivation results in 100,000 crashes per year, with 40,000 injuries and 1,550 fatalities.[16] L. D. Scott's diary study of nurses' drowsy driving over a four-week period showed that 67 percent had at least one such episode, and a small proportion (30 of 895, fewer than 1 percent) experienced drowsy driving after every shift.[17]

In a series of focus groups conducted by Geiger-Brown and colleagues, nurses identified drowsy driving as one of the major drawbacks to working the night shift. "I've had three accidents this year already," one nurse reported. Another said: "I barely make it home by keeping a full bladder and talking to my husband on the cell phone. Sometimes I fall asleep as soon as I pull into the driveway and my husband has to tap on the window to wake me up to come into the house and go to bed."[18] Unfortunately, the strategies that these nurses use to mitigate sleepiness (playing the radio, talking on cell phones, eating) are distractions that increase the risk of a crash over and above that caused by their drowsiness.

The risk of needle-stick injury also increases with extended work hours. In Trinkoff and colleagues' longitudinal study of registered nurses, the risk of needle-stick injury significantly increased when shifts were 12.5 hours or longer compared with eight hours. Nurses who rotated shifts also had more needle-stick injuries than those who worked days only.[19]

Sleep Deprivation Increases Risk of Disease

Nurses are at risk for injury not just on the job or after work. Sleep researchers are also beginning to uncover some root physiological causes for the increased burden of chronic diseases among those experiencing sleep deprivation. When sleep is lost, the body, under increased sympathetic burden, produces neurohormones such as cortisol, and this causes endothelial dysfunction, which in turn produces pro-inflammatory cytokines.[20] These physiologic changes have been linked to increased risk of chronic disorders such as cardiovascular disease (hypertension, stroke, heart disease) and metabolic diseases such as diabetes and obesity. Unhealthy work schedules (working off-shifts or long hours) can also contribute to disease susceptibility by reducing the opportunity or motivation to engage in health-promoting behaviors such as exercise and healthy eating, or by promoting the use of stimulants such as nicotine and caffeine in order to remain alert.

Neurocognitive Consequences of Sleep Deprivation

Nursing is cognitively complex and requires moment-to-moment decision making in a work environment fraught with noise, interruptions, and competing demands. Alertness is the most basic condition for neural functioning; all higher-level cognitive functions presume adequate alertness. Yet inadequate sleep generates predictable changes in neurocognition that decrease alertness. Acute or chronic sleep loss is associated with many deficits in neurobehavioral functioning, such as reduced vigilance, reaction time, memory, psychomotor coordination, information processing, and decision-making ability.[21]

The functional problems that come from sleep deprivation are cumulative, so that a nurse working several long shifts with little sleep will experience a linear decrease in vigilance. This occurs despite the fact that nurses may not subjectively feel any sleepier on the second or third day than on the first day. H. P. A. Van Dongen and colleagues conducted a carefully controlled laboratory study of the effects of chronic partial sleep restriction (four or six hours of sleep allowed per night over fourteen days) on neurocognitive functions and sleepiness.[22] The researchers found that after an increase in sleepiness during the first day of sleep restriction, subjects' *perceptions* of sleepiness changed little, despite clear decreases in neurocognitive performance. They also found that as the hours and days of sleep deprivation increased, behavioral alertness and executive functioning abilities decreased.

Not surprisingly, sleep-deprived nurses, as well as others who are sleep-deprived, are generally unable to accurately judge their own level of impairment. Furthermore, getting one really good night's sleep after a stretch of sleep-deprived days does not sufficiently restore neurocognitive functioning to baseline levels.[23] As a result, individuals who are chronically sleep-deprived will continue to show unstable performance on tasks. For example, when intense concentration is required, the task may start off well, but as time goes on, errors can creep in. The longer the task takes, the more likely it is that a nurse will make an error of omission or commission. Yet because this does not happen to the nurse 100 percent of the time, the nurse may be falsely reassured that he or she is able to work safely in a sleep-deprived state. When tasks take place under time pressure, a nurse who is slower in processing information is more likely to make errors. Nurses who are fatigued may also have to slow down to preserve the accuracy of their work.

Microsleep and Poor Sleep Affect Flexibility and Coping

Adding to all these problems is the condition known as microsleep. The brain is organized into neural columns that communicate information from the senses to the central nervous system, through a stimulus gate, and to the higher cortical regions. These neural columns can activate or deactivate, going "on" or "off." They will spontaneously shut down after a period of sustained activity. But the brain doesn't shut them down like a switch that turns off all visible signs of activity. Therefore, when a nurse is sleep-deprived, he or she might look wide awake, but portions of these neural columns are shut down and no longer processing information. This is known as microsleep, and it occurs in episodes lasting from five hundred milliseconds up to three to five seconds.[24] The nurse may not recognize any impairment while microsleep is occurring but can nonetheless make errors during microsleep episodes. The level of functional impairment that occurs during sleep deprivation is similar to that for alcohol intoxication: after about nineteen to twenty-one hours of sustained wakefulness, some individuals will be functionally "drunk," that is, with a level of psychomotor functioning equivalent to that produced by a blood alcohol level of 0.08 percent.[25] When determining whether a person is driving while drunk, most U.S. states use this level as a legal standard.

Poor sleep can also compromise situational awareness. Nurses who experience inadequate sleep may misperceive some monitoring activities or fail to recognize subtle signs of patient deterioration. Poor sleep also leads to the loss of cognitive flexibility—the ability to shift between tasks that have different cognitive demands. Long work hours also affect verbal learning and visual memory as well as alertness and concentration.[26] Ellen O'Shea found that nurses ranked distraction and being tired or exhausted in the top three perceived causes of medication errors.[27]

Poor sleep also affects nurses' ability to cope with the interruptions that are one of the constant components of their job. Nurses are continually interrupted, for example, by physicians, patient call bells, other staff members, and requests from patients' family members, among many other things. When the interruptions occur, nurses must be able to remember interventions that need to be completed and find the time to go back and complete them—all of which affects the ability to deliver safe care.[28]

While the lay public is generally unaware of the extent of nurses' cognitive work, they do highly value the nurse's empathic presence, which also can deteriorate with sleep deprivation. Loss of sleep is associated with irritability, anxiety, and depression, as well as impaired interpersonal communication. What this may translate into is a lack of empathy in dealing with patients or other colleagues.

How the Nursing Profession Has Responded

Failure of Nursing Education to Address the Problem of Sleep Deprivation

Nurses are taught that along with caring and empathy, they have a professional mandate to advocate for their patients. Yet in most nursing schools there is little emphasis on the way sleep affects nurses' ability to do so, just as there is little emphasis on other aspects of sleep in the curriculum. Rather than connecting nurses' sleep to their ability to care about and advocate for patients, many nursing schools almost seem to emphasize the opposite. Nurses who work long hours may be perceived as more dedicated than those who do not. In addition, as nursing shifts have increased from eight hours to twelve, the duration of many students' clinical rotations has similarly increased so that students can "get used to it." Although nursing schools highlight the importance of critical thinking, there has been little discussion about the wisdom of switching many nursing positions to shifts of twelve or more hours a day from eight hours. In the United States, for example, it is little known that European nurses typically work thirty-seven-hour weeks and are often prohibited from working twelve-hour shifts.

Setting Work-Hour Limits

Although the health care industry has not regulated nurses' work hours and relies on the professionalism of the nurse to come to work well rested, it has begun to recognize this problem in regard to physicians. In 2003 the Accreditation Council for Graduate Medical Education (ACGME) began limiting resident physicians to eighty hours per week in order to promote improved rest and performance.[29] Preliminary data thus far indicate that the workloads of health providers who don't have work hour limits (such as nurses and attending physicians) may have increased to compensate for residents' work hour limits.

If work hour limits are important for physicians, they should be just as important for nurses, whose knowledge, judgment, and actions are necessary for ensuring patient safety and quality of care. The Institute of Medicine (IOM) in 2004 recommended that nursing hours be limited to no more than twelve in a twenty-four-hour period and no more than sixty hours in seven days. Yet, these limits are regularly exceeded.[30] Moreover, research indicates that these work hour limits may not be stringent enough to prevent patient care errors or episodes of drowsy driving and other adverse consequences.[31] Because people are unable to evaluate accurately their ability to work when sleep-deprived, mandatory work hour limits for nurses should be considered. While most nurses dislike and lobby for bans on *mandatory* overtime, many feel there is no problem if a nurse *volunteers* to work for sixteen or even twenty-four hours at a time. Physiological imperatives, however, do not change because overtime hours are voluntary rather than mandatory. In addition, for the purposes of restricting nurses' hours, it is not useful to draw a distinction between voluntary and mandatory overtime. Real restrictions on nurses' hours are needed. Unfortunately, some unions have not put a great deal of support behind such measures, and sometimes even oppose them, because some nurses like to work longer hours provided they are voluntary. Nevertheless, the body's physiologic requirements for sleep must be respected in order to maintain health, vigilance, optimal practice, and safety for patients.

Promoting Healthy Schedules

Several approaches to improving sleep in workers have been found to be highly successful. In a worksite intervention to prevent "occupational jet lag" for shift workers, sleep improved significantly in the treatment group when sleep hygiene education was provided in combination with exercise.[32] In another study, shift work education was given to all workers in U.S. Saturn auto manufacturing plants. Although outcomes were proprietary, the company expanded the program, finding that it was also cost-effective.[33] Although nurses who start new positions may receive an extensive orientation to the job, this generally does not include information on coping with schedules or different work shifts, or on how to obtain sufficient levels of quality sleep. At this writing, researchers at the National Institute for Occupational Safety and Health (NIOSH) have designed an evidence-based sleep hygiene training program for health care workers, focusing on nurses, that will be accessible on-line at no cost.

In addition to modifying schedules, napping is an important option that some facilities are exploring, although many workplaces still will not allow nurses to take naps while on the job, even during breaks. Despite this, if workdays are extended, the opportunity to nap can improve alertness levels and reduce sleepiness. Emergency room nurses who took a forty-minute nap in the middle of a twelve-hour shift also showed improved performance for at least three hours following the nap.[34] In a qualitative study of nurses' napping during the night shift, Diana McMillan found that nurses subjectively experienced increased alertness after brief naps, and they took extra care to ensure that patients were well supervised by competent staff prior to napping.[35]

Unfortunately, the culture of most nursing workplaces currently prohibits or is strongly opposed to napping. One advocate of workplace napping suggests that evidence-based information about the benefits will be applied only when employers' attitudes change from viewing a nap as "sleeping on the job" to "napping at the break."[36] Although naps for night shift nurses are a standard practice in Japan,[37] formal napping programs are uncommon for nurses in U.S. hospitals, but we believe it could be of great benefit.

Nursing Organizations' Responses to Sleep Deprivation and Fatigue

The American Nurses Association (ANA) issued two position statements on schedules and fatigue in 2006, one that designates the employer's role and another that addresses the nurse's responsibility to avoid working when fatigued.[38] The employer is "encouraged" to "establish policies and procedures that promote healthy nursing work hours" that maintain the safety of both nurses and patients. This requires establishing work schedules that provide an opportunity for "adequate rest and recuperation," "sufficient compensation" (to reduce the motivation to take on extra jobs or work hours), and safe staffing levels.[39] This policy recognizes that the health care system needs to promote optimal choices for nurses. The employee position statement says that "regardless of the hours worked," nurses have the responsibility "to carefully consider their level of fatigue" before accepting any work hours over and above the regularly scheduled workdays. Furthermore, a nurse has the "right and obligation to refuse an assignment if impaired by fatigue."[40]

Although these statements are a step in the right direction, the ANA doesn't acknowledge the leverage an employer has over an employee when it comes to scheduling. By focusing only on work hours assigned in excess of the designated schedule, the organization avoids having to acknowledge that even regularly scheduled assignments of twelve hours can lead to impairment due to fatigue.

This position paper also doesn't address the fact that employers and employees view sleep as private behavior; nor does it recognize the link between current nursing schedules and lack of sleep opportunity. By asking nurses to judge their ability to sleep when they are getting inadequate sleep in the first place, it ignores research that documents how difficult it is for people to accurately assess their own levels of sleepiness.

Although some nursing organizations—such as the American Society of Peri-Anesthesia Nurses (ASPAN)—have tried to develop guidelines to assess fatigue or to identify when practice may become unsafe, there are currently no reliable, objective tools that can measure whether someone has had enough sleep to work safely. Without such measures, the prudent approach is to assume that nurses' long schedules mean that they are often sleep-deprived and in need of more rest. Managers, supervisors, and peers should be alert for subtle signs of sleep deprivation (yawning, low motivation, irritability, or changing moods) and ask the nurse about these observations with regard to their sleep. Nurses who are excessively sleepy need to be given an opportunity to obtain the necessary sleep.

Since nurses are often required to work more than their scheduled hours, many nursing organizations and unions have fought for limitations on mandatory overtime as a safety remedy. Most laws limit such hours to sixteen per month, and some include provisions that allow nurses to express choices as to when the hours take place. Nevertheless, although such laws are an important restriction on unlimited overtime requirements, they can still lead to problematic work schedules. For example, overtime laws can be circumvented through other scheduling practices, such as on-call requirements.

Another opportunity for scheduling flexibility may be found in hiring older, experienced nurses or those with other time demands such as child and family responsibilities, who may be unwilling or unable to work twelve hours at a stretch, for shorter workdays. In addition, there also may be nurses with disabilities who physically cannot withstand extended-hour positions but could return to work if the day length was diminished. To reengage them in nursing might require new scheduling paradigms (such as four-hour days or work schedules coinciding with elementary school hours). The flexibility that has been a hallmark of nursing positions can be leveraged to improve care by promoting schedule choices for nurses that fit their home and lifestyle demands while maintaining their health and ability to continue working as nurses. For the safety of both patients and workers, hospitals and other health care organizations need to reconsider current scheduling practices.

As hospitals and policymakers consider sleep deprivation issues, it will be helpful to listen to the voices of nurses themselves. In Alison Trinkoff's Nursing Worklife and Health Study surveys, one nurse commented: "We are working longer and harder than a human being should be subjected to. You will have no nurses left if this continues."[41] Mary Foley, past president of the American Nurses Association, noted in 2001 that the major reason for the growing shortage of nurses was working conditions, especially the "epidemic use of overtime."[42] Nursing shortages have also created an ongoing vicious cycle, as the turnover of nurses leads to staffing shortages, which employers may try to address by further increasing work hours.[43] Although the economic crisis that began in 2008 has led some nurses to work in nursing longer than they intended, once the economy improves and these nurses retire, scheduling practices could again exacerbate ongoing nursing shortages. To promote patient safety, it is important to pay attention to the growing body of empirical information that supports the need to improve nursing work schedules. If we are to maintain an adequate supply of nurses for current health care needs as well as for the future, we must promote and ensure adequate sleep for nurses.

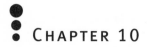

CHAPTER 10

Wounds That Don't Heal

Nurses' Experience with Medication Errors

Linda A. Treiber and Jackie H. Jones

Medical errors have been the topic of much research, much publication, and much public concern.[1] Because nurses administer the vast majority of medications, they inevitably make the majority of these administration mistakes. Yet there is little understanding of the complex occupational and personal trauma suffered by the practitioner who makes an error if that person is a nurse.

We know from studies of physicians that new doctors are supposed to "forgive and remember" their mistakes, provided they learn how to avoid them in the future.[2] But unlike physicians, who have formalized this practice, nurses have no such process. Nurses tend to suffer in silence after such events. Up until the recent focus on systems as causes of errors, nurses were blamed, disciplined, deemed incompetent by peers and supervisors, and sometimes discharged after making a medication administration error. Even now, there is little support for nurses who make such errors. Institutions continue to write nurses up. Like all health care workers who make clinical errors, nurses are at risk of becoming "second victims" in that they can experience emotional trauma long after the event.[3] They may feel personally responsible for the error and believe that they have failed in their duty to the patient.[4]

What happens to a nurse's professional identity when she or he makes a medication error? How does the nurse respond to the occupational and personal trauma induced by the error? As both registered nurses and academics, we (the authors) sought to find answers to this and other questions surrounding the problem of medication errors. Throughout our own careers, we have made mistakes, prevented mistakes from happening, and identified those of others. As onetime staff nurses, managers, and educators, we have stood in the shoes of those we study. Because of this, we decided to ask nurses to describe errors in an anonymous way in hopes of making sense of these events. We also asked them to describe how they felt about their mistakes. Not surprisingly, we found that nurses who make medication errors suffer emotional wounds. These are wounds that do not heal. Their internalized feelings of self-blame tended to last throughout their careers. But we also found that nurses learned a great deal from their mistakes.

Our study was based on 158 written accounts of errors from a random sample of registered nurses. We asked them to describe their medication errors in largely open-ended terms with questions like these: Have you ever made a medication error? What happened? Why did it happen? How did you feel? These simple questions led us to a deeper examination of how nurses made sense of errors and still continued their professional careers. They offered many examples of self-identified errors and the ways in which others exposed their mistakes. Most important, we discovered how deeply their fears were felt.

Nurses often revealed individualized responses and solutions. In other words, they tended to see their errors as individual mistakes rather than the fault of the system. This is not to say that they shouldered 100 percent of the blame. They did not. Their error accounts often indicated that the actions of pharmacists and other nurses, as well as technologies, workloads, distractions, time pressures, and their own inexperience, contributed to making the error. Even so, many attempted to make sense of their mistakes and to soldier on, but with a memory of feeling devastated that remained long after the event. We also found that nurses sought to learn from their mistakes and, as a result, developed personal rules for avoiding errors.

Background of the Medication Error Problem

Despite intense scrutiny, we don't really know the scope of the problem. Differing definitions and reporting methods are only a few of the factors that make measuring medication errors problematic.[5] It is therefore no surprise that attempts to assign blame are everywhere. But what constitutes an error? And just who is at fault? For example, if the automated medication dispensing machine gives the wrong drug, the nurse is supposed to notice it. But if she or he actually gives the medication, is it solely the nurse's fault?

What about the context? Can nurses be held accountable if the number of patients simply makes it impossible to provide adequate care for them all? Or if the medication administration record contains errors or is incomprehensible?

One of the most challenging issues in accurate assessment is that we rely on a system of voluntary reporting. Most errors are usually small and produce little harm. Only the more serious, that is, harm-causing, errors are consistently reported, because they are too large to ignore.[6] This not only makes quantification difficult but also undermines our ability to address the underlying causes of errors. While there is much publicity about medication errors, the role that nurses play in stopping them is often obscured. Although nurses make many of these errors, the International Council of Nurses has estimated that nurses are also responsible for preventing approximately 86 percent of errors made by physicians, pharmacists, and others by intervening before they can occur.[7]

Although a great deal of proscriptive literature has come out of organizations such as the Joint Commission and the Institute of Medicine, the recommendations may seem unrealistic, given the realities of frontline nursing. Too often the voice and involvement of frontline nurses in formal quality-improvement processes is minimal.[8] As a result, their wisdom, intimate knowledge of practice environments, and clinical expertise have largely been overlooked.

Although following the "five rights" of medication administration (right patient, right medication, right time, right route, and right dose) sounds quite simple, in reality the administration of medications is far more complex than is commonly realized. In addition to knowing about the medication itself (what it is, what it does, why the patient is getting it, correct dosages, the contraindications to receiving it, and potential side effects), the nurse must also know how to administer medications in multiple ways: by mouth, intravenously (IV), into a muscle, topically, or subcutaneously (that is, under the patient's skin). Thus, to administer a medication intravenously, the nurse must know whether it is to be given by IV push (the medication solution is pushed directly into the patient's circulatory system, typically over one to five minutes), IV piggyback (a small bag of medication solution is infused typically over thirty to sixty minutes), or by continuous infusion. If medication is to be given by IV push, the nurse must know if it needs to be diluted, with what to dilute it, how much diluent to use, and how fast it can be pushed. If by piggyback, she or he must know over what period of time it can be infused and how to operate the infusion pump. Many medications entail specific nursing considerations that must be known prior to administration. For example, the nurse must check the coagulation lab values before giving heparin.

Thus, medication administration is a complicated process requiring considerable nursing skill. Institutional policies and procedures can make these complex tasks more difficult. For example, almost all institutions have standardized medication administration schedules. Generally, the majority of the daily medications are administered at 9 AM. While attempting to administer all of these at the appropriate time, a nurse usually encounters numerous distractions and interruptions. Most hospital nurses carry an institutionally provided cell phone or pager. During administration, the nurse might therefore be called by doctors, laboratory personnel, medical reception, or any of the patients (or their families) for whom she or he is caring. This opens the door to error.

Nurses also deal with a number of varied technologies designed to reduce medication errors. Unfortunately, these technologies can also fail to function properly, leading to unintended negative consequences. Whereas in the past, nurses were able to access medications simply by opening a locked drawer in the patient's room, today's automated dispensing cabinets (ADCs) feature a time-consuming sign-on system. Most nursing units have more than one ADC located in different places on the hospital unit. In the event of unanticipated use, inadequate stocking, or drawers that won't open, it is not uncommon for a nurse to have to go to two, three, or more machines to retrieve the medications for a single patient. To add to the problem, nurses are expected to retrieve medications for each patient, administer those medications, then return and retrieve another patient's medications. This frequently requires waiting in line. Barcoded medication administration (BCMA) systems are also sometimes flawed. Research has found that problems with BCMA include malfunctioning scanners, unreadable barcodes, lost connectivity, failing batteries, unreadable patient wristbands, and non-barcoded medications.[9]

Nurses are frustrated when technologies take time away from patients.[10] Also, the time required to utilize technologies properly can make an inherently risky enterprise increasingly fraught with opportunities for error. Research estimates that 40 percent of a nurse's day is unavailable to patients because of increased expectations related to things such as documentation, new procedures, and new technologies.[11] As a result, nurses are forced to create workarounds to meet the needs of their patients.[12] Given these complex situational contexts, it is surprising that more errors are not made. What happens when nurses do make medication administration errors? We wanted to know more about how nurses handle these events.

The Research Study

Our study was based on a subset of responses to open-ended survey questions mailed to a random sample of registered nurses in our state. Nurses were asked, "Have you ever made a medication administration error?" We analyzed the responses of those nurses who replied yes to this question and/or described making an error. The surveys were anonymous, unless the nurse voluntarily chose to provide additional information. Those who responded were given the option of completing the survey on paper or on-line at a secure site.

To analyze the error accounts, we systematically identified key themes within each. We confirmed these themes with each other and cross-checked data for emerging patterns. The resultant categories were often interrelated and sometimes overlapped. Although the medication errors were voluntarily disclosed, we still wondered how candid nurses could be when their personal and professional liability was on the line. In light of our own experiences, their stories rang true. We believe that the accounts accurately illustrated both severe and non-severe errors.

The nurses in our study were demographically comparable to the national nursing population. Of the 158 respondents, 87 percent were female. In terms of race and ethnicity, 84 percent were white; 9 percent were black or African American; 2 percent Mexican American, Puerto Rican, or other Hispanic; and 2 percent Asian. The remaining respondents were Native American or indicated "other" race. The majority (65 percent) worked in hospitals. The remainder worked in a variety of other settings, including public health, long-term care, home health, education, or other venues. Only 7 percent indicated that they were no longer working in nursing. There was a considerable range in experience levels, from one year to over forty-eight years, with a mean of twenty-one years.

As we describe in this chapter, we identified several key patterns. First, there was a distinct "I'm to blame but . . ." theme, with the nurse admitting responsibility while faulting other health care providers, including other nurses, the pharmacy, or doctors. Many blamed their own inexperience or "being new," and a few had tried to cover up their mistakes. Another identified theme was that nurses were clearly frustrated with technologies and regulations. Not only did technologies and rules take time away from patient care, but also they were seen by some as increasing the opportunity for error. Third, we identified a theme of feeling devastated, characterized by gut-level responses to errors. Strong emotions were identified by nurses, including fear for their patients and themselves. These visceral responses were often seemingly unconnected to the severity of the error and the passage of time. Finally, we identified a "lessons learned" theme, with nurses supplying evidence that they had learned from their mistakes. Many described how they personally had found ways to avoid future errors. Here we develop these key themes.

Who or What Is at Fault?

The first major pattern we identified was the "I'm to blame . . . but" theme. In other words, nurses acknowledged that making a medication error was ultimately their fault but pointed to external causes as well. In addition to accepting self-blame, some described how working several night shifts in a row, being new, or having a high patient-to-nurse ratio was also culpable. Others noted multiple distractions, being floated to a new area, understaffing, and having to administer too many medications to too many acutely ill patients as reasons for errors. The fact that nurses tolerate these extremes in their attempt to care for their patients has been documented previously.[13] In fact, these scenarios play themselves out in nursing environments with numbing regularity. Nurses also frequently reported that no one was available to support them during times when support was badly needed or when they were completely overwhelmed. As one registered nurse, a woman with thirty-three years' experience, stated, they "just have to cope."

> *Researcher:* What factors contributed to the medication error? Why did it happen, in your opinion?
> *Participant:* High census with high acuity. No one to help, just have to cope. Called everyone to come help—they won't—tired. Don't blame them. Manager won't help. Call over her head—sure—but it takes time you don't have and who is going to come? Some desk jockey who doesn't know what to do.

Regardless of the factors that contributed to making an error, our nurses often considered themselves negligent and incompetent after the event. This is consistent with other studies.[14] The nurses believed that they should be able to do the job right regardless of the challenges presented by their environment. In failure, they often described themselves as "stupid" "ashamed," and "incompetent." But in doing so, they became the "second victims" of the mistake by internalizing guilt and blame.

Error stories were commonly framed in terms of the "five rights" mandate that guides medication administration. It seemed clear that the nurses had internalized these "rights" from the first semester of nursing school. Still, there was no consistent definition of when failure to follow the five rights was actually an error. Giving a medication late violated the "right time" rule—but how late is "too late," and thus a five rights violation? And was it still an error when a nurse obtained an order for the medication after the fact? This was not always clear.

In one account, a nurse with one year of experience mixed up the patients' names, violating the "right patient" rule. She identified multiple reasons why the error happened (for example, patient overload, being in a hurry, being a new graduate), but ultimately she blamed herself for not checking the armband:

> *Researcher:* Please describe the error. Reveal as much as you are comfortable with.
>
> *Participant:* I had 2 patients in the same room that were receiving the same IV antibiotic (same dosage as well) @ the same time, but I mixed up the names.
>
> *Researcher:* How did you feel when you made a medication error?
>
> *Participant:* Stupid that I did not check the name to the armband, but relieved that no harm was done.
>
> *Researcher:* What factors contributed to the medication error? Why did it happen, in your opinion?
>
> *Participant:* High patient load—overwhelmed and in a hurry—improper training for a new grad—admit that it was totally my fault for not checking the armbands though.

Even when other health care workers were also at fault, nurses blamed themselves. For example, this nurse, a woman with sixteen years' experience, blamed both the pharmacy and herself:

> *Participant:* The dosage dispensed by our pharmacy tech was incorrect (lower than prescribed and I did not check the label against the written order). The patient had already been discharged by the time the error was caught and therefore did not receive the fully prescribed dose.
>
> *Researcher:* How did you feel when you made a medication error?
>
> *Participant:* First & foremost, I felt horrible that the problem for which the med was prescribed might not be alleviated due to not enough med given. (I did later call the patient, to come in for more drug). Secondly, I felt really, really stupid and inadequate that I didn't take the time to check the order
>
> *Researcher:* What factors contributed to the medication error? Why did it happen, in your opinion?
>
> *Participant:* It was extremely busy, short staffed. I just grabbed the medicine (checked for the right patient name & drug, but not the dose).

Another nurse, with ten years' experience, described how she gave the wrong, similar-sounding IV medication, incorrectly released by the pharmacy. Afterwards, she feared that the patient could have an adverse reaction and was upset with herself for "not being thorough." When asked why it had happened, she pointed to the pharmacy's mistake but then accepted personal responsibility:

> *Researcher:* Please describe the error. Reveal as much as you are comfortable with.
>
> *Participant:* IV antibiotic bag had right label & name, to right patient . . . but the vial attached to bag wasn't the right antibiotic— instead of Ceftriaxone it was [the antibiotic] Cefizox.
>
> *Researcher:* How did you feel when you made a medication error?
>
> *Participant:* Fear that the patient may have adverse reaction. Upset at myself for not being thorough.
>
> *Researcher:* What factors contributed to the medication error? Why did it happen, in your opinion?
>
> *Participant:* The pharmacist releasing the medication didn't double-check and I didn't check the vial but just focused on the label.

When pharmacy departments make mistakes, nurses are supposed to catch them. We found this pattern at all levels of nursing skill, including a nurse with thirty years' experience who administers anesthesia:

> I am a CRNA [certified registered nurse anesthetist]and responsible for life-altering medications. I always check the medication and know the patient and the appropriate dose. Over 30 years, I have seen an increase in the pharmacy stocking errors—wrong medications. The last I remember occurred just a month ago, when I obtained my narcotic package and checked the drugs. What I usually have supplied is Midazolam [preoperative sedative] 1mg/ml/5ml bottles. What pharmacy supplied was 5mg/ml/5ml bottles. A potential for overdose. The pharmacy tech I spoke to on the phone said to "just return it" and she would "take care of it."

Covering Up

Relatively few nurses admitted to covering up medication errors, although several said that this was their first instinct. One wrote: "I was a new nurse and I was very upset. I wanted to cover it up because I was afraid to get fired, but I knew I had to tell." When nurses discovered their errors, fears for patients were paramount, followed closely by concerns for their professional security. We also unexpectedly found that physicians could be important allies for nurses who made errors by giving orders to cover mistakes after the fact. For example, a nurse with thirty-four years' experience wrote that she had given the pain medication Demerol to the wrong patient and then obtained a doctor's order for that drug retrospectively. She blamed the error on staffing and isolation: "[I was the] only RN on floor—gave Demerol to wrong pt. but MD gave me an order for it after I told him about it." Another nurse described covering over several errors:

> *Researcher:* Please describe the error. Reveal as much as you feel comfortable with.
> *Participant:* Gave a Benadryl [antihistamine] to a patient by mistake, I did not report it. Gave the wrong dose of insulin, and did report it. I gave a double dose of Solu-medrol [steroid], because another nurse gave the drug, and did not check it off on the order sheet. The doctor rewrote the order for the dose that I gave.
> *Researcher:* How did you feel when you made a medication error?
> *Participant:* I felt ill and questioned my ability as a nurse.

The fact that nurses reported these incidents when asked about medication errors indicates that they still considered them mistakes, even though they had received a doctor's order for the medication afterwards. It was not clear in these accounts whether or not the drugs prescribed after the fact were appropriate for the patients.

Rules, Technologies, and Time

Our research showed that nurses were ambivalent about technologies and the organizational rules that govern care delivery. One registered nurse, a woman with twenty-two years' experience, told us that efforts to decrease errors were counterproductive for nurses:

> Some of the Joint Commission [a hospital accrediting organization] directives are ridiculous! They treat nurses like incompetent idiots! It's insulting. If hospitals would discipline or fire incompetent nurses instead of imposing new rules and routines that make med passes slow and stressful we would all be better off.

Consistent with previous research,[15] others told us about glitches and problems created by computer technologies, particularly when there was not enough time to recheck medication orders. One RN, a woman with sixteen years' experience, recounted:

In the facility where I work, we reorder the next "cycle" of meds for each patient in the computer. Frequently, the computer will change the dosage from what's actually ordered (a glitch in the program?). If you don't recheck what the computer orders against the original order, errors are made.

Another nurse with ten years' experience feared the potential for errors in the place where she worked, owing to mistakes in the pharmacy-generated medication administration records:

I feel the hospital that I work at is currently very dangerous and at high risk for med errors. The pharmacy is very much the weak link and I am constantly finding mistakes and spend a lot of extra time checking my meds and MARS [Medication Administration Records] for errors. I feel that it is very unsafe and would not [come] myself or [let] my family [come] to this hospital.

A new graduate described a situation in which Internet access had been discontinued but not replaced with access to the necessary information found in a drug reference book:

I find it beneficial to have current drug book handy . . . no, you don't always have time to look at it, but it needs to be available. Also, the hospital I did work at took away internet privileges due to internet surfing, but I was not able to look up meds not found in the drug book.

Thus, technologies and rules seemingly designed to help nurses were not always effective in decreasing errors and detracted from their ability to function as professionals. Looking back on her error, a registered nurse with twenty-six years' experience doubted the value of technology without concomitant nursing diligence:

Researcher: Please add any additional comments or thoughts you have about why/how medication errors occur.
Participant: Barcode med administration would not have helped in my error. Barcode med administration is important but the nurse must always be diligent and stay focused.

Devastation

Along with the individualization of blame, we found that nurses felt devastated by their mistakes. Making a medication error seemed to result in an indelible mark, with ensuing emotions of guilt, fear, panic, and distress. We liken it to a wound that doesn't heal.

The raw emotion is evident in this account related by a nurse with over five years' experience who mistakenly gave the wrong dose of IV chemotherapy:

> *Researcher:* Please describe the error. Reveal as much as you feel comfortable with.
>
> *Participant:* Gave Vincristine IV [anti-cancer chemotherapy drug given intravenously] to a leukemia pediatric patient. There is no antidote. We had always received 1 mg vials . . . the 5 mg vials were mixed with 1 mg. . . . As I went to dispose of vial, I reread it and it was 5 mg. Physician immediately notified. Family was told. Child became very ill within 48–72 hours. Although it did not impact the length of time child lived, it made him acutely ill. I was devastated.

With a mistake of this magnitude it was not surprising that she would feel this way. It is the type of event that you would remember the rest of your life. Yet nurses expressed deep emotional devastation over errors that we considered relatively minor. For example, giving a vitamin to the wrong patient or giving one unit of insulin instead of two, while not serious, still made the nurses involved feel miserable. Statements such as "I felt sick . . . terrible, horrible, scared" after the error was realized were frequently expressed. A visceral, gut-wrenching reaction was noted for a variety of errors, not necessarily proportional to the severity of the error or harm to the patient. Nurses were aware that anything less than perfection has the potential to hurt the patient. It is not surprising, given the emphasis on "virtue scripts" (being good and kind) in nursing, that they would see this as a moral failing.[16]

Several participants indicated that they had considered leaving nursing after making an error. One was a nurse with thirty years' experience:

> *Researcher:* Please describe the error. Reveal as much as you are comfortable with.
>
> *Participant:* IV overdose in an emergency situation resulted in hypotension but no other harm.
>
> *Researcher:* How did you feel when you made a medication error?
>
> *Participant:* Horrible, scared, afraid, wanted to leave nursing, then I told myself I would not ever let it happen again.

Because we asked nurses to tell us about any error that happened at any time during their career, we sometimes received accounts of mistakes that happened years ago. Even over time, the visceral memory remained fresh.

Nurses who made errors thirty years before were as upset by them as nurses who had made recent errors. Time had done little to assuage the pain and guilt. This led us to question: Should the nurse who makes an error ever forget the pain? Remembering an error is important, but what about still feeling sick over it some twenty years later? Because the visceral memory remained, we now examine the positive and negative functions of such emotional memories.

Lessons Learned

How do nurses go on being nurses after an error event? To make sense of errors in their professional lives, nurses developed what we call "lessons learned." These often took the form of personal rules. Frequently that lesson was stated as simply, "I now know I need to follow the five rights," but other lessons were more elaborate. These rules were crucial to how the nurses were able to continue in the face of shame and guilt.

Thus, a nurse with twenty-six years' experience who made an error while a different patient was talking to her developed a "no talking" rule:

> I gave meds to the wrong patient because I was pouring the meds for another patient in a four-bed room and the wrong patient was talking to me—I just walked over to him and gave him the wrong meds. . . . We had to monitor his VS [vital signs] closely x 24 hr. I was familiar with these patients and didn't check armbands—it was an automatic thing to go to the patient I was talking to. I tell patients now and have for years not to talk to a nurse while she is giving meds.

Different errors often led to similar rules. Several nurses developed "slow down/triple-check" rules to deal with time pressure errors, including one male RN with several years' experience:

> *Researcher:* Please describe the error. Reveal as much as you are comfortable with.
>
> *Participant:* High patient to nurse ratio, started a drip diprivan [used in anesthesia] @ the NS [normal saline] rate and NS @ the diprivan rate. I double-checked rates prior to leaving the room and caught my error. No harm was done (In a big hurry, very busy).
>
> *Researcher:* How did you feel when you made a medication error?
>
> *Participant:* I could not believe I had made such a huge error. I learned to slow down no matter what the circumstances. I now triple-check when giving meds, but staffing is still a huge issue and I now feel

like patient satisfaction has to suffer because I have slowed down my pace which means longer wait times.

A more experienced (twenty-seven years) nurse offered similar advice:

There were two patients in a semi-private room and I gave each one the other's medication. It taught me a valuable lesson—it is now force of habit to double- and even triple-check the five rights of giving medication.

Even after years of working, once an error was made, many nurses were devastated. Another RN developed similar personal rules about double-checking:

Researcher: How did you feel when you made a medication error? Please let us know.

Participant: Like the end of the world. It was my first med error in twenty-five years' experience. It took a month to get over the depression and I still check and recheck everything after six months.

Researcher: What factors contributed to the medication error? Why did it happen, in your opinion?

Participant: A lot of loud noise & crying children. I drew up med and held hysterical child then gave without checking.

Rules were developed for actual errors as well as near-misses. A "near-miss" error was recounted by a nurse with sixteen years' experience who, distracted by his supervisor, subsequently developed a "no distractions" rule for avoiding future errors:

[I was] distracted by my supervisor while I was drawing up multiple medications at one time. I did not label them as I drew them, and thus had two syringes each with the same volume, and no way to know which was which. Meds were discarded and I learned to never be distracted, no matter who was seeking my attention. I also now label and draw up meds one at a time.

The "lessons learned" themes were most often listed when an error happened early in the nurse's career. Novices make mistakes. Being new was excused and understood, but only to a point. New graduates often felt that because they were not being properly mentored, they had to learn the hard way. One young woman, an RN with two years' experience, told us:

I think the experienced nurse was just expecting me to do all the charting to gain experience in doing that, but I had no way of realizing she'd already given the drug because she hadn't said so. I made it a personal priority to only chart what I'd done, what I'd seen, etc. from that point on. Even if I was covering for another nurse on break, I'd chart what I did for her/his patient myself.

In summary, personal rules were useful but individually based. The "lessons learned" always reflected a nurse's own personal behavior and did not address the systems in which the nurses were embedded. While double- and triple-checking medications might help avoid errors, these solutions rely on individual initiative and consume inordinate amounts of valuable time. We never found a rule that said "I went out and changed the system" as a result of a mistake. Instead of fixing problems, the "lessons learned" reflected personal adaptation strategies needed to survive.

Nurses' Suggestions for Decreasing Errors

The nurses in our study offered few concrete solutions for change. Because of the "I'm to blame" aspect of the accounts, it was clear that nurses held themselves responsible first and foremost. That they pointed to their own human error even when distracted, physically tired, or rushed owing to understaffing was evident. Even when others had shared in the culpability, the internalization was clear. Their emotions of shame and fear remained strong. We questioned how to use these feelings in a practical way.

To provide an answer, we first examined nurses' voices in terms of what was explicitly as well as implicitly stated. Not surprisingly, our research led us to examine the role of health information technologies and bureaucratic regulations in decreasing errors. Are more rules and procedures the answer? While the official party line might be that technologies are wonderful, nurses complained that they were slowed down by them and that they increased the potential for mistakes. In situations in which speed and efficiency were at a premium, following some procedures was perceived as interfering with the pace of work on a busy hospital floor. We concluded that technologies can be helpful but only if they function properly, if nurses believe in them, and if nurses use them as designed. The downside is that safety technologies may be cumbersome, depersonalizing, or just not practical. They can also be dangerous.

Another issue was time. It was clear that nurses wanted enough time to follow the five rights without feeling rushed or distracted. The time aspect is closely intertwined with technologies and rules designed to eliminate mistakes. Nurses expressed the desire to exercise professional judgment over and above bureaucratic rules. Likewise, nurses called for fairness in a nonpunitive environment. For example, as described previously, when nurses were forbid-den to access the Internet as a punitive measure, this signaled a lack of trust. The existence of many error-preventing technologies and rules implies a lack of faith in the ability of nurses to provide safe care without them.

We also found that nurses realized that the buck stopped with them. Indeed, administrators and physicians as well as nurses place the primary responsibility for patient safety on nurses. This responsibility was readily accepted and even embraced. Nurses are keenly aware that they are the last line of defense in catching medication errors. As one nurse in our study said, "Nurses in their role as gatekeepers are expected to protect patients." Another nurse, a man, called for a change in the nursing culture of perfection:

> *Participant:* I've been doing this 36 years. I'm way beyond the "perfec-tion ideology" pitched in schools of nursing, which is neither real-istic nor appropriate. I make errors at intervals, probably <1 percent of meds given [and] often corrected before administration. The unrealistic expectation of perfection needs to be replaced by a cul-ture that defines difference between normal human error and prob-lematic levels of error and promotes learned practice modification.

As the sociologist Dana Weinberg has noted, the inability of nurses to articulate and defend their skills effectively has been problematic, particularly in times of threatened cost cutting.[17] Nursing education is based on a model of punitive discipline similar to that found in the military and the church.[18] This likely leads to a tendency to handle problems privately. It is possible that nurses tend to keep solutions to problems private as well, or at least to share with only a trusted few others.

While no one advocates a laissez-faire attitude toward medication errors, it is unlikely that blame with consequent feelings of devastation and loss of self-esteem is productive. In fact, these same attitudes may lead to a failure to disclose, hence handicapping us in our ability to develop realistic solutions. Although it is possible that the ongoing feeling of devastation serves a posi-tive function in making nurses more vigilant, this could also lead the nurse to question her or his abilities in negative ways. Indeed, it could also cause nurses to leave nursing altogether. To address this problem, we believe that there needs to be institutionalized support for "second victims." Such orga-nizationally based programs have the potential to decrease personal trauma and the likelihood of continued adverse personal and occupational effects.[19]

More openness about these devastating emotional wounds might lessen their impact, while the important lessons remain. Still, these lessons were deeply individualized. We discovered a pattern: that of nurses remaining out on a limb, each fighting the good fight, but more or less alone. Like medicine, nursing can be seen as an "error-ridden activity" in which opportunities for mistakes lie at every turn.[20] Yet there is little help for nurses when mistakes are made. Our findings indicate that instead of trying to change the system, they internalized guilt and vowed to redouble their personal efforts. Although we found simultaneous self-blame and finger-pointing in the accounts, we generally did not find a commitment to structural change. We believe that this is because the nurses felt impotent, assuming that they lacked the power to effect such changes.

We think that utilization of "lessons learned" on a widespread institutional level might help. The institutionalization of sharing and transmitting personal rules in a medication error grand rounds or a review setting could empower participants. Small group sessions to discuss these issues of errors and near-misses in a supportive fashion could help nurses develop realistic solutions. Other groups of health care workers have benefited from this sort of approach.

Having said that, we also need to ask: Can we take a system error view more seriously? Are medication administration errors caused by bad people or by bad systems? If we want to improve things, we must realize that there is shared culpability. Completely failing to discipline nurses who make serious errors is reckless and does nothing to protect the public against dangerous individuals. No one wants this. Yet simply relying on the error-free imperative alone is not sound policy. Many years' experience has proven that it doesn't work. We believe that the major focus must lie at an organizational or system level—in part because, until the system is "fixed," there can be no "fix" for the problem of medication error, and in part because nurses themselves often do not focus on the system level. Perhaps it is a sense of duty that compels nurses to continue to try to do more with less. Perhaps it goes further than that. Like the doctor who keeps pulling people out of the river because he doesn't have time to go upstream to see who is pushing them all in,[21] nurses don't have time to change the conditions in which they work. They are too busy helping patients get well.

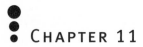

CHAPTER 11

On Teams, Teamwork, and Team Intelligence

Suzanne Gordon

The mystery that motivates this book is why more than a decade's worth of time, energy, and resources devoted to patient safety have not produced as much progress as many anticipated. Other chapters have discussed a number of factors that negatively impact patient safety. This chapter looks at how the failure to construct a robust concept of teams, teamwork, and team intelligence contributes to the slow pace of patient safety improvement. To explore teamwork and team intelligence, in the following pages I first examine inter- and intraprofessional hierarchies and rivalries, then show how professional self-definitions prevent cooperation and coordination, before looking at the way teams are defined, constructed, and maintained.

As a journalist who has been observing nurses, doctors, and other health care workers in hospitals and other settings for over a quarter of a century, I have spent years interviewing them and watching them do their work. Trained as a literary critic, I have taken the workplace as text. Since the first moment I entered the hospital setting to study nursing work in the late 1980s, what I have read in that text has been as disturbing as it has been enlightening.

When, to write my first book on nursing, *Life Support: Three Nurses on the Front Lines,* I followed three registered nurses at the Beth Israel Hospital in Boston in the late 1980s, I was surprised to find a workplace still dominated by status hierarchies and behaviors that the social movements of the 1960s and 1970s had helped to delegitimize. Hospital employees, it seemed, had never heard of, and certainly had never addressed, the concept of "hostile workplace." They complained but didn't seem to do much about some of the communication problems I observed. Even at Beth Israel—which was then a mecca for nursing—incivility, disrespect, one-upmanship (or womanship) were enacted in front of my eyes as I watched members of the so-called health care team do their work. As I listened to nurses and doctors, and later aides, or janitors, or home health workers talk, I could palpably feel their demoralization, anger, and resentment at being continually misunderstood and implicitly or explicitly put down by members of another profession. I had not yet read the literature on teamwork. Nonetheless, to me as an outsider with a front-row seat on hospital culture, it was crystal clear that for all the incessant talk of teamwork, there was absolutely no infrastructure being laid down for it in this and most other health care settings.

In the late 1980s there was little discussion of how poor communication among health care workers led to patient deaths or preventable complications as there is today. But it was pretty evident to me. In fact it took me only a few minutes to see how upset and off-track "team members" got when confronted with disrespect or incivility from those with whom they worked. Nurses would routinely come to me and tell me that they'd just had a nasty encounter with a doctor and angrily demand that I write about it in my book.

Oh, that will really help, I thought. This book will come out in, maybe, five years, and I doubt the physicians whom nurses complained about would read it.

RNs weren't the only unhappy ones. Doctors would complain to me about nurses who advertised themselves as "the patient's advocate." "So what does that make me," an irate surgeon demanded, "the patient's enemy?" Even physical therapists and social workers expressed annoyance at nurses' attempt to put a lock on "caring." To them, too, the notion that nursing is "the caring profession" suggested that other professional and occupational groups were the opposite.

I began my work writing about and observing nursing, convinced that nurses were the victims—of doctors, of the media, of administrators—and my oh-so-righteous anger was directed at those groups. I looked through nurses' eyes and saw the slights they experienced, the putdowns they contended with, and the hubris of medicine, and found it far from the "game" that the psychiatrist Leonard Stein wrote about in his two essays "The Doctor-Nurse Game" and "The Doctor-Nurse Game Revisited."[1] And I bristled with them and for them. But gradually I came to see that very few who work in health care have learned how to communicate in other than hierarchical or dyadic terms. Nurses, doctors, physical therapists (PTs), occupational therapists (OTs), social workers—take your pick—are schooled in nurse-to-patient, doctor-to-patient, PT- to-patient communication. In the silos in which they are trained, their education and socialization include a focus on working as a dyad but very little on how to deal with the team. From the actors whom medical and nursing schools hire to play the standardized patient or family member, to the objective structured clinical examinations (OSCEs), or simulators used in nursing and medical schools, people learn how to dance in twos but not in lines, squares, or rounds. RNs may claim to be communicators par excellence, but they are no better at team communication than anyone else on the professional or occupational ladder. As if to prove it, these so-called great communicators have as their professional mantra that "nurses eat their young." In fact, their sense of insult and injury—particularly from doctors—and their attempt to claim their own "caring" corner of the health care universe may lead some nurses, just like everyone else, to make bad communication even worse.

Although the situation is slowly changing (more on this later), neither teamwork theories, skills, nor team intelligence is taught in most nursing or medical education programs. Or if it is, it is taught in the most perfunctory manner. Sitting and listening to a lecture together does not make nursing and medical students understand each other, particularly when the aspirations, which often ground the professions, make teamwork seem like a mission impossible. It is not simply that doctors and nurses and other health care professionals are educated in silos. It almost seems that they are educated in fortresses and socialized to view other professionals or those in other occupations as members of an opposing team, or even of an invading army.

Doctors are socialized to give orders to nurses, not to work with them and view them as colleagues. The buck-stops-here, captain-of-the-ship ethos of medicine leads to a not so hidden agenda in which some physicians seem far more concerned about asserting status and authority over others than is healthy for them, their patients, or their co-workers. In her book *Of Two Minds,* the anthropologist T. M. Luhrmann carefully explains that the socialization of doctors attaches importance to the minute details of costume and image. "Every hospital I was in had an implicit dress code in which doctors looked like one another and emphatically not like nurses."[2]

This kind of battle for authority doesn't take place just between doctors and nurses. It can also occur between physicians. In a tragic example, Peter Pronovost, in his book *Safe Patients, Smart Hospitals,* describes what can happen to patients because of hierarchy within the medical profession. Although

Pronovost is a world-famous patient safety pioneer at Johns Hopkins, as the intensive care physician on call he was unable to persuade a surgeon to attend to a patient on his ICU who was experiencing disastrous complications only hours after her operation. Because of the mostly unwritten rules of medicine, he could not effectively challenge the surgeon's decisions and rescue the patient. As a result, a patient who came into the hospital relatively healthy, and was supposed to stay for only a few days, ended up losing both kidneys, being on dialysis, and remaining in the hospital for six months and a rehab facility for a year.[3]

The aviation safety movement has defined the team leader as someone who has developed what is called "mature authority." The team leader is someone who must make sure all team members can do their job efficiently and effectively. This revolutionary concept of leadership makes a distinction between a team leader, or director, and an institutional star, or prima donna. A team leader recognizes that other team members exist as entities that are separate from the higher-level player. Under this definition of mature leadership, a surgeon would not be chosen to lead a team if he could not make sure that those construed as below him—such as the director of the ICU, not to mention nurses and nursing assistants—are able to do their job of protecting patients

Health care, however, maintains an immature view of leadership. Like an infant who cannot conceptualize people as anything but an extension of himself, many health care professionals are carefully taught to view the occupational or professional group as on a lower rung of the ladder, not as separate from but as extensions of those above them. Just as physicians in the nineteenth century conceptualized nurses as little more than an inanimate tool in the physician's armamentarium, the contemporary MD views many team members as "physician extenders," allied health professionals, the "doctor's eyes and ears." Thus in 2002, in a celebration of Nurses Week at the medical college of the South Carolina Medical Center, the director, Dr. John Heffner, lauded nurses because "they amplify by their daily presence the value of our brief daily patient encounters."[4]

The same definitions of the "professional-as-other," as Sartre might have put it, apply to the professional who is conceptualized as the other. Nurses who boast four-year BSN degrees, for example, are taught to refer to nurses who have associate degrees from community colleges as "technical, not professional, nurses." As the dean of one university nursing program put it, they are "our educated hands and feet." The four-year nurse, by contrast, has "critical thinking and decision-making skills," while the two-year nurse apparently has none. Licensed practical nurses (LPNs) and nursing assistants are even less than lower extremities, allegedly having no skills or thinking ability whatsoever, and thus deserve to be relegated to the status of the "nurse extender."

As nursing, like other professional groups, breaks into even more educational shards, we now have clinical nurse leaders who earn BSN degrees after entering nursing school with a four-year degree in another subject. The American Association of Colleges of Nursing—the group that pioneered this new "role"—deems that graduates who have just left nursing school and have no practice experience at all are equipped to be the "leaders" of veteran floor nurses. Today many so-called advanced practice nurses (APNs) also have no significant experience in practice. Nonetheless, equipped with a master's degree and the title APN, they are declared to be advanced in their practice. So what does that make floor nurses with many years of actual practice experience—retarded and inferior? None of these splinter groups are conceptualized as different from—but rather always better than—the group to which they compare themselves.

All of this fragmentation has been exacerbated by the demand of payers, educators, and policymakers that the professions justify their existence (and thus the money they receive). As payers try to secure cheaper services, this encourages professionals and nonprofessionals alike to try to usurp territory that traditionally belonged to another professional or occupational group. Nurses asked to justify their existence do so by distinguishing themselves from "medicine." To legitimate their claim to payment and status, they insist that they provide more holistic care than physicians, and criticize a narrow "medical model," which according to many nurses is at the root of a number of our health care woes. Nursing, RNs insist, represents "the solution" to medicine's limitations and the most significant health care problems.

Once medicine is put firmly back in its silo and the door is shut and locked, registered nurses then define themselves against LPNs, who return the favor by arguing that RNs no longer have the time to deliver hands-on care and so can no longer truthfully lay claim to holism. Nurse practitioners for their part, look up the ladder, seeking the title of "Doctor." Physicians go ballistic and try to establish physician assistant programs. Pharmacists pursue the Pharm.D. degree (doctorate) and are rewarded with the proliferation of pharmacy techs and, in the United States, by drug benefit management programs that try to put them out of business entirely.

Each time a professional or a profession plants a stake in the ground of patient care, it seems to separate that profession or professional from others with whom that profession should be able to work collaboratively. And if things are bad for those we consider highly skilled professional workers, they are absolutely abysmal for nonprofessional, so-called lower-level, "unskilled" workers—who are viewed as utterly without skills, mindless, and invisible, with nothing to contribute to patient care except their ability to follow the orders of a higher-level group. If we are trying to create a whole out of the sum of its parts, it is hard to imagine doing so within the current definitions of professional and occupational identity and authority.

The Joint Commission believes that "improving communication requires a systems approach, including the creation of a culture that emphasizes open communication as a crucial component of safe, quality care."[5] It now demands an end to "behaviors that undermine a culture of safety" and insists that to prove they have mastered the "elements of performance . . . [l]eaders establish a team approach among all staff at all levels."[6] While this new attention to teamwork is heartening, what I continue to observe in the health care setting does not suggest much movement on the teamwork front.

Are Health Care "Teams" Really Teams?

The Harvard sociologist J. Richard Hackman, who has spent decades describing and analyzing teams, articulates five conditions of successful teamwork: "The team must be a real team, rather than a team in name only; it has a compelling direction for its work; it has an enabling structure that facilitates teamwork; it operates within a supportive organizational context; and it has expert teamwork coaching."[7] Simply accomplishing a particular task or set of tasks—performing an activity or activities—is not enough, Hackman cautions, to qualify as a successful team. To be effective, a team or workgroup must satisfy three other requirements:

1. It must produce an output that "meets the standards of quantity, quality, and timeliness of the people who receive, review, and/or use that output."
2. The process through which that output is produced must enhance "the capability of members to work together interdependently in the future."
3. The process through which the team or group works must contribute "to the growth and personal well-being of team members."[8]

Do we see anything resembling this in most hospitals today?

Let's take Hackman's definition point by point, though not always in his order.

First, the team must be a real team, rather than a team in name only.

In spite of all the intelligence chatter about teamwork and the "team," in health care there seems to be little precision even in defining the concept of a team. Most frequently, teams are implicitly defined as a group composed of members of the same discipline, for example, the physician "team" that rounds in the morning. Or we have a team of nurses, pharmacists, and so on. Sometimes, though certainly not always, teams in health care are defined as excluding other disciplines. People in one discipline sometimes actually consider themselves exempt from working or collaborating with another, particularly if that discipline has a lower status. Even when a "team" of multiple disciplines is gathered, little effort is made to help these people—who have, as we know so well, been trained in silos and in opposition to one another—work together effectively.

Let me give two examples of this definition of the "team" and "team-work." In one instance a physician expressed frustration with a nurse who seemed—that is, to him—inexplicably disturbed about his decision to prolong the life of a terminally ill patient. "Why didn't she understand that the patient had explicitly stated his desire to hang on until a relative could arrive to see him in two days' time?" he wondered. "After all, we discussed it with the team."

When I asked who, precisely, constituted the team, he said, as if it were obvious, "Well, the interns, residents, and med students." So routine was this definition of the team (recall the conversation Bonnie O'Connor and I cited in chapter 3) that this man, who has exceptional emotional intelligence, did not understand the nurse's frustration. Of course she was frustrated. She did not have the critical information that would help her understand the "team's" plan because she was not conceptualized as one of its members.

Or consider how one ICU nurse dealt with a resident who had made a mistake and ordered the wrong dressing for a patient. The dressing had been applied. Concerned about being chastised by his attending at morning rounds, the resident asked the nurse to change the dressing. This request couldn't have come at a worse time, the RN thought. It was shift change, and she was caring for a very critical patient. As she was about to explain all this to the resident, she thought angrily: "Why should I tell him anything. These residents are always asking us to clean up their messes." She informed him that she could not do the dressing change. He insisted. She declined once again. The conflict escalated, and the nurse manager—who had no training in managing such conflicts—was notified about the dispute. She scolded the RN, who then lost faith in the manager, whom she described as "taking the doctor's side." The RN reports that she found it very difficult to work with the resident after that and literally felt sick whenever she saw him.

Another unwritten definition of the team is a stable group of people who have worked together over time and have thus earned one another's trust. To work as "teammates," one person has demonstrated to another that he or she is a competent professional. Nurses often proudly proclaim that they have no problem working as team members with physicians. The teamwork is great between her and Dr. X, the nurse will boast, because she has worked with that physician for twenty years and earned his trust. (I have rarely heard a physician express his or her belief that doctors should earn the trust or respect of nurses or other non-physician staff.)

Trust established over time applies to those in health care both in the inter- and intradisciplinary context. As noted earlier, one of the mantras in nursing is that "nurses eat their young." This generally refers to more experienced nurses who do not support, listen to, or accord respect and civility to the new kid on the block, who may be a newly minted nurse or simply a recent recruit to their work unit. (Although physicians would argue that they are routinely eaten up in training, they have no similar mantra.)

In this definition of "the team," establishing teamwork involves a constant process of proving that one has "the right stuff." This quest for approval may be unending if one is in a lower-status discipline or occupation. The same need to "win trust," however, occurs among members of the same discipline or occupation when a new person enters the group. Rather than welcoming the new recruit, members of the established group often put that person through the kind of hazing that seems to be as common in health care as it is in boot camp or college fraternities and sororities.

When team building includes this kind of hazing, or even bullying, team members may become so stressed that they are unable to perform up to par.[9] These definitions of teams and teamwork significantly impact patient safety. Pity the poor patient who is dependent on an intern who not only has been up for thirty hours but also has just been scolded by an attending during morning rounds for making a mistake (the kind of mistake that is essential to the learning process). Or the poor patient who is cared for by Dr. X and a nurse she has worked with for only a few days or even weeks. Or the new nurse whose RN colleagues are showing him who's boss on the unit. If teamwork is a matter of years spent earning the trust of a higher-status professional, patients will not be safe under the kinds of conditions that are all too common in health care—in which people work with people with whom they have never worked before.

Finally, there is perhaps the most common definition of the word "team"—that is, a group of people who happen to be assigned to the same patient or work on the same unit or in the same space or location. This team exists only because a group of discrete individuals happen to work on the same person or task. Indeed, this kind of team is not really created or constructed. It is simply declared into existence because of the serendipity of location, assignment, or employment. The members of this kind of team are, as I have written elsewhere, "intimate strangers," engaged in "parallel play" around a patient or activity.[10] The primary concern is with individual—not team—competence, responsibility, or authority. People are preoccupied with getting their own job done, or with how others help—or hinder—them as they execute their work.

On teams engaged in this kind of parallel play there is little awareness or acknowledgment that people take pride in what they consider to be their own work. Nor is there much acknowledgment of the sense of responsibility and risk that they bear. An example of this is the physician who insists that the nurse is his or her "extender" and that the MD—not the RN—is responsible for the patient because "the buck stops here." This ignores the fact that the nurse considers the patient to be "her" responsibility and that she has an ethical and even financial stake in the outcome of patient care. This pattern trickles down the entire health care ladder. Registered nurses, for example, argue that their licenses are on the line when they delegate tasks to nurses' aides, conceptualized as "nurse extenders," and thus viewed as having no stake in patient care.

Although this is by no means an exhaustive list of team definitions, to function on any of the kinds of "teams" I have described requires individual knowledge of a particular subject matter or the skill involved in performing a set of discrete tasks. Or it requires the ability to execute the "orders" of a higher-level group. It does not require either emotional intelligence or what I call team intelligence. In fact, I would argue that its implicit commitment to toxic hierarchy often defeats genuine teamwork.

The kind of teamwork Hackman analyzes—the kind that is necessary in the modern, high-tech health care universe—involves a very different set of skills and a different kind of awareness. To paraphrase Lorelei Lingard, it involves the ability to negotiate and navigate multiple, interconnected relationships, situations, and activities, usually quite rapidly.[11] This in turn involves the willingness to grant credibility to people with whom one may never have come into contact, or to whom, because of status considerations, credibility is usually denied.

For a team leader and members to maneuver in the high-stakes world of contemporary health care, credibility and legitimacy cannot depend on where the person stands in a particular hierarchy, or on what Paolo Freire would have called the authority of status. It must instead be based on the recognition that this person—by virtue of the kinds of education and experience he has had, skills he has mastered, and tacit knowledge he has acquired (to Freire, the "authority of knowledge")—is a potential resource. Credibility allows both team members and the team leader the opportunity to gather, solicit, and share important information that will be central to decision making, as well as in preventing, managing, and containing threats to patient safety.

To create this kind of credibility, not only individuals but institutions as well have to have what I call "team intelligence." As Hackman puts it, a condition of teamwork is that the team "operates within a supportive organizational context."

In a large and complex institution like a hospital, people have to believe that the institution has enough intelligence to hire the right people for the job, to give them the right kind of orientation and education to do it, and to ensure the right kind of working conditions that will make it possible to do a job that people can believe in. With this confidence, a team leader or member will be able to reach out for—not merely receive—information across boundaries of class, gender, ethnicity, nationality, and status.

But in most health care institutions there is little attempt to construct the kind of supportive infrastructure that encourages and sustains teamwork—or what Hackman delineates as condition number three, "an enabling structure that facilitates teamwork," which follows condition number two, that the team have "a compelling direction for its work."

On hospital teams that are "teams in name only," we do not see even a minimal attempt to create the "enabling structures" that follow from this shared sense of direction. To name only a few, the kinds of structures that enable teamwork include the following.

The team leader and members must be flexible so that a group that includes one occupation or discipline can expand to accommodate new members of that occupation or discipline as well as members of other occupations or disciplines. This is critical if they are to assemble teams quickly out of groups and individuals with whom they have not worked before. Whether they are quickly assembled teams or long-standing working groups, the central task of team formation in the modern hospital or health care institution involves creating teams across boundaries of status, gender, ethnicity, religion, class, and discipline or occupation. Some understanding of the problems of power in the workplace is critical. To create teamwork, team members and leaders must engage in the basics, which include:

- Introducing themselves to one another so they can identify and find one another (here, knowing everyone's first and last names and function is essential).[12]
- Knowing one another's jobs, rhythms, and imperatives and understanding how they intersect.
- Sharing not only common goals but also information.
- Listening to one another and acknowledging and respecting one another's concerns.
- Viewing one another as resources, not competitors or obstacles.
- Cross-monitoring one another so as to prevent, manage, and contain error.
- Engaging in team learning and teaching.
- Together recognizing and coping with any obstacles or barriers to teamwork.
- Placing team mission—in this case safe patient care—over considerations of status and false authority.
- Publicly acknowledging the roles and contributions of other teammates.

Constructing the Team out of a Collection of Individuals

The biggest challenge of teamwork is knowing how to turn a collection of individuals into a high-functioning team. To do this, the first component of team construction seems so obvious it almost goes without saying: making introductions. It is impossible for people to function as a team if they aren't introduced to one another, can't find one another, don't have the faintest notion of what their job is in connection to the jobs of others, and are unaware of the team's goals and priorities.

To see what happens when the basic structures of teamwork are not established, I invite you to follow me as I observe morning rounds in a major northeastern teaching hospital.

This particular gathering is part of an experiment, created in collaboration with the dean of a nursing school and the chief nursing officer of the hospital—one that proudly trumpets its Magnet status. One of the teams of doctors that assembles each morning now includes "an attending nurse"—an advanced practice nurse with a master's degree and some standing in the institution. Each morning she joins an attending physician. Staff nurses also join the rounds. The job of the "attending nurse" is to help floor nurses "find their voice" and integrate nursing concerns into the medical plan of care. With the help of the attending nurse, floor nurses supposedly engage more fully with a group of doctors in training—medical students and residents—as the physicians determine the plan of care. The attending nurse will help the attending physician to understand nursing issues, and this, it is suggested, will help physicians in training better appreciate nursing concerns.

As the chief nurse officer described this experiment to me, she said that it was already a "win-win." It had gained physician buy-in because "physicians don't receive as many pages from RNs asking, 'Doctor, what do you want me to do about . . . ?'" Plus, she told me, doctors and doctors in training were now much more attentive to nurses and willing to learn from them.

Enthusiastic about this experiment, I observed the group on one particular morning in the spring of 2010. The "team" included a pharmacist and two nurses—the bedside RN caring for the patient the group would be discussing first, and an RN who acted as "group leader," who would be taking notes on all the patients' plans of care. The team leader, Dr. S, stood in a crowded, cramped hallway outside a patient's room and began the "learning/ teaching experience." A man and a woman in long white lab coats—two residents—joined us along with a younger man and woman in short white lab coats, the medical students. The attending did not verify whether people in the group knew one another and made no introductions; the doctors in training were not introduced to the bedside nurses or to me, a journalist invited to participate in the rounds.

As Dr. S discussed a series of patients, she stood with her back to the two nurses and addressed the residents and med students. For the next fifteen minutes her stance never altered. She never turned to include them in the conversation. The attending nurse stood alongside the doctors and did not suggest that the two nurses move in front of the doctor and join the team circle. The two bedside nurses stood on tiptoe or craned their necks in an effort to hear what the doctor was saying to the residents and medical students.

Dr. S led off with a discussion about the patient—an older Italian man— who had been admitted with a serious neurological problem. At one point the bedside nurse responsible for the patient mentioned that the old man spoke little English. Indeed, he didn't even speak formal Italian but rather spoke a dialect. Perhaps, she offered rather tentatively, a translator would be in order.

Almost before she'd finished her sentence, the medical student interjected: "Oh, his English isn't such a problem. With my Spanish and his English we did fine this morning." Neither the attending nurse nor Dr. S backed up the RN, and she said nothing further about translation.

As the "team" continued to talk about this man, the nurses were constantly leaving to tend to other patients. There had been no adjustment in staffing to accommodate their patient load, nor was there any attempt to juggle the order of patients under discussion so that RNs could have uninterrupted time when their patient was being discussed. The RNs were thus far too busy to listen or contribute to the entire discussion, and were constantly missing opportunities to teach and learn. Since the attending nurse was actually the director of a different service and worked neither on the unit nor with the patients under discussion, she could not fill in the blanks.

As the group of doctors moved down the hall to talk to the Italian man they had been discussing, I paused for a moment with the two nurses. I was curious about the team leader's failure to make introductions. Maybe I was wrong and introductions were unnecessary because everyone knew one another very well. I asked the two nurses if they knew the names of the med students or residents or if the residents and med students knew their names. No, they replied, they didn't know the names of the doctors in training and doubted the doctors in training knew theirs. They rotate in and out, one nurse said of the doctors. We sometimes recognize them—the residents, that is—because there are photos of the residents (but not the med students) at the nurses' station. But nurses and residents are never formally introduced. Moreover, there are no pictures of the nurses on the unit. For the entire time they were talking, neither the nurses nor the doctors knew the name of person to whom they were speaking—unless they could decipher the small print on their badges, several of which were turned around and couldn't be read at all.

I rejoined the "team" as they talked to the patient in question outside his room. The doctors were asking him what he understood about his condition, how he felt, and what his primary care doctor had told him. The old man could barely understand a word. This fractured—and ultimately failed—attempt at communication went on for a good five minutes more. (I checked my watch.) Finally, I interjected. Since I speak Italian, I proposed, perhaps I might be able to translate. The physicians jumped at the offer. I moved closer to the old man and was then bombarded by requests from the med students (including the one whose Spanish had helped him communicate so well earlier that morning), the residents, and the attending. Ask him if he knows the name of his primary care physician. He couldn't remember. Does his wife know? Yes, she does, she'll be in later in the morning. What's her name and phone number? He told me, I translated, and they wrote it down. Does she speak English? No, not really, the patient grimaced. What about his kids? Oh, he has five of them, they all speak English. Was there a phone number for one they could call? He gave it to me, and I translated.

Then the doctors turned to how the old man was feeling. *Cosi-cosi*—so-so. He felt a little dizzy. So they talked some more. The translation was not easy going. I am not really fluent in Italian, and he spoke in a heavy dialect. Even a professional medical translator might have had difficulty. Though helpful in the breach, I was definitely not the right person for the job. What was needed was someone who not only could decipher the dialect but understood medical language as well. Surprisingly, no one expressed any concern that my serving as translator violated the patient's right to a professional medical translator as well as his right to privacy—a right clearly articulated on Patient's Bill of Rights posters plastered all over the hospital.

After I'd finished translating, the team leader moved on to another patient.

Case Analysis

To build a team that is more than one in name only, one needs a leader who is not a leader in name only. According to Hackman, among many others, that leader needs expertise in coaching and teaching. As defined in the CRM model used in aviation (see chapter 3), the role of the team leader is to make sure each and every member of the team can do his or her job efficiently and effectively, while the job of team members is inquiry, advocacy, and assertion.[13] In this particular instance, the team leader made no introductions, did not explain the function of different players, and, throughout her encounters with staff, asserted her status rather than the integrity of the team and of each and every member. Some people were greeted respectfully (according to the traditional medical definitions of respect, which comprise last name and title). Some were not. Some were not even named or greeted at all. Some were talked to face-to-face. Others were relegated to the sidelines. This behavior on the part of the "team leader" did not create a team that crossed boundaries. Given the signals she sent, it would be hard to imagine that nurses felt good about themselves, or that this team could function interdependently on other occasions.

Not only was the physician giving clear messages to excluded "teammates," but also she was teaching and reinforcing the hidden curriculum of medicine that places status above concerns for patient care. That she did this while participating in an experiment whose goal was to address status inequalities demonstrates how profoundly this concern continues to be embedded in medical culture.

This case is hardly an isolated one. About six months before I observed this experiment in teamwork, I was asked to consult with a rehabilitation unit in a teaching hospital. Staff from different disciplines—PTs, OTs, nurses, physicians, speech therapists, and others—were finding it hard to work together to care for patients who had been admitted after major motor vehicle accidents, strokes, and other serious trauma. As I sat in on staff meetings, it became clear to me that, as Hackman would put it, this was a team in name only and that none of the prerequisites for teamwork were in play. This became apparent in a meeting I observed in which a nurse manager, resident, and attending physician were discussing a patient's case.

As the resident was presenting the case, he explained why he wanted to prescribe one drug, while the nurse caring for the patient disagreed and suggested another. What should he do, he asked the attending? Without hesitating, she replied: "Well, you know, this is a rehab unit so we really pride ourselves on teamwork. But the dark side of teamwork is that the nurse will have her own ideas. So remember. You're the doctor and you're in charge."

The nurse manager did not say a word. There was no pharmacist present to discuss the merits of these medications. When it came to establishing the structures that facilitate teamwork, no one present seemed to notice that in only a matter of seconds, the attending had dashed any hope of creating the infrastructure necessary to support effective teamwork.

In the two examples I've cited, it is the physician leader who lacks team intelligence—the ability to help establish the infrastructure of teamwork and coach team members. Under their leadership, team members did not seem to feel comfortable inquiring, advocating, or asserting. Nurses also acquiesced to this state of affairs. The attending nurse did not play a leadership role in standing up for lower-status team members.

On the rehab unit, teamwork was difficult not only interprofessionally but intraprofessionally as well. Thus a nurse manager was unable to coach one of her nursing staff effectively, who became a particular target of concern. This nurse seemed deliberately to countermand decisions other team members had made—sometimes endangering patients as a result.

When I interviewed the RN, she seemed convinced that everything she did for patients was right and that she could not trust other "team members" to share the same intensity of concern for patients. Nurses, she informed me, are patient advocates, and no patient on the unit could have a better, more devoted advocate than she was. Indeed, she seemed to believe that her co-workers were out to endanger "her" patients. For her, patient advocacy was an individual practice, not a collective one that could include professionals in other disciplines.

Sharing and/or Requesting Information

Establishing and maintaining a team is impossible if team members regard one another with such suspicion. Mutual wariness precludes the kind of information sharing that is crucial to the effective execution of a common mission. In aviation, for example, the captain briefs the first officer about the flight and soon thereafter briefs flight attendants before the plane leaves the ground. This process includes not only a discussion of what potential threats or problems are expected but also, as CRM has evolved into threat and error management (TEM), a discussion of how to manage those threats. This process is much more effective if the team leader or team member shares information directly. Thus a captain who has real team intelligence will do more than conduct his initial briefing with the purser—that is, the head flight attendant—but will take the time to brief all the flight attendants. This ensures that relevant information is not lost in translation.

Teamwork demands not only sharing information but also requesting it. This is particularly important when status hierarchies are involved. It is the rule, rather than the exception, that people who have been socialized to believe that they are "subordinates" dealing with a "superior" will be reluctant to cross status boundaries and will fear reprisals if they do. They will be unlikely to tell "superiors" that there is a problem or that the superior is about to make a very bad mistake if they have been socialized to defer to those status hierarchies. That is why, when information or input is offered, someone with team intelligence will acknowledge it, consider it, and thank the person for his or her effort. Even if that information is incorrect or inaccurately interpreted, or the concern is unwarranted, someone with team intelligence will express gratitude for the information and the concern.

Supporting, Cross-Monitoring, and Situational Awareness

If a team, as Hackman puts it, is an entity that "has a compelling direction for its work" and operates in a supportive organizational context, then someone has to do the directing and the supporting. To direct and support, however, demands at least a rudimentary working knowledge of the jobs and roles of other team players. It will certainly be difficult to lead the team if one has no understanding at all of the work that other players do. In health care, it seems to be the rule rather than the exception to assign a leadership role—whether administrative or clinical—to people who lack even the vaguest understanding of the roles that members of their team are supposed to play. Thus a chief resident at a major teaching hospital involved in a series of highly publicized patient safety initiatives recently asked the dean of its nursing school to explain what nurses do. This physician was truly baffled by the presence of nurses in the institution. To grasp the significance of his ignorance, just imagine a hockey coach who confesses that he isn't sure what the goalie does.

This kind of ignorance of the work of team members who have traditionally had lower status is often rationalized because the higher-status worker considers the lower-status one to be doing "mindless" work. Someone who considers himself or herself to be a superior will be unlikely to listen to, learn from, or view such "mindless" workers as resources. If, to protect patients, the "mindless" or "unskilled" worker persists in speaking up, that persistence can lead to accusations of "insubordination" or disciplinary actions. As cases cited elsewhere in this book make clear, if a lower-level worker is disciplined for pursuing a legitimate concern about patient care, this will send a very distinct message to all workers in all institutions.

The establishment of a structure that supports the kind of team that can include many players at many different ranks is at the core of two other critical components of teamwork: cross-monitoring and the maintenance of situational awareness.

Teamwork requires cross-monitoring. This involves being aware of what someone else needs to do and know in order to accomplish his or her job.

Consider the following examples. First, my colleague Patrick Mendenhall is a pilot with Delta Airlines. He had a medical problem that forced him to quit flying for several years. When he had been cleared to return to the cockpit, he immediately put his long experience with CRM to use. Every time he worked with a new captain, he informed his team leader that he'd been off work for a few years and asked him or her, "Please watch my back."

I recently observed another exquisite example of cross-monitoring when I was having lunch in a Brazilian restaurant in New York. While I was waiting for my order, four men at a table behind me were also waiting for theirs. As I sat and read, the waiter responsible for both tables began to clear away dirty dishes from tables in the front of the restaurant. Hands full, he headed back toward the kitchen. Just as he was about to pass us, a busboy deposited a tray with the four men's piping-hot food on a tray stand. The waiter looked down at the hot foot and then at his hands. He clearly realized that he could not take the dirty dishes back to the kitchen and simultaneously dole out the plates to the men waiting to eat. As he was contemplating this dilemma, another waiter, empty-handed, was heading toward the front of the restaurant. He saw his colleague glance at the tray of plates waiting to be served, recognized the problem, and without either waiter saying a word (the one with the full hands never said, "Hey, I could use a hand here,"), the empty-handed waiter deftly took the plates from his colleague, swiveled on his heels, and headed back to the kitchen. Our waiter, hands free now, passed out the plates of food to his customers, who contentedly began to eat. These waiters understood the demands of each other's work, which allowed them to cross-monitor each other and thus detect problems and help address them.

These waiters also had what is known as "situational awareness." In aviation, making sure that crew members maintain situational awareness is the nonnegotiable ground of safety. As defined in aviation, situational awareness is "the accurate perception and understanding of all the factors and conditions . . . that affect safety before, during, and after the flight."[14] It means being aware of the big picture, of what is going on around you, as well as what is going on in your particular job, crisis, or emergency. Situational awareness is critical to preventing, managing, and containing error. That's because crises and emergencies put situational awareness in great jeopardy. Eastern Airlines Flight 401 crashed in the Everglades in 1972 because three very smart pilots—a captain, flight engineer, and first officer—were so focused on a fifty-nine-cent green light that had malfunctioned that no one was paying attention to flying the plane or to the fact that it was losing altitude, something they realized only seconds before the plane crashed in a swamp and all lost their lives.

Practicing the skills of cross-monitoring and situational awareness leads to an *organized* team, one that can better respond in the disorganizing, almost hurricane-like winds of an emergency. The two waiters who had such skill in cross-monitoring and situational awareness during normal activities will presumably be able to become hyperorganized during an emergency.

In contrast, consider this example of a "team rounds" at another major northeastern teaching hospital, where Ross Koppel and I had been invited to observe a morning "reporting in" session.

A resident, an acute care nurse practitioner, and a "charge nurse" were "sharing" the responsibility for this activity. A few bedside nurses were also present, as was a "discharge nurse." Both the charge nurse and the discharge nurse were clearly senior to the other nurses. All had gathered around a conference table in a room off the main unit. The bedside nurses had come to report about their patients and were constantly moving in and out of the room as patients were discussed. No nurse introduced herself as she presented details about her patient (whose name was, of course, always given). Sometimes nurses left after presenting the information about their patient and returned later after the group had moved on to other patients. If the idea was to learn about the patients and to share knowledge so as to improve or better coordinate care, this peek-a-boo process prevented such learning. The nurses could stay for only a few minutes because they had to attend to their patients.

No nurse brought with her any chart or paperwork about the patient. Therefore, nurses were reliant on their memory. Occasionally one indicated that she was not certain about a specific figure (such as blood pressure) but seemed confident of the general trend. Sometimes a nurse was not sure about, for example, the specifics of a patient's dialysis schedule and indicated that she would check on it later. While the charge nurse listened to the nurses' reports, the senior resident spent most of his time with his cell phone glued to his ear, as he received reports about the patients' tests, procedures, or transfers to or from the OR or to a different unit. Only rarely could he listen to what the nurse describing her patient's condition had to say. When, in a rare moment off the phone, he was paying attention, he scribbled his notes on a single sheet of paper. That small sheet contained all of the names of patients on the unit and an overview of their medical condition, procedures, tests, and medications. On this sheet the resident also wrote additional notes about forthcoming events and issues. Because his writing was so small and, far more important, the available space for notes so limited, we worried about the possibility for errors in reading the handwritten notes.

The charge nurse was the key record keeper and often moved the session from patient to patient. The charge nurse maintained a notebook that allocated approximately one eighth of a page to each patient for that shift. Interestingly, her entries in those small squares appeared to vary by preferences and by what she deemed was salient, given her years of experience; for example, one patient would receive a "room air" notation, or another "dialysis at 4 PM," or another "probable discharge by Thursday." To these observers the process seemed remarkably unstructured.

The discharge nurse also recorded her notes on a copy of the sheet of paper the senior resident used. Later she transferred her notes into the computer for the resource allocation records. Presumably the same issues of limited space for recording information and the small script could lead to errors of interpretation or omission.

What was most interesting was how little discussion there was about a series of patients with very complex conditions. No report or discussion of any patient exceeded four minutes, and each was fractured by nurses leaving or entering the room, or the resident being paged or on the phone. Although the resident was the ostensible team leader, there was little to no conversation or reflection between him and either the nurse practitioner or the charge nurse. Also, because there was no "protected time" for the nurses to present their cases, they were clearly in a great hurry to return to their patients on the ward.

The interactions we observed in this setting, as in so many others, were characterized by a total lack of cross-monitoring and situational awareness. One could perhaps attribute the problems in teamwork here to status, to lack of coaching, or to many other factors. To us, one of the underlying problems that created a chaotic rather than an orderly discussion of patient care was the intensification of work. The resident, who was supposed to be the team leader, had to juggle too many cases. This in turn created a constant stream of interruptions. The nurses also had too many patients to attend to and could not stay in the room. With each additional patient being discussed, the interruptions escalated, either from the phone or from trips in and out of the room, which in turn created greater distractions and more opportunity for error, not to mention less opportunity to teach and learn.

All of this, in turn, pointed to the failure of the institution to support teamwork. Clearly, the institution had created no sheltered time in which people could reflect on the job at hand, plan, and refine care. Although we now know that the human brain is in fact very poor at multitasking, sheltered time has become an increasingly scarce commodity in the health care world of today. Like the doctors and nurses in the rounds we observed, many in health care are forced to be more concerned with what is going on outside or apart from the activity at hand than they are with it.

The acceptance and/or creation of this kind of relentless work intensi-fication is a sign of a lack of institutional support for teamwork. Provid-ing support for teamwork necessitates an awareness of the obstacles that can get in the way of doing one's work effectively and efficiently. Work intensification—asking people to do more and more with less and less—is a recipe for error as well as an impediment to institutional learning.[15] When workers complain about this kind of intensification, dismissing their con-cerns by asking them to "work smarter, not harder" is a clear demonstration that those in authority are not listening attentively and seriously considering obstacles to team effectiveness and thus patient safety.

As stated earlier, in discussing effective teams, Hackman and his colleagues insist that getting the job done is not the ultimate criterion by which we judge a high-functioning team. Obviously output is important, but if a group "burns itself up performing one of its tasks, . . . or alienated or deskilled its members, then its success must be questioned." It is worth reiterating Hack-man's message that a team is effective "to the degree to which the group experience contributes to the growth and personal well-being of team members."[16] Many contemporary managers repeat a common slogan, "There is no 'I' in the word 'team.'" On the contrary, a team is, in fact, composed of a group of "I"s doing their "I" work in the service of a shared goal or mission. To manage a team in a way that permits little recognition of the individuals on it and thus little growth suggests a lack of team intelligence and a narrow understanding of the meaning of teamwork.

Rather than suggesting that participation on a team should involve the deliberate self-effacement of an individual member, team leaders and members should understand that being on a team always involves acknowledging the contributions of all team members.

What Is Missing: Team Intelligence

The examples and issues I have discussed are only the tip of a very large and sturdy iceberg that has been built up over a century in our health care system. It is part of the hidden curriculum and culture of health care—a culture whose content and impact is only now being oh-so-gingerly addressed. There is increasing awareness that the culture of our health care system is part of the problem. Yet—and perhaps this is only to be expected—to some of those who participate in trying to reform the culture, much of it is opaque or even invisible. As Janelle S. Taylor has pointed out, medicine is a culture that fails to see itself *as* a culture.[17]

To create the kind of teamwork that patient safety depends on will, however, require a very detailed understanding of the kinds of obstacles to teamwork I have discussed. Many of these obstacles are subtle. They exist in the interstices, in a gesture or stance in a hallway grouping, a quick comment made during morning rounds, attention distracted by too many pages. If teamwork is to become a reality, these interstices must be studied by observers and researchers who are not so much a part of the culture they are observing that they fail to see its implicit messages in action. These observers and researchers must move into the private spaces that cannot be captured in a broad survey of nurses talking about bad experiences with disruptive doctors, or medical journal articles written by doctors thinking about the games they play with RNs. Nor can they be fully uncovered by accounts of physicians trying single-handedly to change the system and tear down the silos. While they are certainly illuminating and useful, works by such larger-than-life doctors as Atul Gawande or Jerome Groopman risk becoming simply another part of a heroic medical narrative that in a peculiar and fascinating way subverts teamwork as much as these particular physicians tout it.

What is needed in medicine is the kind of systematic study of team relationships—or their absence—that took place in aviation and was central to the creation of the aviation safety movement known as crew resource management. In aviation, sociolinguists, anthropologists, sociologists, and organizational, social, and clinical psychologists, to name only a few, managed to penetrate the private spaces of the airline cockpit and cabin to detect and analyze the ways in which the hidden agenda and socialization of pilots and other airline staff contributed to a culture that defeated safety. Combined with National Transportation Safety Board analyses of crashes and NASA research, these accounts helped to illuminate exactly how teams worked when they existed and didn't when they did not.[18]

Until the same level of scrutiny is applied in health care, we will never understand how subtle messages are delivered and broader goals for team building subverted. Knowledge of how teams work—or don't—is also crucial to building a concept that I believe is central to patient safety efforts. Although the literature on teamwork in health care routinely includes discussions of the need for emotional intelligence, I would argue that another concept—what I have been calling team intelligence—needs to be added to the discourse on teamwork. Deeply influenced by the theories of multiple intelligence generated by the work of Howard Gardner, popularizers of Gardner's work, such as Daniel Goleman, have made the concept of "emotional intelligence" a household term, particularly in management, and now in the health care literature. Talk about the need for teamwork in health care, and the concept of emotional intelligence inevitably crops up. Emotional intelligence (EI) has become such a popular concept that it now comes with its own set of constructs, promises, management tomes, scoring systems and inventories, and, of course, critiques.

While emotional intelligence is certainly an important concept, creating genuine teamwork in health care—or anywhere else, for that matter—requires moving beyond the idea of emotional intelligence to that of team intelligence. The concept of emotional intelligence tends to focus so much on the self in maintaining integrity in relation to and with others that it ignores the team as the central construct. What is key, in a sense, is the integrity of the successful individual, what skill that individual has, what knowledge he or she possesses, how competent he or she is, and how he or she performs alone. In other words, if one imagines emotional intelligence as the hub of a wheel, it is the self that is in the center of that hub, with the spokes of various relationships emanating from it and back to it.

Team intelligence is what allows people to function in the intricate web of what Lorelei Lingard has described as the "collective enactment of multiple threads of activity in which health care may be socio-spatially distributed among multiple organizational units."[19] In other words, it is the team, the collective, that is at the hub, while individuals moving toward the hub of that team and radiating outward and inward make up the whole.

When safety researchers and advocates began to focus on the need for better crew communication in aviation, a common observation was that a lot of very smart people occupying the same space and managing the same problems were making a lot of very stupid decisions. Before the advent of crew resource management, the conventional wisdom was that intelligence naturally resided in the smartest, most qualified person in the room, on the plane, or in the institution. That "smartest person" was invested with the power to identify problems, make decisions, and choose whether or not to involve anyone else in participating, particularly in the case of managing emergencies.

As aviation researchers began to investigate accidents closely, they noticed that the majority of crashes resulted when some of the most proficient pilots in the business were in the cockpit. They were all competent, highly experienced, and had huge reputations. Some were very well liked. Yet when it came to preventing, managing, and containing error, they did poorly. Indeed, all too often, a lot of smart people produced a lot of major catastrophes. To paraphrase Oscar Wilde, who famously stated that a collection of opinions does not constitute a point of view, a collection of the smartest people in their field does not always produce wisdom and adequate action, particularly in the heightened stress of an emergency, and/or when status and authority are perceived as being challenged.

The same is true of emotional intelligence. We constantly see people who may exhibit enormous emotional intelligence—defined in terms of individual skill and competence in dealing with dyadic relationships—fail miserably at creating, mastering, or enhancing teamwork. The attending physicians we met in this chapter may be excellent with patients and with doctors in training. In relationships in which they are the undisputed authority or that do not cross disciplinary boundaries, they may behave in an exemplary fashion. As the leader of a team that includes members of other professional disciplines and demands that the leader pay attention to the concerns of people who have not historically been defined as part of her discipline or tribe, they may, however, fail on every measure of team intelligence. The same may be true of the attending nurse whom we also met. She may be an excellent nurse manager, knowledgeable and attentive and concerned about her staff as well as the staff on the unit where she is engaged in these monthly rounds. Measure her EI quotient, and she may score in the top percentile. When, however, it comes to being one of the leaders of a team in a department where she does not work and where her authority is ambiguous, her score on TI—if one had such a scoring device—might come out in the lowest percentile.

Team intelligence is the behavior that embodies the understanding that most endeavors involved in health care today demand what the cognitive scientist Edwin Hutchins calls "distributed cognition." In systems in which the division of labor necessitates cognitive labor, two kinds of labor are distributed, "the cognition that is the task and the cognition that governs the coordination of the elements of the task."[20] Team intelligence is the mastery of the cognition governing that coordination. It involves being aware not only of what skills and material people have mastered but also of what they don't understand but need to. It means making sure that people speak the same language, share the same goals, have clear expectations, are not subverted by unclarified assumptions, and help one another maintain situational awareness. Being aware of the barriers that might prevent people from sharing important information and insights is also central to team intelligence. Finally, team intelligence involves an appreciation not just of what one needs to do one's own job but of what other people need to do theirs, so that each member of the team can help other team members as they try to carry out their jobs safely and effectively. This concern for the integrity of the team—the whole—is different from a concern with each individual and each individual's professional role. This is why the person or institution that has team intelligence will publicly acknowledge the efforts not merely of those it perceives as team *leaders* but of those who are team *members* and will also encourage the kind of institutional learning that is necessary for safety in any endeavor.[21]

Shifting Awareness

Developing TI necessitates a very different kind of awareness from the kind that individuals cultivate when they live out their occupational or professional lives mastering a particular set of skills, or what is now known in medical (and managerial) jargon as "competencies." It also involves a very different definition of assertion, empowerment, and confidence.

An impressive contemporary example of team intelligence at work was exhibited by Captain Chesley Sullenberger before, during, and after the masterly efforts of the team he led during the safe landing of US Airways Flight 1549 in the Hudson River on January 15, 2009. In almost all discussions of this amazing feat, Sullenberger was credited with being the heroic individual who did it all by himself. Sullenberger himself has staunchly resisted this focus on the solo actor who pulls off an amazing feat of magic. In his autobiography, he emphasizes the roles of his team members and talks in detail about how he, as team leader, worked to bring a collection of individuals who had never worked together before into a cohesive team that was able to join forces to do the seemingly impossible.[22]

Time and again he has refused to take sole credit for the landing and has publicly acknowledged his team members' roles in the event. When the newly elected President Obama invited Sullenberger and his wife to his inauguration five days later, Sullenberger responded with a magnificent display of team intelligence. The captain refused to attend the event unless the entire team of first officer and flight attendants were invited to accompany them. They were, and they went.

In terms of content and activities, health care is clearly different from what goes on in the cockpit or cabin of an airplane. But whether one is performing cardiac surgery or landing a plane with three hundred passengers on board, the underlying issues remain the same. Teamwork is one of the lynchpins of safety. Vulnerable people, who cannot protect themselves, rely on the skill, actions, judgments, and decisions not only of those at the helm but also of those who work with the helmsman. We shall never have safer patient care if we do not conduct a serious discussion of what a health care team is, how it should be led, and how our institutions create and support the intelligence needed to build and maintain it.

Conclusion

Twenty-seven Paradoxes, Ironies, and Challenges of Patient Safety

Ross Koppel, Suzanne Gordon, and Joel Leon Telles

Patient safety efforts are paradoxical. Their successes are usually ephemeral and frequently challenging. Patient safety is an action, not an achieved status. It's the avoidance of errors and creation of routines to maximize safe actions; it's stocking the right items in the right bins. Achieving safe care for patients demands specific actions and constant vigilance both at a worm's-eye view and at a bird's-eye view. Yet despite the sometimes elusive, sometimes clear, and sometimes protean requirements, the consequences of failing to ensure patients' safety are real, costly, and often horrible.

Patient safety is both the absence of harm to patients and the actions we take to prevent harming them. Patient safety is thus both a negative and a positive space. It means we do not make life worse for the patients who are in the care of the medical system; we do what is expected ("standard of care") when we are supposed to do it, and the way we are supposed to do it. And when the standard of care is insufficient for a specific patient, we must take that extra step to avoid causing harm. If we do cause harm, we should report our mistakes in order to fix the error and improve the "standard of care" by learning from the error. Patient safety also means that we structure the office, hospital, and other institutional processes to eliminate known causes of errors, making sure, for example, that children's medicines are not stored on the same shelf as the adults' medicines, gloves are available where needed, sinks and antibacterial hand lotion dispensers are available and functioning. We provide enough oxygen tanks for patients to be able to travel across a large hospital system; we confirm the identity of the patient in front of us; we make sure that caregivers have had enough sleep. And when we cannot prevent errors, we try to manage and contain them effectively.

Hospitals and doctors can't charge patients more money for *not* harming them, but ironically, clinicians and hospitals can sometimes make more money from treating the harm they have caused—a perverse incentive now partly addressed by the U.S. government's decision to deny reimbursement to hospitals for certain avoidable errors: the nonpayment for what are called "never events," surgery.

We must also consider the complexity of care in current health care settings. Patients are treated by many physicians, nurses, therapists, technicians, and so on, whose perspectives and priorities might differ from one another's and the patient's. Laboratory results from scores of tests ordered by different clinicians must return to the ordering clinician and should also be made available to the others. The results must be interpreted, and those interpretations should be explained and recorded in the patient's chart. Hospital patients receive many medications that are ordered by a multiplicity of clinicians, who continually alter them in response to changes in the patient's condition and therapeutic requirements. There are hundreds, perhaps thousands, of hand-offs, notes, reports, memos, and so on. One could reasonably ask: Why are so few patients seriously harmed?

In short, patient safety is often a paradox: something we strive to ensure but cannot achieve by doing any one thing, or even by improving many things. Patient safety requires fixing everything we can think of and many things we do not yet know about. It means we must coordinate many, often complex processes, in addition to maintaining a constant focus on work design, staffing levels, the environment, training, professions, professionalism, management, communications, information technology, regulation, certification, and testing. Patient safety efforts themselves can endanger patients' safety through conflicting or confusing initiatives or onerous reporting requirements. Patient safety requires a synoptic level of understanding from often incomplete, unreliable, and missing data.

Ensuring patient safety is an endless mission on which there has been substantial progress. Health care professionals and administrators have learned a lot and try daily to implement what they have learned. They are often successful in addressing known hazards, and they continue to learn and apply new insights. Rates of several types of hospital-acquired infections, for example, have been declining nationwide. While all must make real-world tradeoffs, these are almost never negotiated with a callous disregard for harming patients.

What we outline in this final chapter must be seen as the *difficulties* of preventing harm to patients, not the *impossibilities*. Although we could enumerate many more than twenty-seven points, we conclude this book with salient or consequential paradoxes, ironies, and challenges essential to achieving patient safety.

1. Patient Safety Easily Falls between the Cracks

Because patient safety is everyone's responsibility, it can become no one's responsibility. Steps needed to ensure patients' safety can slip through the cracks between departments, but also among managers, between doctors and nurses, between nurses and techs, between shifts, and between nurses and transport services. Patient safety thrives best when everyone does everything right in each setting. But even that will not guarantee safe care unless the right things in one place are also the right things in another place. Consider, for example, what would happen if hospital A uses a yellow wristband to denote allergies to opioids while hospital B two blocks away uses that same color wristband to indicate an allergy to penicillin. Patients are often transferred between hospitals, but no one notices conflicts or gaps until something terrible happens. Or take another example: a patient's current medications are listed in alphabetical order by one physician, grouped according to organ systems by another, and listed as they are remembered in yet another office. Worse, the lists are frequently outdated, missing key drugs or dosages, or otherwise incorrect. Reconciling this information becomes onerous if not impossible.

Health care is almost always a complex sequence of events involving multiple actors who are seldom in direct communication with one another. Also, many players are frequently in different segments (or stages) of what we think of as a sequential process.

Handoffs—transferring information from one clinician or department or shift to another—are rich in opportunities to drop or miss essential information. Sometimes the handoffs are structured by careful guidelines and checklists, but often they are informal and dependent wholly or in part on small pieces of paper, memory, and urgency. We have observed handoffs that were interrupted repeatedly by phone calls, pages, requests for information from a colleague, and of course emergencies—some created by the kinds of mistakes noted earlier. Some handoffs are augmented by email or references to patient records that go unseen for hours or longer. Handoffs are constant, because one caregiver cannot possibly provide all care in a 24/7 institution with many shifts, thousands of staff, varieties of expertise, and massive information gathering.

It's not just information that gets lost at handoffs. As recounted in the introduction, at a top hospital, Ross Koppel's wife was moved from major surgery to the hospital floor. Unfortunately, she was left on the gurney where the nurses could not see her. She lay there freezing and dehydrated until he found her. The nurses had been informed that she was "on the way" but did not suspect she had been left by the elevator.

Meanwhile, at another prestigious hospital not long ago, a patient was admitted with a bowel obstruction and in shock. Two weeks into her admission, a nutrition consultant recommended that the patient receive tube feeding (inserting nutrition directly into the stomach). The recommendation sat in the patient's electronic medical record unheeded, while the patient lost considerable weight and developed symptoms of severe malnutrition. Over the next two months, as the patient was moved in and out of that hospital, nurses and doctors insisted that she was "uncooperative" because she wasn't "trying hard enough" to eat. Not until the patient was near death, and after frantic appeals from a physician friend, did a clinician notice that the patient was starving and initiate tube feeding.

2. Patient Safety Risks and Preventive Actions Are Everywhere and Nowhere

Patient safety is the result of almost everything anyone in health care does—or does not do: people washing their hands and washing the floors; surgeons performing complicated operations and workers transporting the patient to the operating room; nurses ensuring the "five rights" of medication administration and physicians considering the patient's many other illnesses and other medications while ordering new medications; workers unloading sterile supplies from a truck; clinicians monitoring patients, whether by using the newest technology or by looking into patients' rooms to ensure that frail and disoriented patients are not trying to climb over bedrails; technicians entering information about new drugs in the pharmacy; data entry clerks typing in names correctly; insurance companies negotiating what treatments will be allowed and at what rates; as well as the patient's family and friends accurately remembering the patient's medications when talking with a nurse or doctor. There are essential patient safety actions in nearly every health care–related activity. Patient safety can't be separated from the rest of health care; there is no distinct set of patient safety actions.

3. Patient Safety Is Not a Thing, a Single Action, or an Attitude; It's an Outcome Obscured by the Paradox of Prevention

As we have said, safety occurs when prevention works. And when prevention works, nothing "remarkable" happens. We benefit from—but do not observe—the absence of unexpected infections, pressure ulcers, or falls; no medications required to counteract an adverse drug reaction; no surgical supplies left in the patient's chest. Here are some other examples of the myriad patient safety actions we avoid:

- We do not give patients treatments intended for other patients.
- We do not cover the barcode on a patient's medicine with a decal reminding the nurse to scan the barcode.
- We do not send patients for a one-hour trip to physical therapy with an oxygen tank that lasts only half an hour.
- We do not lose patients' medical records when they go from one doctor to the next, or from one unit of the hospital to another unit.

And we do thousands of routine things required to avert harm:

- We clean patients' wounds when we should.
- We wash our hands.
- We make sure that the right medications are given to the right person, in the right dosage, at the right time, and via the right route (the "five rights" of medication administration).
- We put up signs so everyone will pay special attention to patients at risk of falls.
- We do thousands of other things that we may or may not fully notice, understand, or have time to accomplish, or can't adequately perform with missing or inappropriate supplies.

The irony, of course, is that nothing happens when we prevent an error. That's Sherlock Holmes's dog that didn't bark: people often forget or do not know that something had to happen to ensure that nothing happens—the kinds of actions and focus required to make prevention work. In other words, the absence of harm requires the presence of prevention.

4. Patient Safety Requires Sweating the Small Stuff Even While We create the "Miracles" of Modern Medicine

What this point means is that small steps toward risk avoidance can be as consequential as the "big" diagnostic and treatment activities. We stop killer infections with extraordinary medications and techniques, but if we fail to refill the antibiotic lotion dispenser, our work may be for naught. We appreciate extraordinary technical skill and scientific mastery; and our culture celebrates the "hero" heart surgeons and physician-researchers. The public and even the profession of medicine, however, rarely celebrate the thousands of actions and routines preceding, accompanying, and following these impressive feats—the small, quotidian tasks that make the "miraculous" possible. As we see throughout this book, it's often the little things that lead to patient harm. But innovative surgeons (like all other people) are so eager to get to the big stuff—the operation—that they might not bother with surgical checklists or make sure they operate on the right kidney. Physicians may employ sophisticated diagnostic tests but ignore the fact that the patient is actually dying from malnutrition. Staff might not notice that a patient whose surgery was successful has not been delivered to her room but lies shivering in a hallway. Hospital cleaning is outsourced, and no one notices that the new cleaning company has stinted on supplies or training.

We are enthralled by dramatic medical advances, but patient safety often resides in the easily overlooked details. The small stuff is often the big thing in patient safety.

5. Patient Safety Can't Be Fully Routinized

In the whirl of activities, and with the difficulty of making the system work with every action, transfer, handoff, and so on, a mistake at any point can result in a patient's receiving the wrong medication or a recommendation's being ignored. This inability to pretest and repair problems is different from the situation in which a lot of other human activities occur. For example, the creators of databases expect errors, use the system to find them, and then fix them so they will not occur again. But each medical event is often new because of the nonroutine nature of medical care. The human body is always adjusting to itself and the environment. And no patient works quite according to the model. Patients are by definition sick. Therefore, unlike a computer program that once fixed stays fixed and will therefore work correctly the next time and every time, patient safety presents unique challenges with each encounter, action, and interaction, even though conditions and patients may appear similar to those from the time before.

6. Patient Safety Is the Result of a Multitude of Tradeoffs

There are always tradeoffs between safety and time, staffing levels, money, training, amount of supervision, quality of supervision, hiring decisions, labor relations, promotion decisions, quality of technology, aggressive and/or proactive management, vigilance and empathy: take your pick or take all of them. Safety is the net result of myriad decisions and nondecisions, evasions, missed cues, grudges, departmental rivalries, professional rivalries, silos, and even efforts at avoiding silos. Administrators and clinicians make decisions that 99.5 percent of the time have the expected and reasonable results. Bad results are sufficiently uncommon that we do not think about the resources required to avoid those unwanted outcomes. Often, however, small misses have catastrophic results. Too frequently, moreover, conflicts and tradeoffs are not obvious even to staff. For example, on one hand, an increasing focus by hospitals on patient satisfaction has two different aims with different consequences for patient safety. When hospitals work on improving the patient's experience, there are changes like faster treatment in the ER, providing comfortable surroundings, and responding quickly to patient requests. On the other hand, when hospitals seek to boost patient satisfaction survey scores—to meet benchmarks and avoid Medicare payment penalties—resources can be diverted from providing the best care. Some hospitals, at the urging of expensive consultants, require nurses and aides to visit each patient room once per hour to announce, "I am here to give you very good care." Why? Because on patient satisfaction surveys, patients are asked if they received "very poor, fair, good, or very good care." Some hospital consultants contend that if patients hear "very good care" hourly, they will choose "very good" care on those survey forms. Alas, this task may take nurses' scarce time away from attending to patients who require the most care, perhaps several visits each hour. In general, efforts to improve the patient *experience* are likely to contribute to safety, while a focus primarily on improving *satisfaction scores* risks diverting resources from patient safety.

Last, we note that the ultimate tradeoff to those with macro-level policy power is between providing medical care or providing safer care versus fewer road repairs, schools, or army bases.

7. Patient Safety Is Pan-hierarchical

Patient safety depends on the actions and beliefs of the person highest on the health care ladder—the chief medical officer, a cardiac surgeon—and the janitor, transport staff, or kitchen worker. One decision or action by any of them can alter a patient's life. An unclean floor can infect a score of patients. The jobs of cleaning staff and their supervisors, however, may have been outsourced to a firm that neither trains its employees nor provides enough supplies for them to work competently. Those in charge of the janitorial staff may have limited commitment to, and understanding of, patient safety, while the hospital retains liability for inadequate cleaning. Studies of hospital-acquired infections (HAI) find that local epidemics are caused by seemingly trivial oversights, for example, inadequate care by the hospital worker who cleans the poles on which IV bags are hung. Similarly, decisions to discharge patients are based on physician-defined "medically necessary care." In contrast, patients may need continued hospitalization because they require "necessary nursing care"—monitoring, arranging follow-up care, and teaching them or their caregivers how to handle new medications or medical devices. Few health care policymakers, insurance company executives, or hospital administrators, however, are attentive to the concept of "necessary follow-up and nursing care."

8. Patient Safety Cannot Be Located within Any One Building, Organization, or Office

Just as patient safety cannot be limited to one stratum in the health care hierarchy, it can't be contained within one organization. If an office or hospital is not sent the necessary documentation of previous treatments, conditions, allergies, antibiotic resistance, and medications, then the patient's care is endangered. Similarly, if a patient is sent to a rehabilitation center or other facility, failure to provide the needed information will negatively affect and delay the patient's care. The risk of readmission to the hospital is dramatically increased for patients released to their families without the needed instructions, medication access, follow-up care, or equipment (or skill in using equipment). Even though the data on the value of continuity of care are unequivocal, care is increasingly fragmented. Equally problematic is the lack of incentives to conduct follow-up care.

9. Patient Safety Is Directly Affected by Policies and Decisions Made by Federal, State, Organizational, Regulatory, and Corporate Powers

When insurance companies set reimbursement limits for procedures or length of stay in the hospital, they directly influence the levels of resources and personnel available for patient safety. When the law and the association of medical schools restrict the number of hours residents can work (so that less exhausted residents will make fewer errors), it affects hospital budgets, training routines, educational procedures, patient care, supervision, the number of handoffs and shifts, and patient outcomes. It ultimately can affect the ability of patients to obtain insurance coverage, and therefore even obtain medical care. When the Medicare and Medicaid programs announced that they would no longer provide reimbursement when certain types of errors (such as wrong-site surgery or slips and falls—those "never events") are made, they were using policy decisions to influence hospital and clinician behavior. Similarly, reimbursement and insurance coverage affect policies that determine which medications are used and under what circumstances, how many nurses are on the floor at any time, the number of available hospital residents, how often a wound dressing will be checked or changed, whether or not a nurse will be available to coordinate post-hospital care, how many visits to a specialist patients are permitted, the cost of co-pays, and what is covered by insurance (or not) in an emergency room visit.

In the health care insurance industry, the amount that does not go to profit, executives, and business expenses is called the "medical loss ratio." To patients and clinicians, the "medical loss ratio" is called medical care.

10. Patient Safety Efforts Are Always Influenced by Economic and Legal Conditions and Policies

Just as patient safety cannot be separated from the overall health care system, it cannot be isolated from the position of the health care system in the larger economy. For example, much medical charting reflects the need to justify billing insurance companies, legal fraud avoidance, and regulations from professional or trade associations and government payers. A surprisingly large percentage of the documentation process and the interaction between patients and doctors is driven by the business requirements of submitting invoices. Physicians and nurses complain proving that a service was provided or appropriate is often more time-consuming than providing the service. For example, ordering a needed test or procedure may require fifteen minutes of the physician's time, spent in working with the electronic medical record and other team members to "justify" the action, entering diagnostic codes on the patient's digital record, and checking to see if the patient's insurance carrier will subsidize the action. These tasks steal time from patient care and might result in mis-codes that live on in digital form forever—often metastasizing to other medical records, causing diagnostic errors, erroneous medication choices, loss of insurance, and injury. Because of the complexity and impact of documentation and coding, hospitals and physicians are usually obliged to hire firms to check their accuracy. Because of all these factors, the system suffers related distractions, inefficiencies, and ironies when

- patients do not receive preventive care because of cost, lack of adequate insurance coverage, or individual concerns (for example, being diagnosed with a preexisting condition that will limit future employment or the ability to obtain affordable insurance);
- doctors must spend hours negotiating treatment decisions with insurance company operatives who receive incentives for rejecting procedures or medications;
- medical decisions depend on local medication formularies based on financial grounds as well as medical evidence;
- some medical decisions (for instance, ordering unneeded tests) are made to avoid possible litigation; and
- politicians require or prohibit medical procedures on the basis of ideology or pharmaceutical corporation lobbying

At the same time, the larger financial, legal, and governmental system can push health care to improve patient safety efforts, such as in quality and patient safety efforts driven by the focus of insurers and the government, and infection reduction efforts driven by public reporting.

11. Patient Safety Is Dependent on "Evidence-Based Medicine" and Its Limitations

"Evidence-based medicine" (EBM) refers to guidelines based on the most recent clinical and statistical research. It turns out, however, that it is often remarkably difficult to generalize from clinical research. Why? Clinical studies usually require researchers to examine a small sample of volunteers with one disease who are taking only one medication. But as we have seen throughout this book, the average patient is an elderly person with co-morbidities taking ten or twelve medications. In other words, it's often very difficult if not impossible to generalize from research based on clinical studies to real-life patients with co-morbidities affecting the heart, kidney, and liver—all organs vulnerable to the usually recommended medications for many illnesses and conditions. Because they address this complexity, we admire thoughtful clinicians who balance possible treatments and the patient's health and wishes along with the many possible outcomes and side effects. It could be argued that if medical practice could be reduced to simple algorithms based on EBM, doctors or other highly trained professionals would not be needed at all.

Another paradox of evidence-based medicine and patient safety is that health care providers often implement a multiplicity of solutions simultaneously, so it is almost impossible to measure what, if anything, helped. Thus we do not have proof of improvement from evidence-based treatment. There are similar confusions and ironies regarding the multiplicity of patient safety initiatives. In hospitals and other facilities, staff sometimes undergo so much initiative fatigue that the push for patient safety can, if misapplied, make patients less safe. Moreover, it is hard to identify which initiatives were effective when many were implemented simultaneously.

12. Patient Safety Requires That We Know about Our Mistakes and the Mistakes of Others

Data about medical errors are worse than sporadic; probably fewer than 2 or 3 percent of errors are known. Why? Patients are sick and often become sicker despite our best efforts. Many patients are taking a dozen or so medications, some of which work in unknown ways with their other medications, and all of which affect their treatment and test results. Some of these may have been newly prescribed medications. Medications and treatments change over the course of hospitalization. Most medications also interact in complex ways with the patients' co-morbidities, underlying conditions, and current illness. Also, physicians will often order exactly the right medication, dose, schedule, and route for the patient's diagnosis, but the diagnosis generating all of that good effort will later turn out to have been incorrect. Sometimes everything is right but the pharmacy dispenses the wrong medication and the error is not noticed. Sometimes we have the right medication for the wrong patient. Added to this complexity is the reality that errors in medical care are freighted with concerns about reputation, liability, insurance premiums, professional status, advancement, and licensing. Even if errors are known to the clinician or his or her colleagues (which, as noted, is infrequently the case), self- and colleague reports of errors are uncommon. And if errors are known to researchers like us, we might be in the dark about whether they are obscured, ignored, or believed to be inconsequential: known errors may be covered up at the bedside, the risk management office, the general counsel's suite, or the insurance company office. Some are subject to legitimate confusion over who did what and when in the chaos of emergencies and highly stressful settings involving many simultaneous actions by numerous individuals.

Another irony here is that improving patient safety requires knowing about errors, but clinicians become more vulnerable and at risk legally when errors are known. As a result, clinicians have an incentive to restrict knowledge of errors to protected personnel and facilities. The more openly clinicians report errors, the more vulnerable they become, and the more tempting it is reduce the reporting that encourages changes to prevent errors.

13. Patient Safety Requires Learning from Our Mistakes, but We Can't Learn from Mistakes We Can't See

How can we learn from the things we can't see? This is not a Zen parable. Recall the joke about the man looking under a lamppost for his lost car keys in the dark, even though he knows he dropped them twenty yards away. When asked why he's looking under the lamppost, he replies, "It's the only place I can see." In looking for evidence on medical errors, we are a lot like that man. Because we know about such a small percentage of all errors made, we focus on the errors we can "see." We ceaselessly scrutinize the area under the lamppost, and develop better and better ways of addressing those problems.

For example, we usually discover surgical instruments left in patients' bodies, wrong-site surgeries, and adult doses given to children. We then increase protections against these types of mistakes by counting instruments before and after surgery, by requiring the surgical team to agree on the surgery site, and by making surgeons sign the body part before operating. We also demand that children's medications and adult doses come in different colors and maybe increase the font size of the label. These steps are helpful and reduce these types of errors.

But what of the other errors that are not so easily discovered—errors that cannot be directly observed but must be found through indirect measures and proxies? How do we find and prevent them? The answer requires investigating many and varied possibilities, using often obscured or proxy measures that suggest (1) an error was made; and then (2) how to intervene to stop such errors henceforth. For example, we examine the rate of post-surgical infections (which we can see) in several units, and then, according to the rate differentials, we examine every aspect of the services involved in the lower infection rates. Is there better communication in those units? Are the surgical areas being cleaned more carefully? Perhaps wound dressings are being changed more frequently or more carefully? Is it the design of the floor or the rooms? Is there something different about the pre- or postoperative procedures? We can extend that logic to all of the other measures of "quality and safety," for example, length of hospital stay for similar problems, number of extra medications or treatments required to address complications, speed of recovery, on so on. In this way we enhance institutional learning and go beyond examining only the reported problems and errors; we are guided to find that which we could not originally see but now know to investigate.

If our indirect measures are too broad, they may point to so many activities and systems that we cannot single out promising targets. Many things affect, for example, "length of stay" in a hospital. More precise measures permit us to focus on specific aspects of patient safety but also increase the risk of missing the cause. Be they direct or indirect, by examining indicators of those errors that are hard to see and seldom reported, we avoid being led astray by focusing on the very small proportion of problems that are easy to see and are frequently reported.

14. Patient Safety Requires That We Acknowledge Our Biases in What We Recognize as Problems

Just as our information about patient safety dangers varies, there is variability in our willingness or ability to recognize the errors we see. What errors we perceive depend on the settings and types of problems (for example, prescribing, dispensing, administering), where the problem occurred, who saw it, the probability that it will be discovered, as well as the opprobrium associated with making that kind of mistake. Our ability to confront problems is also affected by how much harm they caused, how expensive it is for the clinician or institution to address them, and how easy it is to deflect responsibility (for instance, a medication was on the wrong shelf, the referring department gave inadequate data). Staff are less likely to hesitate in reporting errors they see—near-misses—because they knew about them and stopped them. For instance, the wrong patient or medication was sent, but the mistake was caught and prevented. What's not to report? At the same time, serious errors (in particular, errors resulting in a patient's death) are more obvious than others and are thus more likely to be reported. But in most cases we do not notice the errors we made, because if we'd noticed them, we wouldn't have made them. And as noted earlier, almost all hospital patients are very sick, the health care system is complex, the potential causes of an event are many, and staff are all trying very hard under difficult circumstances.

15. Patient Safety Can Be Both Improved and Worsened by the Application of an Industrial Model to Health Care.

We seek to reproduce in health care the efficiencies of industry, of manufacturing, and of other service businesses. Despite what can be learned from industrial system engineering, there are severe limitations to applying a model developed on assembly lines to the care of sick patients. Sick patients are not like yet-to-be assembled automobiles or books at on-line bookstores. Every patient in a hospital and every patient who comes to a doctor or nurse with a problem is *not* working according to the product manual. These patients are "broken." Manufacturing or business models are not primarily designed to fix something that's not working as designed, with often unknown problems and incomplete data, and subject to more variations than most of us can conceive. Patient care is messy, often unpredictable, frequently confusing, and usually ensconced in·unknowns. For the patient, it can involve life-altering consequences. Even the definition of success is stunningly variable, from facilitating a comfortable death, to just keeping the patient alive, to restoring full function. The work requires hundreds or thousands of handoffs and dozens of disciplines. It frequently demands that patients and families comply with complex regimens without medical or nursing supervision. It also means that patients must make decisions about "compliance" that are rational from the clinician's perspective but may seem irrational from the patient's perspective. In addition, as we have argued, trying to reduce medical care to algorithmic routines risks compromising patient safety. That's one reason why clinicians can't give warranties when a patient signs on for an operation, hospital stay, or even routine care—and why it would be a lot easier to take care of people if they weren't sick, or had only one medical problem or took only one medication.

To be clear, there are essential lessons to be learned from the business models brought to health care. Systematizing supply schedules, simplifying processes, and even regularizing many medical procedures and actions have been of great value. Such systems have contributed to increased patient safety, but applied superficially or too broadly will endanger that safety.

16. Patient Safety and Business Cost Center Accounting Are Uneasy Bedfellows

Some of the cost-cutting and tradeoffs beloved of businesses—Toyota Lean Production, Six Sigma, Disney Running Your Hospital, or the Studer Group—are very useful in some health care settings but can be inappropriate for others. The analogy of patients as customers who must be satisfied rather than sick people who need treatment is fraught with problems. Purchasing managers at automobile plants can objectively evaluate the quality of the delivered parts, but evaluating "the product" is a more complex task in health care settings. As noted earlier, many patients are old, most are very sick, and a lot of health care activities occur out of sight. Information about "inputs" and "outputs" may well be incomplete.

And patients are not the only "customers." At community hospitals, doctors who can bring business with them are revenue generators who must not be offended lest they take their marbles (that is, their patients) and go play in another facility. The quality of those physicians' patient workups, and indeed the quality of their work in the hospital, will not easily be questioned. There are unending tales of physicians selecting a particular medical device, treatment, or drug because they were associated with the company offering that item. Other doctors at the hospital may object to that method or device, only to be silenced by those with economic interests. In the overly narrow bean-counting view, if quality and patient safety are seen as cost centers, staff engaged in those activities may well be considered just another financial liability. Medical disciplines have become product lines, and departments of hospitals compete with one another. In a seemingly unrecognized irony, the same consultants who critique medical silos are fostering competing businesses—in other words, silos within silos.

17. Patient Safety Confronts the Conflicts of a "Just Culture"

Our understanding of errors is also linked to our ability to maintain a "just culture"—one in which errors are quickly reported and addressed rather than hidden. Alas, such a culture is often difficult to construct and maintain. We must distinguish between (1) unintentional errors, such as mental slips, misunderstandings, miscommunication, interruptions, lost attention, and the like; and (2) stretching the limits, deliberate errors, intentionally avoiding policy and procedures, or repeated negligence. Often, however, the distinction between actions that are and are not blameworthy is unclear. Workarounds are epidemic, often necessary, and efficacious, if risky; a clinician's desire to help a patient or just finish work will result in "making do." It is not feasible to stop care while awaiting a perfect system that does not need a workaround; systems will always need workarounds. A nurse who has repeatedly called the pharmacy for a needed medication may see little danger in swapping an available dose perceived as identical for one that is on the way. Prior to the use of medication barcode scanning systems (BCMA), a nurse could use the equivalent drug sent by the pharmacy; now the BCMA system issues an alert if the medication is not the precise one in the prescription, and the nurse must override the alert in an apparent safety violation. Or perhaps a physician reprioritizes patients' treatment schedules because of one patient's suddenly worsened condition. Errors can ensue if not all staff are informed of the urgent switch. Beyond the immediate question of attributing blame, most administrators also struggle to maintain accountability. If staff repeatedly violate policy and harm ensues, do those committing such errors deserve comfort or sanctions? What if the staff member simply forgot the appropriate policy and the misstep was unintentional? How do we reconcile the need for accountability with the realities of human frailty and the pressures and complexity of modern health care?

All of these factors, needless to say, are influenced by the regulatory climate around reporting, by local newspaper campaigns that affect an institution's standing in the community, and by the extent to which institutions or persons believe they have been unjustly accused of errors.

18. Patient Safety Requires a "Culture of Safety" That Is More Encompassing Than the Freedom to Report Errors

A "culture of safety" means more than ensuring the ability to report errors without fear of blame or retribution; it means that everyone should focus on safety and on institutional learning—increasing knowledge about errors and prevention across the organization. A culture of safety therefore includes activities such as:

- maintaining a continual focus among staff on identifying potentially dangerous actions or omissions;
- rating managers and team leaders on whether they maintain a nonpunitive environment for errors (focusing on the problem and not the person) and for reporting potentially dangerous actions or omissions;
- ensuring that information is not lost during shift changes and other handoffs;
- keeping relationships positive between teams and among team members;
- maintaining adequate staffing ratios;
- using errors to inform process redesign and other efforts to prevent future risks;
- being able to question authority;
- giving staff and others the freedom to choose to take steps to avoid risk; and
- devoting attention to things beyond or in addition to the intended task at hand

A culture of safety also requires an awareness that social relations (such as between staff and manager, doctor and other clinicians, and clinicians and nonclinicians) often impede the ability or willingness of individuals to communicate effectively about patient safety issues. It must be deeply informed by what we know about how systems work, how people are motivated, and how both institutional culture and individual behavior can be transformed. "Team management" is frequently invoked and seldom observed. Practitioners are taught lessons from airplane cockpit management, which many agree are useful. Yet such lessons may be ignored in the stress of the operating room or the hospital floor. Patient safety, in other words, is dependent on the fabric of the workplace—and on the way all the threads of health care work are woven together. In so many cases, efforts by lower-status workers to alert others of possible errors—per the dicta of the culture of safety—are overridden or ignored by those of higher status. It is equally dangerous when staff hesitate to report possible errors because they anticipate a negative or even a nasty response from superiors.

Last, we must remember that culture is always dynamic. While short-term changes can be effected by design, maintaining a culture is an ongoing process that cannot easily be engineered and will inevitably change in unintended directions. If ensuring safety in dealing with patients is hard, crafting a culture that is responsive to emerging patient safety needs is much harder.

19. A "Culture of Safety" Does Not Make Up for Inadequate Organizational and Mechanical Resources

A culture of safety supplements organizations, it does not repair failures. The culture is a critical prerequisite to achieving patient safety but is not by itself adequate. If dangerous equipment cannot be fixed, if the process is inadequately designed, if risks cannot easily be observed, culture change will not be enough. A culture of safety thus is needed but is insufficient to create the reality of safety. Practices, supply chains, equipment, and maintenance systems need to be devised and implemented to prevent errors; just reporting them does not fix or avert risks. One reason, as noted earlier, is that most errors and their causes are unknown and thus can't be reported. Another is that reporting problems involves profound social, legal, and ethical issues, some of which require nimble and nuanced balancing, for example, distinguishing among errors, preventable errors, and negligence. Yet another is that hierarchical and job security concerns tend to trump institutional goals; and intra- and interdisciplinary conflicts are endemic in organizations operating 24/7 under high stress, with shifting boundaries, many unknowns, and always emerging medical conditions and goals—for example, moving from full restoration of health to avoiding death or total incapacitation—as conditions present themselves and change.

Because it's so easy to focus on people and norms, we often sidestep underlying conditions of workload, shift length, patient acuity levels, staffing policies, training policies, supervisory issues, and a host of other factors that are not under the control of the individuals suffused with the culture of safety.

Last, here are a few key lessons and limitations of a "culture of safety":

- Seek continually to move safety efforts away from reliance on the willingness of staff and toward systematic incorporation into processes not dependent on individual will.
- Explicitly take relations of power, status, and friendship into account in implementing a culture of safety.
- Recognize that there are continual pressures toward cultural change, and much as one would adjust machines and processes in the face of events that move them from their design, there should be an active effort to assess and adapt culture to forces that move the organization away from attitudes and actions that contribute to patient safety and avoid risk.

In sum, an improved "culture of safety" is essential but cannot replace devoting resources to adequate supplies, reasonable workloads and schedules, clear documentation, coherent workflow, and good training. It is necessary but not sufficient.

20. Patient Safety Is Built on Assumptions, and One of Those Assumptions Is That We Know What Others Are Assuming

On the most obvious level, we assume that acronyms are universally understood throughout the health care system; for example, SOB stands for shortness of breath. We not only assume that DNR (do not resuscitate) in a patient's chart is understood, but also, more profoundly, we assume that we know how much care the patient desires when he ultimately deteriorates; how much pain he is willing to tolerate; how important it is to him to speak with his loved ones one last time; how much he fears loss of control, ability to reason, and so on. We have heard many stories of physicians who tell patients they can return to their "normal activities," only to find that the doctor does not know what "normal activities" mean to that particular patient. If normal means taking three buses to work and climbing four flights of stairs to get home, then returning to "normal" may not be such a good idea.

To complicate matters, assumptions are embedded in our efforts to avoid errors. Several years ago, safety advocates came up with the idea of the "red sock," which was to be put on the limb *not* to operate on. The problem was that some clinicians misunderstood the red sock to represent the limb that *should* be cut. Similarly, some physicians and patients are asked to sign the area to be cut. But if one first looks at the patient's other side or other limb, one will not see a note that says "Do *not* cut here," which might be more effective than signing where one should cut. (And in fact, some facilities now mark the area *not* to be cut "Do *not* cut here. See other side or limb.") Each of these problems can be fixed, but an endless number of assumptions—ways in which safety can fail—will remain.

Assumptions underlying handoffs (between physicians, nurses, shifts) remain insufficiently examined. One does not know for sure which or all of the following the clinician is or is not providing:

- news about the case (medicines or treatments)
- the most lethal immediate dangers
- the primary diagnosis
- changes in the diagnosis
- information *not* in the record
- information *not to be trusted* in the record
- the order of what's covered—organ systems, some other protocol
- information dependent on other disciplines or subdisciplines (nurses, pharmacists, surgeons)
- the level of understanding of the other clinicians
- the implicit levels and types of measurement (grams, liters, micrograms, pounds, inches)

More generally, in any interaction between clinicians and patients (or anyone else) there are myriad other assumptions about:

- the patient's or caregiver's level of understanding
- the level of expected family or other support
- the patient's expectations (less pain, total rehabilitation)
- the patient's living conditions
- the efficacy of a specific drug or treatment
- the efficacy of modern medicine
- and perhaps most profoundly, the patient's desire to live or simply not to be abandoned by his or her doctor at the end of life

21. Patient Safety Is Increasingly Dependent on Health Care Information Technology, on the Vendors Who Make It, and on Its Implementation in Diverse Medical Settings.

Health care information technology (HIT) includes systems such as patients' electronic medical records or electronic health records (EMRs/EHRs); computerized provider (or physician) order entry (CPOE), which allows physicians and others to order medications directly via the computer system; the electronic medication administration record (e-MAR) for the nurse to record medications; and electronic prescribing (eRx), which allows physicians to submit prescriptions directly to the patient's pharmacy. HIT is often seen as the panacea for the ills of health care. We are promised that HIT will make care faster, better, safer, universally available, and more clinician-friendly. All of these promises may come true. At the moment, however, they are only foreshadowed, even though some of the technology is in at least its fourth decade of use. HIT currently embodies a mix of progress, frustration, innovation, arrogance, incomprehension, and hope.

There are many reasons why the promises of HIT are as yet unrealized:

- HIT has been oversold with extravagant claims based on little independent empirical data.
- It is designed by firms whose systems communicate only with their own "suite" of products, not with their competitors' systems, since effective data standards and interoperability would limit each vendor's sales.
- HIT costs hundreds of millions of dollars. software and hardware cost about $120 million for a new system for a large hospital, and about five times that figure for implementation, training, configuration, cross-covering of staff, and so on. Because illness, accidents, and pregnancies can't be scheduled around HIT training and implementation needs, the hospital must continue to operate while its core information systems are developed and installed.
- HIT has been without any meaningful regulations. In 1997 the vendors, in cooperation with many clinicians and medical informaticists, convinced regulators that regulation would dampen creativity and limit an infant industry. In economics this is called regulatory capture. For patients and clinicians it often resulted in software that is unresponsive to patient care needs. Generous government funding to encourage the use of HIT (and regulations reducing revenue to medical practices and

hospitals that do not buy the equipment) concentrated on obliging the clinicians to buy from a limited list of software vendors that met certain criteria.

We increasingly see, also, former government policy advisers who created the legal structure that is so generous to HIT vendors now working for those vendors.

22. Patient Safety Is Increasingly Dependent on Machines

Here we are talking not about health care *information* technology but rather the machines that are often directly involved in hands-on patient care: devices that monitor patients' blood pressure and oxygen levels; X-ray and MRI machines; devices that deliver medications directly into the bloodstream (smart pumps); machines that alter the patient's body via radiation treatment, artificial joints or valves, or robotic tools for surgery; and the like. These machines are regulated by the Food and Drug Administration (FDA) and may receive careful attention. But as many recent events have made tragically clear, the use of the machines can be misguided, unsupervised or undersupervised, and based on unjustified faith in the technology. Also, makers of many of the devices avoided regulatory oversight by claiming that their devices were very similar to others that had been approved after careful analysis. Unfortunately, it has become increasingly clear that approval under provisions for "essential similarity" has been granted to devices different enough to harm or kill patients.

As with any essential technology on which we rely, we must understand how that technology is integrated into a complex workplace and meshes with workflow and work organization. The work is dependent on machines but also on not treating the workers as if they were machines.

23. Patient Safety Is Endangered by Exhausted, Sick, or Distracted Caregivers

Administrators and consumers urge clinicians to be (and certainly hope they will be) "competent," "vigilant," and "attentive." But if they are overwhelmed, overworked, exhausted, or overstressed, that competency, vigilance, and attentiveness will be severely challenged. Staffing levels, staff schedules, enforced or even voluntary overtime, the use of back-saving equipment such as lifts for heavy patients, and the availability of sufficient supplies all affect patient care. Hospitals are temples for the application of modern science and extraordinary knowledge, but staff scheduling, enforced nurse overtime (or even voluntary overtime), and intensified workloads can undermine the latest scientific advances by applying the practices of an earlier industrial age. We now know, for example, that the human brain cannot multitask very well, yet we constantly ask clinicians to do just that. The economic benefits of "just in time" nurses and doctors must be weighed against the costs in loss of contextual knowledge, patient safety concerns, or the human cost of such arrangements.

24. Patient Safety Initiatives Can Themselves Impede the Safe Care of Patients

We must balance patient safety initiatives with the problems these initiatives generate in their efforts to achieve patient safety goals. The complexity and number of initiatives can overwhelm staff. Management's well-intended but seemingly relentless stream of new ideas and impressive consultant reports can pose problems for the clinicians and others who must implement their recommendations. Nurses and others frequently report that they are working hard to incorporate the latest initiative when even newer ones are introduced. Because we all want to do something to reduce harm to patients, we develop more and more initiatives. This suggests both action and leadership. But is that the case? And if it is, is it effective? And if it is effective, does it complicate care and take resources away from other patient safety efforts? To frontline workers, initiatives fall like snow in winter. Some contradict earlier initiatives. Cost cutting and staff layoffs interfere with the amount of time that staff can spend on patient care and new initiatives. Both the recent health care reform laws and the prestigious Institute of Medicine tell physicians and hospitals to review all medications at each visit or hospitalization. For physicians this task might represent a large portion of the seven to fifteen minutes slotted per patient. While it is certainly sensible, how is this to be done if the doctor is also supposed to diagnose and treat the presenting problem in such a short amount of time?

Similar rubber-meets-the-road problems emerge with many well-intended initiatives. Here are two examples. First, prescriptions for a large class of medications (such as addictive painkillers) must be printed on special paper that cannot be photocopied or faxed. If the only expeditious way of sending the prescription is via fax, the patient's treatment may be seriously delayed. Second, physicians have traditionally written prescriptions for certain patients indicating that the patient should fill it if the fever worsens or other symptoms emerge. Most electronic prescriptions can't handle that kind of contingency, however. Thus, what is supposed to be a safer and more efficient method of ensuring that the correct prescription is quickly provided to the right patient in fact becomes a barrier to achieving those goals.

25. Patient Safety Is Helped by Coherent Regulation

We think of hospitals, medical devices, and health care professionals as extensively regulated. They are, but often the matrix of regulations resembles a crazy quilt more than an integrated set of guidelines and overseers. Many years ago, hospitals created their own certifying authority, now called the Joint Commission. It establishes rules for safety and procedures such as keeping stairwells free of boxes, recordkeeping and peer-review procedures, labeling rules, medication storage requirements, and so forth. Yet fire safety codes and plumbing and electrical standards are also set by local building authorities and the state department of health. The Center for Medicare and Medicaid Services (CMS), the federal organization that pays over half of all medical expenses, has thousands of rules about what is and is not acceptable. Medical residents may be employees of the hospital, but their hours and training regimes are under the control of the Accreditation Council for Graduate Medical Education (ACGME). Medical devices that involve radiation and X rays are overseen by both the Nuclear Regulatory Commission and the Food and Drug Administration, but most other "medical devices" are primarily under FDA regulations.

State and local medical authorities also license and regulate medical institutions, be they hospitals, clinics, or even physicians' offices, and the CMS has requirements for participation in Medicare and Medicaid. Individual practitioners are licensed by state authorities, often working with state and national professional organizations. A state's licensing of physicians, for example, is generally under the control of the state's medical society. Nurses, respiratory technicians, and pharmacists are licensed on a state level, although the testing may be national. Often there are consequential differences in practice between states. For example, in some states a pharmacist can alter a medication or dose without the physician's participation. In others, the pharmacist must contact the physician before changing a dose or medication.

Hundreds of different insurance companies and other "payers" impose yet another layer of requirements, documentation, and permissions. Fear of liability likewise generates additional steps and procedures, each with attendant costs.

This erratic pattern of regulation is sometimes helpful because it enables one authority to catch or intervene where another may have overlooked a potential hazard. And some regulations harmlessly (and reassuringly) over-lap. Unfortunately, some regulations may conflict or generate significant and unneeded expenses. It is also possible that conflicting regulations may increase the risk of errors, or may provide loopholes that, whether intention-ally or unintentionally, affect patient safety negatively.

26. Ensuring Patient Safety Should Not Put Undue Responsibility on Patients

While it is important to advise patients to be vigilant, ask questions, get a sec-ond opinion, know their medications (doses, shapes, and colors), and demand that clinicians wash their hands on entering the hospital room, among many other things, expecting patients to protect themselves from harm when they are in the hospital is largely unrealistic. As we have repeatedly noted, patients are by definition sick, often old and frail, usually anxious, asleep, in a coma, or impaired by painkillers or other medications. If even the best known physi-cians in the country write newspaper articles about their inability to protect their loved ones from harm when they are at their hospital bedside, how can laypeople hope to protect themselves? Most people lack the knowledge and status to advocate for themselves effectively. Their family members and friends are generally in the same boat, similarly anxious, lacking the neces-sary knowledge, and fearful of clinician retaliation. In a way, demanding that kind of vigilance from patients is another form of outsourcing—this time of responsibility for harm. In this era of consumer empowerment, we must be cognizant of the limits of some of our most cherished myths, such as that of self-help and self-care.

27. Patient Safety Demands a Sense of Humility about What We Know, What Can Be Known, and What Is Known by a Clinician at a Specific Place and Time

The medical model of education and the reality of medical practice require doctors to deal with so many unknowns and ambiguities that they often focus on that which is knowable and can be addressed. Unfortunately, to achieve patient safety we must learn to act in exactly the opposite way: we must fight the premature closure of inquiry, look everywhere we have not considered, and keep an open mind. Renee Fox, the great medical sociolo-gist, noted that doctors must learn to distinguish between what they do not know from what is not known by the profession of medicine. Regrettably, the current litigious and economically stressed environment does not encourage discussing these nuances with patients. While academic medicine is free to explore these issues, the fear of lawsuits and the press of work often limit practicing physicians' willingness to express doubt. Modern tests (labs, MRI, CT scans) help bridge the chasm of uncertainty but can also close minds too quickly. And even if doctors are willing to discuss ambiguities and unknowns, patients often demand a level of certainty and omniscience to alleviate their own worries—or doctors believe they want that. Finally, because insurance companies and other payers require a specific diagnosis and have often prohibited the previously used option of asking for tests to "rule out" a suspected problem, we engender an artificial definitiveness that sometimes generates false diagnoses and treatments.

We already know a good many of the paths that have led and will lead us to safer and better patient care. Myriad other paths are yet unknown, while others are emerging and re-forming as we develop our methods of care, our technology, workflows, funding, understanding of the human body and pharmacology, and our commitment to reducing errors. That commitment inevitably reflects priorities and tradeoffs. We could, for example, require a second nurse to check each dose of every medication (and we do for several classes of drugs). The low yield of that tradeoff—time and resources versus improved safety—would be unacceptable to almost everyone.

But there are also murky paths down which we should proceed with more caution than we currently exercise. We have an overwhelming belief in the power of technology to solve problems, many of which are actually created by those technologies. And some of the errors are made or facilitated by upstream technologies—such as the perpetuation of wrong data from confusing spreadsheets or misidentified patient biological samples. We should of course embrace those technologies that, after serious and objective evaluation, are shown to work. Nevertheless, our powerful desire to reduce errors, the extraordinary hype and marketing of the health care information technology industry, that industry's capture of the regulatory agencies, the regulatory requirements for providers to reduce errors, and our hopes for the ability of HIT to save money have generated outsized expenses, government subsidies, and more than a fair share of marketing overreach.

Likewise, our faith in pharmacology and the vast sums devoted to marketing drugs (to both patients and physicians) leave us vulnerable to less-than-clear thinking about the power of medications and the dangers of adverse drug events.

Many of the solutions to patient safety problems are already known to frontline workers. Although all proposed solutions need to be objectively evaluated, we waste a unique set of insights and generate dissatisfaction, frustration, and additional losses of involvement and creativity if we fail to incorporate their useful suggestions. Our failure to pursue such input and to adopt suggested changes results in higher costs. It sometimes appears easier to go for the newest patient safety initiative than to work with the people who ensure patient safety.

We must continue to research what we are doing and what we could be doing to improve our patients' safety. Such research will guide us to new and better methods and also show us where to search for additional solutions. That patient safety falls between the cracks, and is often ephemeral and paradoxical, means we should encourage and conduct more research, not less.

We must also continue to support the efforts of patient safety workers and teams and of all health care professionals who daily intervene to improve the lives of their patients. They devise safer systems, and they catch thousands of errors and mistakes before they can affect patients. On a systems level, these health care workers have made real progress in reducing errors and other causes of patient harm. Their passion for keeping patients safe is a counter-weight to the increasing ability to harm or overlook patients as advances in medical knowledge, techniques, and technology also grow. Additional test data and more information do not translate to better health care unless they are suffused through a system that provides the needed resources, grants clinicians sufficient time and support to focus on their tasks, and nurtures personnel and leaders who are always cognizant of the dangers as well as the benefits of their work.

Notes

Introduction

1. Rebecca Voelker, "Updated Guidelines Target Reductions in Catheter-Related Bloodstream Infections," *Journal of the American Medical Association* (hereafter *JAMA*) 305, no. 17 (2010): 1753–54; P. J. Pronovost, C. A. Goeschel, E. Colantuoni et al., "Sustaining Reductions in Catheter Related Bloodstream Infections in Michigan Intensive Care Units: Observational Study," *British Medical Journal* (hereafter *BMJ*) 340 (February 4, 2010): c309; P. J. Pronovost, D. M. Cardo, C. A. Goeschel et al., "A Research Framework for Reducing Preventable Patient Harm," *Clin Infect Dis* 52, no. 4 (2010): 507–13; A. Lipitz-Snyderman, D. Steinwachs, D. M. Needham et al., "Impact of a Statewide Intensive Care Unit Quality Improvement Initiative on Hospital Mortality and Length of Stay: Retrospective Comparative Analysis," *BMJ* 342 (January 28, 2011): d219; M. Romig, C. Goeschel, P. Pronovost, and S. M. Berenholtz, "Integrating CUSP and TRIP to Improve Patient Safety," *Hosp Pract* (Minneap) 38, no. 4 (2010): 114–21.

2. Sharona Hoffman and Andy Podgurski, "E-Health Hazards: Provider Liability and Electronic Health Record Systems," *Berkeley Technology Law Journal* 24, no. 4 (2010): 1524–2009.

3. Michael Harrison and Ross Koppel, "Interactive Sociotechnical Analysis: Identifying and Coping with Unintended Consequences of IT Implementation," in *Handbook of Research on Advances in Health Informatics and Electronic Healthcare Applications: Global Adoption and Impact of Information Communication Technologies,* ed. Khalil Khoumbati (Gandhinagar, India: Institute of Information and Communication Technology, 2008); Ross Koppel et al., "Role of Computerized Physician Order Entry Systems in Facilitating Medication Errors," *JAMA* 293, no. 10 (2005): 1197–1203; Ross Koppel, "Defending Computerized Physician Order Entry from Its Supporters," *Journal of Managed Care* 12, no. 7 (2006): 369–70.

4. http://www.ihi.org/IHI/Programs/StrategicInitiatives/TransformingCare AtTheBedside.htm (accessed September 16, 2010).

5. Maggie Lange, "Dirt on the White Coat," *College Hill Independent,* February 14, 2011. Brown University, http://students.brown.edu/College_Hill_Independent/ ?p=4244 (accessed April 25, 2011).

6. Fred Lee, *If Disney Ran Your Hospital: 9 1/2 Things You Would Do Differently* (Bozeman, Montana: Second River Health Care, 2004).

7. Suzanne Gordon and Sioban Nelson, "Nightingale Relevant for Patient Safety Focus," *Morning Sentinel* (Waterville, Me.), August 13, 2010.

1. The Data Model That Nearly Killed Me

1. Steve Lohr, "Technology Gets a Piece of Stimulus," *New York Times,* January 25, 2009.

2. Anne Armstrong-Coben, "The Computer Will See You Now," *New York Times,* March 5, 2009. Dr. Armstrong-Coben describes her professional concerns about computerized medical records.

3. "Summary of Nationwide Health Information Network (NHIN) Request for Information Responses," U.S. Department of Health and Human Services, Office of the National Coordinator for Health Information Technology, June 2005, http://www.hhs.gov/healthit/rfisummaryreport.pdf (accessed March 16, 2009). The report by the National Institutes of Health (NIH) summarizes the responses to a request for information (RFI) concerning the creation of the National Health Information Network.

4. Armstrong-Coben, "The Computer Will See You Now."

5. Conceptual data models describe graphically the medical information (less technical details), for example, the information that an ICU nurse requires to carry out his responsibilities, or that an ER attending physician must obtain to treat her patients. IT personnel use conceptual data models to develop and operate data storage and retrieval systems.

6. Scot M. Silverstein, "Essential Value of Medical Informatics Expertise in High-Risk Areas: An Invasive Cardiology Example," Contemporary Issues in Medical Informatics: Common Examples of Healthcare Information Technology Difficulties (blog), Drexel University, 2007, http://www.ischool.drexel.edu/faculty/ssilverstein/cases/?loc=cases&sloc=Cardiology%20story (accessed March 16, 2009).

7. Shahid N. Shah, "Repeat after Me: Healthcare Data Models Matter," The Healthcare IT Guy (blog), December 22, 2005, http://www.healthcareguy.com/index.php/archives/138 (accessed March 19, 2009); John Carlis and Joseph Maguire, *Mastering Data Modeling: A User-Driven Approach* (Boston: Addison-Wesley, 2001).

8. T. J. Eggebraaten, J. W. Tenner, and J. C. Dubbels, "A Health-Care Data Model Based on the HL7 Reference Information Model," *IBM Systems Journal* 46, no. 1 (2007): 5–18, http://dx.doi.org/10.1147/sj.461.0005. Health Level 7 (www.HL7.org), an open standards group chartered by the American National Standards Institute (ANSI), develops health information standards such as the HL7 Reference Information Model (RIM; http://www.hl7.org/implement/standards/rim.cfm [accessed March 16, 2009]), a conceptual data model.

9. Joseph M. Bugajski, "Data Integration: Fantasies and Facts," *Gartner,* October 3, 2008, http://www.gartner.com/resId=1405370 (accessed March 12, 2009).

2. Too Mean to Clean

1. Prime Minister's Commission on the Future of Nursing and Midwifery in England, 2010, "Front Line Care," http://cnm.independent.gov.uk/wp-content/uploads/2010/03/brochure_report.pdf.

2. R. Porter, "Nineteenth Century Medical Care," in *The Greatest Benefit to Mankind: A Medical History of Humanity from Antiquity to the Present* (London: HarperCollins, 1997), 377–80.

3. V. Smith, "Protestant Regimes," in *Clean: A History of Personal Hygiene and Purity* (Oxford: Oxford University Press, 2007), 216–17.

4. R. Beaglehole and R. Bonita, "Evolution of Epidemiology: Ideas and Methods," in *Public Health at the Crossroads* (Cambridge: Cambridge University Press, 1997), 85–87.

5. Ibid., 87.

6. Ibid.

7. M. Bostridge, "Thorn in the Flesh," in *Florence Nightingale: The Woman and Her Legend* (London: Viking Penguin, 2008), 332–39.

8. G. C. Cook, "Henry Currey FRIBA (1820–1900): Leading Victorian Hospital Architect, and Early Exponent of the "Pavilion Principle," *Postgrad Med J* 78 (2002): 352–59.

9. Bostridge, *Florence Nightingale,* 333–34.

10. Beaglehole and Bonita, *Public Health at the Crossroads,* 87.

11. "The Late Henry Currey," *Journal of the Royal Institute of British Architects* 8 (1901): 113–14.

12. Smith, *Clean,* 216.

13. D. P. Strachan, "Hay Fever, Hygiene and Household Size," *British Medical Journal* 229 (1989): 1259–60; R. J. Settipane and G. A. Settipane, "IgE and the Allergy-Asthma Connection in the 23-Year Follow Up of Brown University Students," *Allergy Asthma Proc* 21 (2000): 221–25.

14. NHS Estates, DH England, *A Matron's Charter: An Action Plan for Cleaner Hospitals* (Leeds: Department of Health, October 2004), www.dh.gov.uk/en/ Publication sandstatistics/ Publications/ PublicationsPolicyAndGuidance/DH_4091506.

15. E. S. Geller, "Actively Caring for the Environment: An Integration of Behaviorism and Humanism," *Environment and Behavior* 27, no. 2 (1995): 184–95; K. T. Huffman, W. F. Grossnickle, J. G. Cope, and K. P. Huffman, "Litter Reduction," *Environment and Behavior* 27 (1995): 153–83.

16. A. Thornton, "Survey of Public Attitudes to Quality of Life and to the Environment: Tracker Survey; A Report to the Department for Environment, Food and Rural Affairs" (London: DEFRA, 2009).

17. A. Kollmuss and J. Agyeman, "Mind the Gap: Why Do People Act Environmentally and What Are the Barriers to Pro-Environmental Behavior?" *Environmental Education Research* 8 (2002): 239–60.

18. The administration of the National Health Service in the United Kingdom is devolved into separate bodies for England, Scotland, Wales, and Northern Ireland.

19. Comptroller and Auditor General, "The Management and Control of Hospital Acquired Infection in Acute NHS Trusts in England" (London: National Audit Office, 2000).

20. National Audit Office, "Reducing Health Care Associated Infections in Hospitals in England," National Audit Office, June 2009, http://www.nao.org.uk/ publications/0809/reducing_healthcare_associated.aspx.

21. M. J. Berens, "*Tribune* Investigation: Unhealthy Hospitals/Infection Epidemic Carves Deadly Path; Poor Hygiene, Overwhelmed Workers Contribute to Thousands of Deaths," *Chicago Tribune,* July 21, 2002.

22. A. B. Zafar, L. A. Gaydos, W. B. Furlong, M. H. Nguyen et al., "Effectiveness of Infection Control Program in Controlling Nosocomial *Clostridrium difficile*," *Am J Infect Control* 26 (1998): 588–93.

23. S. J. Dancer, L. F. White, J. Lamb, E. K. Girvan et al., "Measuring the Effect of Enhanced Cleaning in a UK Hospital: A Prospective Cross-Over Study," *BMC Med* 7 (2009), http://www.ncbi.nlm.nih.gov/[doi]: 10.1186/1741-7015-7-28; P. Pina, P. Guezenec, S. Grosbuis, L. Guyot et al., "An *Acinetobacter baumannii* Outbreak at Versailles Hospital Center," *Pathologie Biologie* 16, no. 6 (2007): 385–94; A. Rampling, S. Wiseman, L. Davis, P. Hyett et al., "Evidence That Hospital Hygiene Is Important in the Control of Methicillin-Resistant *Staphyloccus aureus*," *Journal of Hospital Infection* 49 (2001): 109–16.

24. D. C. Shanson, "Hospital Infection," in *Microbiology in Clinical Practice*, 3rd ed. (Oxford: Butterworth-Heinemann, 1999), 431–36.

25. M. McCartney, "Are Superbug Fears Turning Patients into Hospital Cleaners?" *British Medical Journal* 338 (2009): 729.

26. Rampling et al., "Evidence That Hospital Hygiene Is Important," 112.

27. S. J. Dancer, "Mopping Up Hospital Infection," *Journal of Hospital Infection* 43 (1999): 85.

28. V. Smith, "The Body Beautiful," in *Clean*, 308–52.

29. McCartney, "Are Superbug Fears Turning Patients into Hospital Cleaners?" 729.

30. The derivation of "nosocomial" is from the Greek words *nosus* for disease and *komeion*, meaning to take care of. A term that should apply to any disease contracted under medical care has evolved to mean just those acquired in hospitals and is now used to denote only infection acquired within forty-eight to seventy-two hours of hospital admission. (Time limit definition varies between countries.)

31. National Audit Office, "The Management and Control of Hospital Acquired Infection in Acute NHS Trusts in England" (London: HMSO, February 2000); Centers for Disease Control, "Monitoring Hospital-Acquired Infections to Promote Patient Safety, United States, 1990–1999," *Mortality and Morbidity Weekly Report* 49, no. 8 (2000): 149–53, www.cdc.gov/mmwr/preview/mmwrhtml/mm4908a1.htm; H. Scott, "Hospital-Acquired Infection Rates Continue to Increase," *Br J Nursing* 13 (2004): 825.

32. Z. Kmietowicz, "Hospital Infection Rates in England Out of Control," *BMJ* 320 (2000): 534.

33. National Audit Office, Comptroller and Auditor General, "Improving Patient Care by Reducing the Risk of Hospital Acquired Infection: A Progress Report" (London: National Audit Office, 2005).

34. Department of Health, England, "Towards Cleaner Hospitals and Lower Rates of Infection: A Summary of Action," July 2004, http://www.dh.gov.uk/en/Publicationsandstatistics/Publications/PublicationsPolicyAndGuidance/DH_4085649, www.dh.gov.uk/en/Publicationsandstatistics/Publications.

35. Comptroller and Auditor General, "The Management and Control of Hospital Acquired Infection in Acute NHS Trusts in England" (London: National Audit Office, 2009).

36. Department of Health, "Towards Cleaner Hospitals."

37. D. Green, N. Wigglesworth, T. Keegan, and M. H. Wilcox, "Does Hospital Cleanliness Correlate with Methicillin-Resistant *Staphylococcus aureus* Bacteraemia Rates?" *Journal of Hospital Infection* 64, no. 2 (2006): 184–86.

38. Leeds Teaching Hospitals NHS Trust, *Infection Control Annual Report, 2006–7,* 6, http://www.leedsteachinghospitals.com.

39. C. J. Griffith, R. A. Cooper, C. Davies and M. Lewis, "An Evaluation of Hospital Cleaning Regimes and Standards," *Journal of Hospital Infection* 45, no. 1 (2000): 19–28.

40. House of Lords, "Infection Control," in *Seventh Report of the Committee on Science and Technology,* chap. 6 (London: HMSO, 1998), www.parliament.the-stationery-office.co.uk/pa/ld199798/ldselect/ldsctech/081vii/st0708.htm.

41. S. Davies, "Hospital Contract Cleaning and Infection Control: An Independent Report Commissioned by Unison" (London: Unison, January 2005).

42. " End Private Cleaning in NHS Call," http://news.bbc.co.uk/1/hi/health/7372992.stm.

43. G. Erickcek, S. Houseman, and A. Kalleberg, "The Effects of Temporary Services and Contracting Out on Low-Skilled Workers: Evidence from Auto-Suppliers, Hospitals, and Public Schools," in *Low-Wage American: How Employers Are Reshaping Opportunity in the Workplace,* ed. E. Appelbaum, A. Bernhardt, and R. J. Murnane (New York: Russell Sage Foundation, 2003), 368–406.

44. BBC on-line news, April 29, 2008, http://news.bbc.co.uk/1/hi/health/7372992.stm.

45. Dancer, "Mopping Up Hospital Infection," 85–100; Rampling et al., "Evidence That Hospital Hygiene Is Important," 109–16; G. L. French, J. A. Otter, K. P. Shannon, N. M. T. Adams, D. Watling, and M. J. Parks, "Tackling Contamination of the Hospital Environment by Methicillin-Resistant *Staphylococcus aureus* (MRSA): A Comparison between Conventional Terminal Cleaning and Hydrogen Peroxide Vapour Decontamination," *Journal of Hospital Infection* 57 (2004): 31–37.

46. BBC on-line news, 2008, http://news.bbc.co.uk/1/hi/health/7373595.stm.

47. W. Jensen, "Contracting Out Building Cleaning Services at the National Hospital of Denmark," Organisation for Economic Co-operation and Development (OECD), 1997.

48. S. Domberger, C. Hall, and E. Li, "The Determinants of Price and Quality in Competitively Tendered Contracts," *Economic Journal* 105 (1995): 1454–70.

49. S. Domberger and C. Hall, "Competitive Tendering for Domestic Services: A Comparative Study of Three Hospitals in New South Wales," Australian Government Publishing Service, 1995, 99–13.

50. PEAT report, cited in *Cleaners' Voices: Interviews with Hospital Cleaning Staff,* Unison Communications Unit, January 2005, www.unison.org.uk.

51. Patient Environment Action Teams (British NHS initiative), www.msnpsa.nhs.uk/peat.

52. Unison, *Cleaners' Voices.*

53. Scottish Executive, "The Watt Group Report: A Review of the Outbreak of Salmonella at the Victoria Infirmary, Glasgow, between December 2001 and January 2002 and Lessons That May Be Learned by Both the Victoria Infirmary and

the Wider NHS Family in Scotland," October 2002, http:/www.scotland.gov.uk/library5/health/twgr-00.asp.

54. Auditor General of Scotland, "A Clean Bill of Health? A Review of Domestic Services in Scottish Hospitals," *Audit Scotland* (April 2000), www.audit-scotland.gov.uk.

55. Auditor General for Wales, "The Management of Sickness Absence by NHS Trusts in Wales: Report by Auditor General for Wales," presented to the National Assembly on January 30, 2004, Cardiff.

56. M. Moore, "NHS Hospital Cleaning Firm Bosses Held for 'Blackmailing Illegal Staff,'" *Telegraph,* November 20, 2009, www.telegraph.co.uk/news/uknews/6609041/NHS-hospital-clean.

57. Quotations in this discussion are drawn from Unison, *Cleaner's Voices,* 6, 10–51.

58. Auditor General of Scotland, "Hospital Cleaning: Performance Audit," *Audit Scotland,* 2003, report no AGS/2003/2.

59. Unison, *Cleaner's Voices,* 19.

60. Ibid., 12.

61. V. Curtis, B. Kanki, S. Cousens, I. Diallo et al. "Evidence of Behaviour Change Following a Hygiene Promotion Programme in Burkino Faso," *Bulletin of the World Health Organization* 79 (2001): 518–27, esp. 525.

62. E. Innes, "A Matron's Charter: An Action Plan for Cleaner Hospitals," NHS Estates, DH England, 2004, 9.

63. Chief Medical Officer, England, "Winning Ways: Working Together to Reduce Healthcare Associated Infection in England," Department of Health, December 2003, www.doh.gov.uk/cmo.

3. What Goes without Saying in Patient Safety

1. Ashleigh Merritt and James Klinect, *Defensive Flying for Pilots: An Introduction to Threat and Error Management,* University of Texas Human Factors Research Project 1, LOSA Collaborative, December 12, 2006, http://www.google.com/search?hl=enandq=Threat+and+Error+ManagementandbtnG=Google+Search (accessed October 30, 2007).

2. John K. Lauber, foreword to *Cockpit Resource Management,* ed. Earl L. Weiner, Barbara G. Kanki, and Robert L. Helmreich (Amsterdam: Academic Press, 1993), xvii.

3. Ibid., xv.

4. Suzanne Gordon, interview, 2006.

5. Suzanne Gordon, *Nursing against the Odds: How Health Care Cost Cutting, Media Stereotypes, and Medical Hubris Undermine Nurses and Patient Care* (Ithaca: Cornell University Press, 2006), 30–42.

6. Suzanne Gordon, interview, 2005.

7. Bonnie O'Connor, participant observation, 2003.

8. Kenneth M. Ludmerer, *Time to Heal: American Medical Education from the Turn of the Century to the Era of Managed Care* (New York: Oxford University Press, 1999), 59.

9. Suzanne Gordon and Bonnie O'Connor, participant observation, 2007.

10. Deborah Tannen, *Gender and Discourse* (New York: Oxford University Press, 1994), 22–23.

11. Gordon, *Nursing against the Odds,* 36–54; M. Jeanne Peterson, *The Medical Profession in Mid-Victorian London* (Berkeley: University of California Press, 1978), 184–85.

12. *Times* (London), October 18, 1880, 9.

13. Suzanne Gordon, interview, 2006.

14. Jerome Groopman, *How Doctors Think* (Boston: Houghton Mifflin, 2007), 27–32, emphasis added.

15. Ibid., 32.

16. B. O'Connor, "The Home Birth Movement in the United States," *Journal of Medicine and Philosophy* 18, no. 2 (1993): 147–74.

17. Suzanne Gordon, interview, 2007.

18. An excellent example of this dynamic is found in Thetis M. Group and Joan I. Roberts, *Nursing, Physician Control, and the Medical Monopoly: Historical Perspectives on Gendered Inequality in Roles, Rights, and Range of Practice* (Bloomington: Indiana University Press, 2001).

19. Jacqueline Fawcett, "Nursing qua Nursing: The Connection between Nursing Knowledge and Nursing Shortages," *Journal of Advanced Nursing* 59, no. 1 (2007): 97–99.

20. Sioban Nelson and Suzanne Gordon, *Complexities of Care: Nursing Reconsidered* (Ithaca: Cornell University Press). See American Nurses Association logo for Nurses' Week 2006, with a heart in a hand.

21. Suzanne Gordon, interview, 2000.

22. Suzanne Gordon, interview, 2007.

23. Suzanne Gordon, interview, 2002.

24. Bonnie O'Connor, participant observation, 2000.

25. Bonnie O'Connor, participant observations, 2006–7.

26. Bonnie O'Connor, participant observation, 2010.

27. Lee Ann Runy, "Patient Handoffs," *Hospitals and Health Care News,* http://www.hhnmag.com/hhnmag_app/jsp/articledisplay.jsp?dcrpath=HHNMAG/Article/data/05MAY2008/0805HHN_FEA_Gatefoldanddomain=HHNMAG (accessed November 4, 2010); http://www.ihi.org/IHI/Programs/AudioAndWeb Programs/Effective+Teamwork+as+a+Care+Strategy+SBAR+and+Other+Too ls+for+Improving+Communication+Between+Careg.htm (accessed October 21, 2007).

28. Bonnie O'Connor, participant observation, 2007.

29. Bonnie O'Connor, participant observation, 2007.

30. Suzanne Gordon, interview, 2007.

31. Alan H. Rosenstein. "Nurse-Physician Relationships: Impact on Nurse Satisfaction and Retention," *American Journal of Nursing* 102, no. 6 (2002): 26–34.

32. Suzanne Gordon, interview, 2003.

33. Rosenstein, "Nurse-Physician Relationships."

34. J. Bryan Sexton, Eric J. Thomas, and Robert L. Helmreich, "Error, Stress, and Teamwork in Medicine and Aviation: Cross-Sectional Surveys," *British Medical Journal* 320 (2000): 745–46.

35. Ibid.

36. Gordon, interview, 2007.

37. Sexton, Thomas, and Helmreich, "Error, Stress, and Teamwork."

38. David M. Musson and Robert L. Helmreich, "Team Training and Resource Management in Health Care: Current Issues and Future Directions," *Harvard Health Policy Review* 5, no. 1 (2004): 33.

39. TeamSTEPPS, http://teamstepps.ahrq.gov/ (accessed September 20, 2010).

4. Health Care Information Technology to the Rescue

1. A. Jha et al., "Use of Electronic Health Records in U.S. Hospitals," *N. Engl. J. Med.* 360 (2009): 1628; M. Buntin et al., "The Benefits of Health Information Technology: A Review of the Recent Literature Shows Predominantly Positive Results," *Health Aff* 30 (2011): 464e71.

2. J Sarasohn-Kahn. "Industry Predictions: What Are the Drivers Shaping Health Care IT in 2009?" I-Health, Publication of the California Healthcare Foundation, Dec. 22, 2008; D. Bates, R. Kaushal, and D. Shojania, "Effects of Computerized Physician Order Entry and Clinical Decision Support Systems on Medication Safety: A Systematic Review," *Arch. Int. Med.* 163 (2003): 1409–16.

3. Jha et al., "Use of Electronic Records"; D. Bates, "Physicians and Ambulatory Electronic Health Records," *Health Affairs* 24 (2005): 1180–89.

4. Bridges to Excellence, http://www.bridgestoexcellence.org. (accessed March 16, 2007).

5. Doctor's Office Quality–Information Technology, http://www.qualitynet. org/dcs/ContentServer?cid=1143577170595&pagename=QnetPublic%2FPage%2 FQnetTier2&c=Page (accessed March 16, 2007).

6. Healthcare Information and Management Systems Society, http://www. himssconference.org (accessed May 13, 2011).

7. R. Koppel et al., "Workarounds to Barcode Medication Administration Systems: Their Occurrences, Causes, and Threats to Patient Safety," *Journal of the American Medical Informatics Association* (*JAMIA*) 15 (2008): 408–23; B-T Karsh et al., "Health Information Technology: Fallacies and Sober Realities," *JAMIA* 17 (2010): 617–23; Jha et al., "Use of Electronic Health Records"; Bates, Kaushal, and Shojania, "Effects of Computerized Physician Order"; J. Ash, Z. Stavri, and G. Kuperman, "A Consensus Statement on Considerations for a Successful CPOE Implementation," *JAMIA* 10 (2003): 229–34; A. Bobb et al., "The Epidemiology of Prescribing Errors: The Potential Impact of Computerized Prescriber Order Entry," *Arch. Int. Med.* 164 (2007): 785–92; D. Bates et al., "Reducing the Frequency of Errors in Medicine Using Information Technology," *JAMIA* 8 (2001): 299–308; D. Bates and A. Gawande, "Patient Safety: Improving Safety with Information Technology," *N. Engl. J. Med.* 348 (2003): 2526–34; "Executive Order: Promoting Quality and Efficient Health Care in Federal Government Administered or Sponsored Health Care Programs," the White House, Washington, D.C., August 22, 2006, http://www. whitehouse.gov/news/releases/2006/08/20060822–2.html (accessed May 24, 2007); R. Berger and J. Kichak, "Computerized Physician Order Entry: Helpful or Harmful?" *JAMIA* 11 (2004): 100–103; S. Rosenfeld, C. Bernasek, and D. Mendelson, "Medicare's Next Voyage: Encouraging Physicians to Adopt Health Information Technology," *Health Affairs* 24 (2005): 1138–46; R. Hillestad et al., "Can Electronic Medical Record Systems Transform Health Care? Potential Health Benefits, Savings, and Costs," *Health Affairs* 24 (2005): 1103–17; J. Walker et al., "The Value of Health Care Information Exchange and Interoperability," *Health Affairs Web Exclusive* (2005):

W5–10—W5–18; J. Leviss et al., eds., *H.I.T. or Miss: Lessons Learned from Health Information Technology Implementations* (Chicago: AHIMA Press, 2009).

8. D. Aycock, A. Prasad, and B. Stiber, "A Strategy for Cerner Corporation to Address the HIT Stimulus Plan" (2009), available in "Duke University Fuqua School of Business: Past Papers," students of Professor David Ridley, http://www.ischool.drexel.edu/faculty/ssilverstein/Aycock-Prasad-Stiber-Cerner-2009.pdf (accessed May 13, 2011).

9. Jha et al., "Use of Electronic Records," Centers for Disease Control and Prevention, National Center for Health Statistics, http://www.cdc.gov/nchs/data/hestat/emr_ehr_09/emr_ehr_09.htm (accessed September 20, 2011); American Hospital Association, AHA Annual Survey Database Fiscal Year 2009, http://www.ahadata.com/ahadata/html/AHASurvey.html (accessed September 20, 2011).

10. B-T Karsh et al., "Health Information Technology: Fallacies and Sober Realities"; Leviss et al., "H.I.T. or Miss."

11. B-T Karsh et al., "Health Information Technology: Fallacies and Sober Realities"; J. Sidorov, "It Ain't Necessarily So: The Electronic Health Record and the Unlikely Prospect of Reducing Health Care Costs," *Health Affairs* 25 (July–August 2006): 4, 1079–85; W. Welch et al., "Electronic Health Records in Four Community Physician Practices: Impact on Quality and Cost of Care," *JAMIA* 14 (2007): 320–28; J. Linder et al., "Electronic Health Record Use and the Quality of Ambulatory Care in the United States," *Arch. Int. Med.* 167 (2007): 1400–1405.

12. E. Shortliffe, "Strategic Action in Health Information Technology: Why the Obvious Has Taken So Long," *Health Affairs* 24 (2005): 1222–33.

13. B. Chaudhry et al., "A Systematic Review: Impact of Health Information Technology on Quality, Efficiency, and Costs of Medical Care," *Ann. Intern. Med.* 144 (2006): 742–52.

14. Ibid., 748.

15. Ibid.

16. K. Mandl and I. Kohane, "No Small Change for the Health Information Economy," *N. Engl. J. Med.* 360 (2009): 1278–81.

17. M. Harrison, R. Koppel, and S. Bar-Lev, "Unintended Consequences of Information Technologies in Health Care: An Interactive Sociotechnical Analysis," *JAMIA* 14 (2007): 542–49.

18. Jha et al., "Use of Electronic Records"; J. Aarts and R. Koppel, "Implementing CPOE in American, European, and Australian Hospitals: Lessons from Differing Social, Economic, Governance, and Workplace Environments," *Health Affairs* 28 (March–April 2009): 404–14.

19. B-T Karsh et al., "Health Information Technology: Fallacies and Sober Realities"; Leviss et al., "H.I.T. or Miss."

20. R. Koppel et al., "Role of Computerized Physician Order Entry Systems in Facilitating Medication Errors," *JAMA* 293 (2005): 1197–1203.

21. Ibid.

22. Ibid.

23. Y. Han et al., "Unexpected Increased Mortality after Implementation of a Commercially Sold Computerized Physician Order Entry System," *Pediatrics* 116 (2005): 1506–12; Leviss et al., "H.I.T. or Miss."

24. J. Nebeker et al., "High Rates of Adverse Drug Events in a Highly Computerized Hospital," *Arch. Int. Med.* (2005): 1111–16.

25. R. Shulman et al., "Medication Errors: A Prospective Cohort Study of Hand-Written and Computerised Physician Order Entry in the Intensive Care Unit," *Critical Care* (2005): R516–R521.

26. J. Ash et al., "The Extent and Importance of Unintended Consequences of Computerized Physician Order Entry," *JAMIA* 14 (2007): 415–23; E. Campbell et al., "Types of Unintended Consequences Related to Computerized Provider Order Entry," *J. Am. Med. Info. Assoc.* 13 (2006): 547–56; J. Aarts, J. Ash, and M. Berg, "Extending the Understanding of Computerized Physician Order Entry: Implications for Professional Collaboration, Workflow and Quality of Care," *Int. J. Med. Inf.* 76 (2007): S4–13.

27. D. Bates, "Computerized Physician Order Entry and Medication Errors: Finding a Balance," *J. of Biomedical Informatics* 38 (2005): 259–61.

28. Ibid., 260.

29. C. Nemeth and R. Cook, "Hiding in Plain Sight: What Koppel et al. Tell Us about Healthcare IT," *J. of Biomedical Informatics* 38 (2005): 262–63.

30. Ibid., 262.

31. R. Koppel, "Defending Computerized Physician Order Entry from Its Supporters," *J. Manage. Care* 12 (2006): 369–70; R. Koppel, "What Do We Know about Medication Errors Made via a CPOE System versus Those Made via Handwritten Orders?" *Journal of Critical Care* 9 (2005): 427–28.

32. Ash et al., "Exploring the Unintended Consequences"; Campbell et al., "Types of Unintended Consequences"; Aarts, Ash, and Berg, "Extending the Understanding."

33. Ash et al., "Extent and Importance of Unintended Consequences"; Campbell et al., "Types of Unintended Consequences"; Aarts, Ash, and Berg, "Extending the Understanding."

34. Harrison et al., "Unintended Consequences of Information."

35. J. Metzger et al., "Mixed Results in the Safety Performance of Computerized Physician Order Entry," *Health Affairs* 29 (2010): 655–63.

36. Koppel et al., "Role of Computerized."

37. Koppel et al., Workarounds to Barcode Medication."

38. I-Healthbeat.Org, http://www.ihealthbeat.org/ (accessed October 10, 2010).

39. "Contemporary Issues in Medical Informatics: Common Examples of Healthcare Information Technology Difficulties," http://www.ischool.drexel.edu/faculty/ssilverstein/failurecases (accessed May 13, 2011).

40. Leviss et al. "H.I.T or Miss."

41. J. Demakis et al., "Improving Residents' Compliance with Standards of Ambulatory Care: Results from the VA Cooperative Study on Computerized Reminders," *JAMA* 284 (2000): 1411–16.

42. Koppel et al., "Workarounds to Barcode Medication."

6. Excluded Actors in Patient Safety

1. Nurses' names are fictitious.

2. Interview with Beth Jones, April 16, 2008.

3. Interview with Rick Brooks, August 27, 2008.

4. J. S. Carroll and Amy C. Edmondson, "Leading Organizational Learning in Health Care," *Quality Safe Health Care* 11 (2002): 51–56; Amy C. Edmondson,

"Learning from Failure in Health Care: Frequent Opportunities, Pervasive Barriers," *Quality Safe Health Care* 13 (2004): 3–9.

5. Carroll and Edmondson, "Leading Organizational Learning," 54.

6. Edmondson, "Learning from Failure," 6.

7. Interview with Carol Porter, September 15, 2009.

8. Ibid.

9. Edmondson, "Learning from Failure," 5.

10. Irene Jansen and Janice Murray, "Environmental Cleaning and Health-care-Associated Infections," *Healthcare Papers* 9 (March 2009): 38–43, http://www.longwoods.com/product.php?productid=20925 (accessed December 29, 2009).

11. Interview with Dan Zuberi, May 3, 2010.

12. Ibid.

13. Rosalind Stanwell-Smith, "Hard Work: Life in Low-Pay Britain," *Journal of the Royal Society of Medicine* 96 (June 2003): 307–8.

14. Institute for Health Care Improvement website, http://www.ihi.org/ihi (accessed May 18, 2009).

15. Edmondson, "Learning from Failure," 5.

16. Interview with Dr. George Thibault, August 27, 2008.

17. Debra Draper, Laurie Felland, Alison Liebhaber, and Lori Melichar, "The Role of Nurses in Hospital Quality Improvement," *HSC* 3 (March 2008): 7.

18. Krishna Collie, memo, September 4, 2009.

19. Interview with Ross Koppel, February 8, 2010.

20. Anita L. Tucker and Amy C. Edmondson, "Why Hospitals Don't Learn from Failures: Organizational and Psychological Dynamics That Inhibit System Change," *California Management Review* 45, no. 2 (2003): 55–72.

21. John le Carré, *Absolute Friends* (Boston: Little, Brown, 2003), 273.

22. David Dickinson, *Changing the Course of AIDS: Peer Education in South Africa and Its Lessons for the Global Crisis* (Ithaca: Cornell University Press, 2009).

23. Erving Goffman, *The Presentation of Self in Everyday Life* (New York: Double-day Anchor, 1959), 17–76.

24. Interview with union leader; interview with Diane Sommers, April 6, 2007.

25. Quoted in Stanwell-Smith, "Hard Work," 308.

26. Suzanne Gordon, Patrick Mendenhall, and Bonnie O'Connor, "Come Fly With Me," unpublished manuscript.

27. Interview with staff nurse at a Massachusetts hospital, November 15, 2008.

28. John Hagel III, John Seely Brown, and Lang Davison, "The 2009 Shift Index Measuring the Forces of Long-Term Change," Deloitte Center for the Edge, 2009.

29. Christopher P. Nemeth, *Improving Healthcare Team Communication: Building on Lessons from Aviation and Aerospace* (Aldershot: Ashgate, 2008).

30. Interview with Keith Hagy, director of engineering and aerospace safety, ALPA, May 5, 2008.

31. Ibid.

32. The Committee for Interns and Residents (CIR) is a member of SEIU (Service Employees International Union).

33. Gordon, Mendenhall, and O'Connor, "Come Fly With Me."

34. Suzanne Gordon, "More on Texas," http://www.suzannegordon.com/?m=201002 (accessed February 24, 2010).

35. Interview with the director of labor relations at a northeastern hospital, April 23, 2009.

36. Peter Lazes, Donna Havens, and Pete Carlson, "Engaging Front-Line Staff: How Are They Engaged in Change Work?" paper presented at the Sloan Industry Studies Conference, June 15, 2009.

37. Ibid.

38. For a fuller discussion, see Mike Rose, *The Mind at Work: Valuing the Intelligence of the American Worker* (New York: Penguin, 2005).

39. Interview with Kamilla Kohn Radberg, October 14, 2009.

40. Interview with nurse at a northeastern teaching hospital, June 13, 2009.

41. Draper, Felland, Liebhaber, and Melichar, "Role of Nurses in Hospital Quality Improvement," 4.

42. Ibid., 5.

43. Interview with the CNO at a northeastern teaching hospital, February 8, 2008.

44. Suzanne Gordon, "Institutional Obstacles to RN Unionization: How 'Vote No' Thinking Is Deeply Embedded in the Nursing Profession," Working USA 12, no. 2 (2009): 279–97.

45. Interview with supervisor, Lutheran Medical Center, Brooklyn, N.Y., January 19, 2009.

46. Interview, March 4, 2009.

47. Interview with unit manager, Lutheran Medical Center, Brooklyn, N.Y., January 19, 2009.

48. Interview with a physician at a Massachusetts teaching hospital, March 9, 2009.

49. Interview with a staff nurse and union representative at a Massachusetts hospital, July 5, 2009.

50. Interview with Cathy Stoddart, January 13, 2009.

51. Interview with David Schildmeier, director of communications, Massachusetts Nurses Association, May 19, 2008.

52. Ibid.

53. Interview with Michael Chacon, March 24, 2008.

54. Interview with Janet McCarthy, September 20, 2009.

55. Suzanne Gordon, John Buchanan, and Tanya Bretherton, *Safety in Numbers: Nurse-to-Patient Ratios and the Future of Health Care* (Ithaca: Cornell University Press, 2008).

56. Interview with Neal Bisno, president of SEIU Healthcare Pennsylvania, September 21, 2009.

57. Interview with Rick Brooks, August 27, 2008.

58. Interview with Alison Trinkoff, March 15, 2009.

59. Interview with Maimonides Medical Center's NYSNA representative, July 20, 2010.

60. All quotations are from Rajiv Jain et al. "Veterans Affairs Initiative to Prevent Methicillin-Resistant *Staphylococcus aureus* Infections," *New England Journal of Medicine* 364, no. 15 (2011): 1419.

61. Robert Reich, *The Work of Nations: Preparing Ourselves for 21st Century Capitalism* (New York: Vintage, 1992).

7. Nursing as Patient Safety Net

1. Shizuko Y. Fagerhaugh et al., *Hazards in Hospital Care: Ensuring Patient Safety* (San Francisco: Jossey-Bass, 1987).

2. Carl-Ardy Dubois, Martin McKee, and Ellen Nolte, eds., *Human Resources for Health in Europe* (Maidenhead: Open University Press, 2006).

3. Lucian L. Leape et al., "Promoting Patient Safety by Preventing Medical Error," *Journal of the American Medical Association* (hereafter *JAMA*) 280 (1998): 1444–47.

4. Institute of Medicine, *To Err Is Human: Building a Safer Health System* (Washington, D.C.: National Academy Press, 1999).

5. See www.ihi.org for specifics.

6. Sean P. Clarke, Carol Raphael, and Joanne Disch, "Challenges and Directions for Nursing in the Pay-for-Performance Movement," *Policy, Politics, and Nursing Practice* 9, no. 2 (2008): 127–34.

7. E. Carol Polifroni, John McNulty, and Lynn Allchin, "Medication Errors: More Basic Than a System Issue," *Journal of Nursing Education* 42, no. 10 (2003): 455–58.

8. Michael I. Harrison, Ross Koppel, and Shirly Bar-Lev, "Unintended Consequences of Information Technologies in Health Care: An Interactive Sociotechnical Analysis," *Journal of the American Medical Informatics Association* 14 (2005): 542–49; Ross Koppel et al., "Role of Computerized Physician Order Entry Systems in Facilitating Medication Errors," *JAMA* 293 (2005): 1197–1203; Ross Koppel et al., "Workarounds to Barcode Administration Systems: Their Occurrences, Causes, and Threats to Patient Safety," *Journal of the American Medical Informatics Association* 15 (2008): 408–23.

9. Linda Perlstein, *Tested: One American School Struggles to Make the Grade* (New York: Holt, 2007).

10. Robin Youngson, "Improving Quality: Leadership and Culture Change," New Zealand Ministry of Health, http://www.newhealth.govt.nz/epiqual/publications/improvingquality.pdf (accessed May 15, 2011).

11. David Ganz et al., "The Effect of a Quality Improvement Initiative on the Quality of Other Aspects of Health Care: The Law of Unintended Consequences?" *Medical Care* 45, no. 1 (2007): 8–18.

12. Diana J. Mason, "Unintended Consequences," *American Journal of Nursing* 108, no. 4 (2008): 7.

13. Lillee S. Gelinas and David Y.-H. Loh, "The Effect of Workforce Issues on Patient Safety," *Nursing Economics* 22, no. 5 (2004): 266–72, 279.

14. Sean P. Clarke, "Failure to Rescue: Lessons from Missed Opportunities in Care," *Nursing Inquiry* 11, no. 2 (2004): 67–71; Sean P. Clarke and Linda H. Aiken, "Failure to Rescue," *American Journal of Nursing* 103, no. 1 (2003): 42–47; Sean P. Clarke and Linda H. Aiken, "Failure to Rescue," in *Nursing Leadership: A Concise Encyclopedia,* ed. Harriet R. Feldman (New York: Springer, 2008), 224–25.

15. Nicola Cooper, Kirsty Forrest, and Paul Cramp, "Patients at Risk," in *Essential Guide to Acute Care,* ed. Nicola Cooper, Kirsty Forrest, and Paul Cramp, (Malden, Mass.: Blackwell, 2006), 1–13.

16. Michael Buist and Rinaldo Bellomo, "MET: The Medical Emergency Team or the Medical Education Team?" *Critical Care and Resuscitation* 6 (2004): 88–91.

17. Corinne Grimes et al., "Developing Rapid Response Teams: Best Practices through Collaboration," *Clinical Nurse Specialist* 21, no. 2 (2007): 85–92.

18. Linda H. Aiken, Sean P. Clarke, and Douglas M. Sloane, "Hospital Restructuring: Does It Adversely Affect Care and Outcomes?" *Journal of Health and Human Service Administration* 23, no. 4 (2001): 416–40.

19. Daniel Allen, "Wisdom from Tragedy," *Nursing Standard* 20, no. 52 (2006): 16–19.

20. Linda H. Aiken et al., "Hospital Nurse Staffing and Patient Mortality, Nurse Burnout, and Job Dissatisfaction," *JAMA* 288 (2002): 1987–93; Linda H. Aiken et al., "Education Levels of Hospital Nurses and Surgical Patient Mortality," *JAMA* 290 (2003): 1617–23; Jack Needleman, "Nurse Staffing Levels and the Quality of Care in Hospitals," *New England Journal of Medicine* 346 (2002): 1715–22.

21. Paul S. Chan et al., "Delayed Time to Defibrillation after In-Hospital Cardiac Arrest," *New England Journal of Medicine* 358 (2008): 9–17; Mary Ann Peberdy et al., "Survival from In-Hospital Cardiac Arrest during Nights and Weekends," *JAMA* 299, no. 7 (2008): 785–92.

22. Clarke and Aiken, "Failure to Rescue."

23. "Determination by Sheriff I. G. McColl in Respect of the Inquiry into the Death of Marlene Patricia Wightman," Sheriffdom of Lothian and Borders at Edinburgh, 2009, http://www.scotcourts.gov.uk/opinions/wightman.html (accessed May 15, 2011).

24. Kaiser Permanente of Colorado, "SBAR Technique for Communication: A Situational Briefing Model," Institute for Healthcare Improvement, http://www.ihi.org/IHI/Topics/PatientSafety/SafetyGeneral/Tools/SBARTechniqueforCommunicationASituationalBriefingModel.htm (accessed May 15, 2011).

25. Annie Chellel, Debbie Higgs, and Julie Scholes, "An Evaluation of the Contribution of Critical Care Outreach to the Clinical Management of the Critically Ill Ward Patient in Two Acute NHS Trusts," *Nursing in Critical Care* 11, no. 1 (2006): 42–51.

26. Bradford D. Winters, Julius Pham, and Peter J. Pronovost, "Rapid Response Teams: Walk, Don't Run," *JAMA* 296 (2006): 1645–48.

27. Paul S. Chan et al., "Rapid Response Teams: A Systematic Review and Meta-Analysis," *Archives of Internal Medicine* 170, no. 1 (2010): 18–26.

28. Institute of Medicine, *Crossing the Quality Chasm: A New Health System for the 21st Century* (Washington, D.C.: National Academies Press, 2001); Institute of Medicine, *Keeping Patients Safe: Transforming the Work Environments of Nurses* (Washington, D.C.: National Academies Press, 2004).

29. Institute of Medicine, *Crossing the Quality Chasm.*

30. Institute of Medicine, *Keeping Patients Safe.*

31. Sean P. Clarke and Nancy E. Donaldson, "Nurse Staffing and Patient Care Quality and Safety," in *Patient Safety and Quality: An Evidence-Based Handbook for Nurses,* AHRQ Publication no. 08–0043 (Rockville, Md.: Agency for Healthcare Research and Quality, 2008), http://www.ahrq.gov/qual/nurseshdbk/ (accessed May 15, 2011); Robert L. Kane et al., *Nursing Staffing and Quality of Patient Care,* Evidence Report/Technology Assessment no. 151 (Rockville, Md.: Agency for Healthcare Research and Quality, 2007).

32. Sean P. Clarke, "Staffing the Organization for Excellence," in *From Front Office to Front Line: Essential Issues for Health Care Leaders* (Oakbrook Terrace, Ill.: Joint Commission on Accreditation of Healthcare Organizations, 2005), 113–44.

33. Suzanne Gordon, John Buchanan, and Tanya Bretherton, *The Perfect Number? Nurse-To-Patient Ratios and the Future of Health Care* (Ithaca: Cornell University Press, 2008).

34. Gelinas and Loh, "The Effect of Workforce Issues."

35. Sean P. Clarke, "Research on Nurse Staffing and Its Outcomes: The Challenges and Risks of Grasping at Shadows," in *The Complexities Of Care: Nursing Reconsidered,* ed. Sioban Nelson and Suzanne Gordon (Ithaca: Cornell University Press, 2006), 161–84.

36. Virginia S. Cleland, *The Economics of Nursing* (Norwalk, Conn.: Appleton and Lange, 1990).

37. Anita L. Tucker, "The Impact of Operational Failures on Hospital Nurses and Their Patients," *Journal of Operations Management* 22 (2004): 151–69; Anita L. Tucker and Steven J. Spear, "Operational Failures and Interruptions in Hospital Nursing," *Health Services Research* 41, no. 3, pt. 1 (2006): 643–62.

38. Sean P. Clarke, "Nurse Staffing in Acute Care Settings: Research Perspectives and Practice Implications," *Joint Commission Journal on Quality and Patient Safety* 33, no. 11, Supplement (2007): 30–44.

39. Sue Kirk et al., "Evaluating Safety Culture," in *Patient Safety: Research into Practice,* ed. Kieran Walshe and Ruth Boaden (Berkshire: Open University Press, 2006), 173–84.

40. Ibid.

8. Physicians, Sleep Deprivation, and Safety

1. Institute of Medicine, *To Err Is Human: Building a Safer Health System,* ed. L. T. Kohn, J. M. Corrigan, and M. S. Donaldson (Washington, D.C.: National Academy Press, 1999).

2. C. P. Landrigan et al., "Interns' Compliance with Accreditation Council for Graduate Medical Education Work-Hour Limits," *Journal of the American Medical Association* (hereafter *JAMA*) 296 (2006): 1063–70; C. P. Landrigan et al., "Effects of the Accreditation Council for Graduate Medical Education Duty Hour Limits on Sleep, Work Hours, and Safety," *Pediatrics* 122 (2008): 250–58.

3. I. Philibert, "Sleep Loss and Performance in Residents and Nonphysicians: a Meta-Analytic Examination," *Sleep* 28 (2005): 1392–1402; C. P. Landrigan et al., "Effect of Reducing Interns' Work Hours on Serious Medical Errors in Intensive Care Units," *New England Journal of Medicine* (hereafter *N. Engl. J. Med.*) 351 (2004): 1838–48; S. W. Lockley et al., "Effect of Reducing Interns' Weekly Work Hours on Sleep and Attentional Failures," *N. Engl. J. Med* 351 (2004): 1829–37; L. K. Barger et al., "Extended Work Shifts and the Risk of Motor Vehicle Crashes among Interns," *N. Engl. J. Med.* 352 (2005): 125–34; N. T. Ayas et al., "Extended Work Duration and the Risk of Self-Reported Percutaneous Injuries in Interns," *JAMA* 296 (2006): 1055–62; Institute of Medicine of the National Academies, *Resident Duty Hours: Enhancing Sleep, Supervision, and Safety,* ed. C. Ulmer, D. M. Wolman, and M. M. E. Johns (Washington, D.C.: National Academies Press, 2008), 1–322.

4. Institute of Medicine of the National Academies, *Resident Duty Hours.*

5. Landrigan et al., "Interns' Compliance with Accreditation Council"; Landrigan et al., "Effects of the Accreditation Council."

6. British Medical Association, "Time's Up: A Guide on the EWTD for Junior Doctors," 2004, http://www.bma.org.uk/.

7. J. Rasmussen and A. Jensen, "Mental Procedures in Real-Life Tasks: A Case Study of Electronic Trouble Shooting," *Ergonomics* 17 (1974): 293–307.

8. Landrigan et al., "Interns' Compliance with Accreditation Council."

9. Institute of Medicine, *To Err Is Human.*

10. J. Reason, *Human Error* (Cambridge: Cambridge University Press, 1990).

11. A. E. Rogers et al., "The Working Hours of Hospital Staff Nurses and Patient Safety," *Health Aff.* (Millwood) 23 (2004): 202–12.

12. Ibid.

13. H. Babkoff, T. Caspy, and M. Mikulincer, "Subjective Sleepiness Ratings: The Effects of Sleep Deprivation, Circadian Rhythmicity and Cognitive Performance," *Sleep* 14 (1991): 534–39; D. J. Dijk, J. F. Duffy, and C. A. Czeisler, "Circadian and Sleep/Wake Dependent Aspects of Subjective Alertness and Cognitive Performance," *Journal of Sleep Research* 1 (1992): 112–17; M. P. Johnson et al., "Short-Term Memory, Alertness and Performance: A Reappraisal of Their Relationship to Body Temperature," *Journal of Sleep Research* 1 (1992): 24–29; W. P. Colquhoun, P. Hamilton, and R. S. Edwards, "Effects of Circadian Rhythm, Sleep Deprivation, and Fatigue on Watchkeeping Performance during the Night Hours," in *Experimental Studies of Shiftwork,* ed. P. Colquhoun et al. (Opladen: Westdeutscher Verlag, 1975), 20–28; G. Hildebrandt, W. Rohmert, and J. Rutenfranz, "The Influence of Fatigue and Rest Period on the Circadian Variation of Error Frequency in Shift Workers (Engine Drivers)," in Colquhoun et al., *Experimental Studies of Shiftwork,* 174–87.

14. J. E. Fröberg et al., "Circadian Rhythms of Catecholamine Excretion, Shooting Range Performance and Self-Ratings of Fatigue during Sleep Deprivation," *Biological Psychology* 2 (1975): 175–88; T. Åkerstedt and J. E. Fröberg, "Psychophysiological Circadian Rhythms in Women during 72 h of Sleep Deprivation," *Waking and Sleeping* 1 (1977): 387–94; T. Åkerstedt and M. Gillberg, "Effects of Sleep Deprivation on Memory and Sleep Latencies in Connection with Repeated Awakenings from Sleep," *Psychophysiology* 16 (1979): 49–52; T. Åkerstedt et al., "Melatonin Excretion, Body Temperature and Subjective Arousal during 64 Hours of Sleep Deprivation," *Psychoneuroendocrinology* 4 (1979): 219–25; G. S. Richardson et al., "Circadian Variation of Sleep Tendency in Elderly and Young Adult Subjects," *Sleep* 5 (1982): S82–S94; J. K. Wyatt et al., "Circadian Temperature and Melatonin Rhythms, Sleep, and Neurobehavioral Function in Humans Living on a 20-h Day," *American Journal of Physiology: Regulatory, Integrative, and Comparative Physiology* 277 (1999): R1152–R1163.

15. D. C. Klein, R. Y. Moore, and S. M. Reppert, *Suprachiasmatic Nucleus: The Mind's Clock* (New York: Oxford University Press, 1991).

16. Dijk, Duffy, and Czeisler, "Circadian and Sleep/Wake Dependent Aspects"; Johnson et al., "Short-Term Memory, Alertness and Performance"; C. A. Czeisler, D. J. Dijk, and J. F. Duffy, "Entrained Phase of the Circadian Pacemaker Serves to Stabilize Alertness and Performance throughout the Habitual Waking Day," in *Sleep Onset: Normal and Abnormal Processes,* ed. R. D. Ogilvie and J. R. Harsh (Washington, D.C.: American Psychological Association, 1994), 89–110; C. A. Czeisler et al., "Stability, Precision, and Near-24-Hour Period of the Human Circadian Pacemaker," *Science* 284 (1999): 2177–81; M. A. Carskadon et al., "Intrinsic Circadian Period of

Adolescent Humans Measured in Conditions of Forced Desynchrony," *Neuroscience Letters* 260 (1999): 129–32; M. A. Carskadon and W. C. Dement, "Sleep Studies on a 90-Minute Day," *Electroencephalography and Clinical Neurophysiology* 39 (1975): 145–55; M. Carskadon and W. Dement, "Sleepiness and Sleep State on a 90-Min Schedule," *Physchophysiology* 14 (1977): 127–33.

17. Czeisler et al., "Stability, Precision"; Carskadon et al., "Intrinsic Circadian Period"; D. G. M. Beersma and A. E. Hiddinga, "No Impact of Physical Activity on the Period of the Circadian Pacemaker in Humans," *Chronobiology International* 15 (1998): 49–57; E. B. Klerman et al., "Simulations of Light Effects on the Human Circadian Pacemaker: Implications for Assessment of Intrinsic Period," *American Journal of Physiology* 270 (1996): R271–R82; S. S. Campbell, D. Dawson, and J. Zulley, "When the Human Circadian System Is Caught Napping: Evidence for Endogenous Rhythms Close to 24 Hours," *Sleep* 16 (1993): 638–640.

18. Dijk, Duffy, and Czeisler, "Circadian and Sleep/Wake Dependent Aspects"; Johnson et al., "Short-Term Memory, Alertness and Performance"; Czeisler, Dijk, and Duffy, "Entrained Phase of the Circadian Pacemaker"; Carskadon et al., "Intrinsic Circadian Period"; M. E. Jewett, "Models of Circadian and Homeostatic Regulation of Human Performance and Alertness" (Ph.D. diss., Harvard University, 1997), 1–276; D. J. Dijk et al., "Variation of Electroencephalographic Activity during Non-Rapid Eye Movement and Rapid Eye Movement Sleep with Phase of Circadian Melatonin Rhythm in Humans," *J. Physiol.* (London) 505, no. 3 (1997): 851–58.

19. C. A. Czeisler, "Human Circadian Physiology: Internal Organization of Temperature, Sleep-Wake, and Neuroendocrine Rhythms Monitored in an Environment Free of Time Cues" (Ph.D. diss., Stanford University, 1978), 1–346; C. A. Czeisler et al., "Human Sleep: Its Duration and Organization Depend on Its Circadian Phase," *Science* 210 (1980): 1264–67; S. H. Strogatz, R. E. Kronauer, and C. A. Czeisler, "Circadian Pacemaker Interferes with Sleep Onset at Specific Times Each Day: Role in Insomnia," *American Journal of Physiology* 253 (1987): R172–R78; S. H. Strogatz, R. E. Kronauer, and C. A. Czeisler, "Circadian Regulation Dominates Homeostatic Control of Sleep Length and Prior Wake Length in Humans," *Sleep* 9 (1986): 353–64; D. J. Dijk and C. A. Czeisler, "Contribution of the Circadian Pacemaker and the Sleep Homeostat to Sleep Propensity, Sleep Structure, Electroencephalographic Slow Waves, and Sleep Spindle Activity in Humans," *Journal of Neuroscience* 15 (1995): 3526–38.

20. W. P. Colquhoun, P. Hamilton, and R. S. Edwards, "Effects of Circadian Rhythm, Sleep Deprivation, and Fatigue on Watchkeeping Performance during the Night Hours," in P. Colquhoun, S. Folkard, P. Knauth, and J. Rutenfranz, *Experimental Studies of Shiftwork* (Opladen: Westdeutscher Verlag, 1975), 20–28; R. C. Friedman, J. T. Bigger, and D. S. Kornfield, "The Intern and Sleep Loss," *N. Engl. J. Med.* 285 (1971): 201–3; T. Åkerstedt, L. Torsvall, and M. Gillberg, "Sleep-Wake Disturbances in Shift Work: Implications of Sleep Loss and Circadian Rhythms," *Sleep Research* 12 (1983): 359; S. Vidacek, L. Kaliterna, and B. R. Vic-Vidacek, "Productivity on a Weekly Rotating Shift System: Circadian Adjustment and Sleep Deprivation Effects?" *Ergonomics* 29 (1986): 1583–90.

21. R. T. Wilkinson, "Sleep Deprivation: Performance Tests for Partial and Selective Sleep Deprivation," *Prog. Clin. Psychol.* 8 (1969): 28–43; J. Aschoff et al., "The Influence of Sleep Interruption and of Sleep Deprivation on Circadian Rhythms

in Human Performance," in *Aspects of Human Efficiency: Diurnal Rhythm and Loss of Sleep,* ed. W. E. Colquhoun (London: English University Press, 1972); W. C. Dement, "Sleep Deprivation and the Organization of the Behavioral States," in *Sleep and the Maturing Nervous System,* ed. C. D. Clemente, D. P. Purpura, and F. E. Mayer (New York: Academic Press, 1972), 319–61; Åkerstedt et al., "Melatonin Excretion, Body Temperature and Subjective Arousal."

22. Babkoff, Caspy, and Mikulincer, "Subjective Sleepiness Ratings"; Fröberg et al., "Circadian Rhythms of Catecholamine Excretion"; Åkerstedt et al., "Melatonin Excretion, Body Temperature, and Subjective Arousal"; D. F. Dinges, "The Nature of Sleepiness: Causes, Contexts, and Consequences," in *Perspectives in Behavioral Medicine: Eating, Sleeping, and Sex,* ed. A. J. Stunkard and A. Baum (Hillsdale, N.J.: Lawrence Erlbaum Associates, 1989), 147–79; M. A. Carskadon and W. C. Dement, "Multiple Sleep Latency Tests during the Constant Routine," *Sleep* 15 (1992): 396–99; J. J. Pilcher and A. I. Huffcutt, "Effects of Sleep Deprivation on Performance: A Meta-Analysis," *Sleep* 19 (1996): 318–26; I. Lorenzo et al., "Effect of Total Sleep Deprivation on Reaction Time and Waking EEG Activity in Man," *Sleep* 18 (1995): 346–54; M. Koslowsky and H. Babkoff, "Meta-Analysis of the Relationship between Total Sleep Deprivation and Performance," *Chronobiology International* 9 (1992): 132–36; L. C. Johnson, "Sleep Deprivation and Performance," in *Biological Rhythms, Sleep, and Performance,* ed. W. B. Webb (New York: John Wiley and Sons, 1982), 111–41; R. T. Wilkinson, "Effects of Up to 60 Hours' Sleep Deprivation on Different Types of Work," *Ergonomics* 7 (1972): 175–86; R. G. Angus, R. J. Heslegrave, and W. S. Myles, "Effects of Prolonged Sleep Deprivation, with and without Chronic Physical Exercise, on Mood and Performance," *Psychophysiology* 22 (1985): 276–82.

23. Department of Transportation, Federal Motor Carrier Safety Administration, *Federal Register* 65, no. 85, (2000): 25541–611.

24. M. A. Carskadon and W. C. Dement, "Cumulative Effects of Sleep Restriction on Daytime Sleepiness," *Psychophysiology* 18 (1981): 107–13; M. A. Carskadon and T. Roth, "Sleep Restriction," in *Sleep, Sleepiness, and Performance,* ed. T. H. Monk (New York: John Wiley and Sons, 1991), 155–67; M. Gillberg and T. Åkerstedt, "Sleep Restriction and SWS-Suppression: Effects on Daytime Alertness and Night-Time Recovery," *Journal of Sleep Research* 3 (1994): 144–51; C. Lafrance et al., "Daytime Vigilance after Morning Bright Light Exposure in Volunteers Subjected to Sleep Restriction," *Physiology and Behavior* 63 (1998): 803–10; M. Blagrove, C. Alexander, and J. A. Horne, "The Effects of Chronic Sleep Reduction on the Performance of Cognitive Tasks Sensitive to Sleep Deprivation," *Applied Cognitive Psychology* 9 (1995): 21–40; D. P. Brunner, D. J. Dijk, and A. A. Borbély, "Repeated Partial Sleep Deprivation Progressively Changes the EEG during Sleep and Wakefulness," *Sleep* 16 (1993): 100–113; D. P. Brunner et al., "Effect of Partial Sleep Deprivation on Sleep Stages and EEG Power Spectra: Evidence for Non-REM and REM Sleep Homeostasis," *Electroencephalography and Clinical Neurophysiology* 75 (1990): 492–99.

25. D. F. Dinges, G. Maislin, A. Kuo, M. M. Carlin, J. W. Powell, H. Van Dongen, and J. Mullington, "Chronic Sleep Restriction: Neurobehavioral Effects of 4hr, 6hr, and 8 Hr TIB," *Sleep* 22, Supplement (1999): S115.

26. D. F. Dinges, "Are You Awake? Cognitive Performance and Reverie during the Hypnopompic State," in *Sleep and Cognition,* ed. R. Bootzin, J. Kihlstrom,

and D. Schacter (Washington, D.C.: American Psychological Association, 1990), 159–75.

27. S. Folkard and T. Åkerstedt, "A Three-Process Model of the Regulation of Alertness-Sleepiness," in *Sleep, Arousal, and Performance,* ed. R. J. Broughton and R. D. Ogilvie (Boston: Birkhäuser, 1992), 11–26; P. Achermann et al., "Time Course of Sleep Inertia after Nighttime and Daytime Sleep Episodes," *Archives Italiennes de Biologie* 134 (1995): 109–9; M. E. Jewett and R. E. Kronauer, "Interactive Mathematical Models of Subjective Alertness and Cognitive Throughput in Humans," *Journal of Biological Rhythms* 14 (1999): 588–97.

28. D. F. Dinges, "Sleep Inertia," in *Encyclopedia of Sleep and Dreaming,* ed. M. A. Carskadon (New York: Macmillan, 1993), 553–54.

29. Folkard and Åkerstedt, "A Three-Process Model"; Achermann et al., "Time Course of Sleep Inertia"; Jewett and Kronauer, "Interactive Mathematical Models"; Dinges, "Sleep Inertia."

30. J. Ribak et al., "Diurnal Rhythmicity and Air Force Flight Accidents Due to Pilot Error," *Aviation, Space, and Environmental Medicine* 54 (1983): 1096–99.

31. A. T. Wertz et al., "Effects of Sleep Inertia on Cognition," *JAMA* 295 (2006): 163–64.

32. D. F. Dinges, "An Overview of Sleepiness and Accidents," *Journal of Sleep Research* 4, Supplement 2 (1995): 4–14; B. Bjerner, A. Holm, and A. Swensson, "Diurnal Variation in Mental Performance: A Study of Three-Shift Workers," *British Journal of Industrial Medicine* 12 (1955): 103–10.

33. Bjerner, Holm, and Swensson, "Diurnal Variation in Mental Performance"; G. Hildebrandt, W. Rohmert, and J. Rutenfranz, "12 and 24 h Rhythms in Error Frequency of Locomotive Drivers and the Influence of Tiredness," *International Journal of Chronobiology* 2 (1974): 175–80; Dinges, "Overview of Sleepiness and Accidents"; M. R. Rosekind, P. H. Gander, L. J. Connell, and E. L. Co, *Crew Factors in Flight Operations X: Alertness Management in Flight Operations* (U.S. DOT, 1999).

34. C. A. Czeisler et al., "Entrainment of Human Circadian Rhythms by Light-Dark Cycles: A Reassessment," *Photochemistry and Photobiology* 34 (1981): 239–47; C. A. Czeisler et al., "Bright Light Resets the Human Circadian Pacemaker Independent of the Timing of the Sleep-Wake Cycle," *Science* 233 (1986): 667–71; D. J. Dijk et al., "Reduction of Human Sleep Duration after Bright Light Exposure in the Morning," *Neuroscience Letters* 73 (1987): 181–86; J. Broadway, J. Arendt, and S. Folkard, "Bright Light Phase Shifts the Human Melatonin Rhythm during the Antarctic Winter," *Neuroscience Letters* 79 (1987): 185–89; A. J. Lewy et al., "Antidepressant and Circadian Phase-Shifting Effects of Light," *Science* 235 (1987): 352–354; D. J. Kennaway et al., "Phase Delay of the Rhythm of 6-Sulphatoxy Melatonin Excretion by Artificial Light," *Journal of Pineal Research* 4 (1987): 315–20; K. Honma and S. Honma, "A Human Phase Response Curve for Bright Light Pulses," *Jpn. J. Psychiatry Neurol.* 42 (1988): 167–68; C. A. Czeisler et al., "Bright Light Induction of Strong (Type 0) Resetting of the Human Circadian Pacemaker," *Science* 244 (1989): 1328–33; D. J. Dijk et al., "Bright Morning Light Advances the Human Circadian System without Affecting NREM Sleep Homeostasis," *American Journal of Physiology* 256 (1989): R106–R11; M. Drennan, D. F. Kripke, and J. C. Gillin, "Bright Light Can Delay Human Temperature Rhythm Independent of Sleep," *American Journal of Physiology* 257 (1989): R136–

266NOTES TO PAGE 158

R41; M. Clodoré et al., "Psychophysiological Effects of Early Morning Bright Light Exposure in Young Adults," Psychoneuroendocrinology 15 (1990): 193–205; T. L. Shanahan and C. A. Czeisler, "Light Exposure Induces Equivalent Phase Shifts of the Endogenous Circadian Rhythms of Circulating Plasma Melatonin and Core Body Temperature in Men," J. Clin. Endocrinol. Metab. 73 (1991): 227–35; M. E. Jewett, R. E. Kronauer, and C. A. Czeisler, "Light-Induced Suppression of Endogenous Circadian Amplitude in Humans," Nature 350 (1991): 59–62; M. Buresová et al., "Early Morning Bright Light Phase Advances the Human Circadian Pacemaker within One Day," Neuroscience Letters 121 (1991): 47–50; D. S. Minors, J. M. Waterhouse, and A. Wirz-Justice, "A Human Phase-Response Curve to Light," Neuroscience Letters 133 (1991): 36–40; D. Dawson, L. Lack, and M. Morris, "Phase Resetting of the Human Circadian Pacemaker with Use of a Single Pulse of Bright Light," Chronobiology International 10 (1993): 94–102; E. Van Cauter et al., "Preliminary Studies on the Immediate Phase-Shifting Effects of Light and Exercise on the Human Circadian Clock," Journal of Biological Rhythms 8 (1993): S99–S108; J. Foret et al., "Effect of Morning Bright Light on Body Temperature, Plasma Cortisol and Wrist Motility Measured during 24 Hours of Constant Conditions," Neurosci. Lett. 155 (1993): 155–58; J. S. Allan and C. A. Czeisler, "Persistence of the Circadian Thyrotropin Rhythm under Constant Conditions and after Light-Induced Shifts of Circadian Phase," J. Clin. Endocrinol. Metab. 79 (1994): 508–12; C. A. Czeisler, "The Effect of Light on the Human Circadian Pacemaker," in Circadian Clocks and Their Adjustment, ed. J. M. Waterhouse, Ciba Foundation Symposium 183 (Chichester: John Wiley and Sons, 1995), 254–302; J. M. Zeitzer, R. E. Kronauer, and C. A. Czeisler, "Photopic Transduction Implicated in Human Circadian Entrainment," Neurosci. Lett. 232 (1997): 135–38; M. E. Jewett et al., "Human Circadian Pacemaker Is Sensitive to Light throughout Subjective Day without Evidence of Transients," American Journal of Physiology 273 (1997): R1800–R1809; C. A. Czeisler and K. P. Wright Jr., "Influence of Light on Circadian Rhythmicity in Humans," in Neurobiology of Sleep and Circadian Rhythms, ed. F. W. Turek and P. C. Zee (New York: Marcel Dekker, 1999), 149–80; T. L. Shanahan et al., "Melatonin Rhythm Observed throughout a Three-Cycle Bright-Light Stimulus Designed to Reset the Human Circadian Pacemaker," Journal of Biological Rhythms 14 (1999): 237–53; R. E. Kronauer and C. A. Czeisler, "Understanding the Use of Light to Control the Circadian Pacemaker in Humans," in Light and Biological Rhythms in Man, ed. L. Wetterberg, 63rd ed. (Oxford: Pergamon Press, 1993), 217–36; R. E. Kronauer, M. E. Jewett, and C. A. Czeisler, "Commentary: The Human Circadian Response to Light; Strong and Weak Resetting," Journal of Biological Rhythms 8 (1993): 351–60.

35. F. G. Benedict, "Studies in Body Temperature I: Influence of the Inversion of the Daily Routine; the Temperature of Night-Workers," American Journal of Physiology 11 (1904): 145–69; P. Patkai, T. Åkerstedt, and K. Pettersson, "Field Studies of Shiftwork I: Temporal Patterns in Psychophysiological Activation in Permanent Night Workers," Ergonomics 20 (1977): 611–19; M. J. Paley and D. I. Tepas, "Fatigue and the Shiftworker: Firefighters Working on a Rotating Shift Schedule," Human Factors 36 (1994): 269–84.

36. T. Åkerstedt, "Sleepiness as a Consequence of Shift Work," Sleep 11 (1988): 17–34.

37. S. Folkard and J. Barton, "Does the 'Forbidden Zone' for Sleep Onset Influence Morning Shift Sleep Duration?" *Ergonomics* 36 (1993): 85–91.

38. National Highway Traffic Safety Administration, "The NHTSA & NCSDR Program to Combat Drowsy Driving: Report to the House and Senate Appropriations Committees Describing Collaboration between National Highway Traffic Safety Administration and National Center on Sleep Disorders Research," National Heart, Lung and Blood Institute, National Institutes of Health, 1999.

39. V. L. Neale, T. A. Dingus, S. G. Klauer, J. Sudweeks, and M. Goodman, "An Overview of the 100-Car Naturalistic Study and Findings," National Highway Traffic Safety Administration. In *Proceedings of the International Technical Conference on Enhanced Safety of Vehicles,* June 6–9, 2005, Washington, DC.

40. National Transportation Safety Board, *Safety Study: Fatigue, Alcohol, Other Drugs, and Medical Factors in Fatal-to-the-Driver Heavy Truck Crashes,* vol. 1 (Washington, D.C.: National Transportation Safety Board, 1990), 1–181.

41. Barger et al., "Extended Work Shifts."

42. L. Di Lorenzo et al., "Effect of Shift Work on Body Mass Index: Results of a Study Performed in 319 Glucose-Tolerant Men Working in a Southern Italian Industry," *Int. J. Obes. Relat. Metab. Disord.* 27 (2003): 1353–58.

43. K. J. Vener, S. Szabo, and J. G. Moore, "The Effect of Shift Work on Gastrointestinal (GI) Function: A Review," *Chronobiologia* 16 (1989): 421–39; A. Knutsson, "Health Disorders of Shift Workers," *Occup. Med.* (London) 53 (2003): 103–8.

44. Knutsson, "Health Disorders of Shift Workers"; I. Kawachi et al., "Prospective Study of Shift Work and Risk of Coronary Heart Disease in Women," *Circulation* 92 (1995): 3178–82; A. Knutsson et al., "Increased Risk of Ischaemic Heart Disease in Shift Workers," *Lancet* 2 (1986): 89–92; A. Knutsson et al., "Shiftwork and Myocardial Infarction: A Case-Control Study," *Occupational and Environmental Medicine* 56 (1999): 46–50; L. Tenkanen et al., "Shift Work, Occupation and Coronary Heart Disease over 6 Years of Follow-Up in the Helsinki Heart Study," *Scand. J. Work, Environ. Health* 23 (1997): 257–65; T. S. Kristensen, "Cardiovascular Diseases and the Work Environment: A Critical Review of the Epidemiologic Literature on Nonchemical Factors," *Scand. J. Work, Environ. Health* 15 (1989): 165–79.

45. S. Davis, D. K. Mirick, and R. G. Stevens, "Night Shift Work, Light at Night, and Risk of Breast Cancer," *J. Natl. Cancer Inst.* 93 (2001): 1557–62; E. S. Schernhammer et al., "Rotating Night Shifts and Risk of Breast Cancer in Women Participating in the Nurses' Health Study," *J. Natl. Cancer Inst.* 93 (2001): 1563–68.

46. World Health Organization International Agency for Research on Cancer, *IARC Monographs on the Evaluation of Carcinogenic Risk to Humans,* vol. 98, *Painting, Firefighting, and Shiftwork,* (Lyon, France: WHO Press, 2010), 561–765.

47. W. H. Bunch et al., "The Stresses of the Surgical Residency," *Journal of Surgical Research* 53, no. 3 (1992): 268–71.

48. R. C. Friedman, J. T. Bigger, and D. S. Kornfield, "The Intern and Sleep Loss," *N. Engl. J. Med.* 285 (1971): 201–3; R. C. Friedman, D. S. Kornfeld, and T. J. Bigger, "Psychological Problems Associated with Sleep Deprivation in Interns," *Journal of Medical Education* 48 (1973): 436–41.

49. C. V. Ford and D. K. Wentz, "The Internship Year: A Study of Sleep, Mood States, and Psychophysiologic Parameters," *Southern Medical Journal* 77 (1984): 1435–42.

50. C. P. West et al., "Association of Perceived Medical Errors with Resident Distress and Empathy: A Prospective Longitudinal Study," *JAMA* 296 (2006): 1071–78; A.M. Fahrenkopf et al., "Rates of Medication Errors among Depressed and Burnt Out Residents: Prospective Cohort Study," *BMJ* 336 (2008): 488–91.

51. K. H. Sharp et al., "Alterations of Temperature, Sleepiness, Mood, and Performance in Residents Are Not Associated with Changes in Sulfatoxymelatonin Excretion," *Journal of Pineal Research* 5 (1988): 499–512.

52. Fahrenkopf et al., "Rates of Medication Errors among Depressed and Burnt Out Residents."

53. R. K Reznick and J. R. Folse, "Effect of Sleep Deprivation on the Performance of Surgical Residents," *American Journal of Surgery* 154 (1987): 520–25; E. J. Bartle et al., "The Effects of Acute Sleep Deprivation during Residency Training," *Surgery* 104 (1988): 311–16; T. F. Deaconson et al., "Sleep Deprivation and Resident Performance," *JAMA* 260 (1988): 1721–27.

54. M. R. Hawkins et al., "Sleep and Nutritional Deprivation and Performance of House Officers," *Journal of Medical Education* 60 (1985): 530–35; L. R. Lewittes and V. W. Marshall, "Fatigue and Concerns about Quality of Care among Ontario Interns and Residents," *Canadian Medical Association Journal* 140 (1989): 21–24; J. Beatty, S. K. Ahern, and R. Katz, "Sleep Deprivation and the Vigilance of Anesthesiologists during Simulated Surgery," in *Vigilance: Theory, Operational Performance, and Physiological Correlates,* ed. R. Mackie (New York: Plenum Press, 1977), 511–27; K. J. Klose, G. L. Wallace-Barnhill, and N. W. B. Craythorne, "Performance Test Results for Anesthesia Residents over a Five-Day Week Including On-Call Duty," *Anesthesiology* 63 (1985): A485; V. Narang and J. R. D. Laycock, "Psychomotor Testing of On-Call Anaesthetists," *Anaesthesia* 41 (1986): 868–69; R. P. Hart et al., "Effect of Sleep Deprivation on First-Year Residents' Response Times, Memory, and Mood," *Journal of Medical Education* 62 (1987): 940–42; D. I. Orton and J. H. Gruzelier, "Adverse Changes in Mood and Cognitive Performance of House Officers after Night Duty," *British Medical Journal* 298 (1989): 21–23.

55. R. C. Friedman, J. T. Bigger, and D. S. Kornfield, "The Intern and Sleep Loss," 201–3; R. C. Friedman, D. S. Kornfeld, and T. J. Bigger, "Psychological Problems Associated with Sleep Deprivation in Interns," *Journal of Medical Education* 48 (1973): 436–41.

56. I. J. Deary and R. Tait, "Effects of Sleep Disruption on Cognitive Performance and Mood in Medical House Officers," *British Medical Journal* 295 (1987): 1513–16; T. Lingenfelser et al., "Young Hospital Doctors after Night Duty: Their Task-Specific Cognitive Status and Emotional Condition," *Medical Education* 28 (1994): 566–72.

57. N. J. Taffinder et al., "Effect of Sleep Deprivation on Surgeons' Dexterity on Laparoscopy Simulators," *Lancet* 352 (1998): 1191.

58. T. P. Grantcharov et al., "Laparoscopic Performance after One Night on Call in a Surgical Department: Prospective Study," *British Medical Journal* 323 (2001): 1222–23; B. J. Eastridge et al., "Effect of Sleep Deprivation on the Performance of Simulated Laparoscopic Surgical Skill," *American Journal of Surgery* 186 (2003): 169–74.

59. J. T. Arnedt et al., "Neurobehavioral Performance of Residents after Heavy Night Call vs. after Alcohol Ingestion," *JAMA* 294 (2005): 1025–33.

60. I. Philibert, "Sleep Loss and Performance in Residents and Nonphysicians," *Sleep* 28 (2005): 1392–1402.

61. Barger et al., "Extended Work Shifts."

62. N. T. Ayas et al., "Extended Work Duration and the Risk of Self-Reported Percutaneous Injuries in Interns," *JAMA* 296 (2006): 1055–62.

63. L. K. Barger et al., "Impact of Extended-Duration Shifts on Medical Errors, Adverse Events, and Attentional Failures," *PLoS Med.* 3 (2006): e487.

64. Landrigan et al., "Effect of Reducing Interns' Work Hours"; Lockley et al., "Effect of Reducing Interns' Weekly Work Hours."

65. Landrigan et al., "Effect of Reducing Interns' Work Hours," 1845.

66. K. G. Volpp et al., "Mortality among Patients in VA Hospitals in the First 2 Years Following ACGME Resident Duty Hour Reform," *JAMA* 298 (2007): 984–92; K. D. Shetty and J. Bhattacharya, "Changes in Hospital Mortality Associated with Residency Work-Hour Regulations," *Ann. Intern. Med.* 147 (2007): 73–80.

67. Volpp et al., "Mortality among Hospitalized Medicare Beneficiaries in the First 2 Years Following ACGME Resident Duty Hour Reform."

68. Landrigan et al., "Interns' Compliance with Accreditation Council."

69. Federal Motor Carrier Safety Administration, "The Revised Hours of Service Regulations," Washington, D.C., August 31, 2005; Federal Aviation Administration, "Pilot Flight Time and Rest," 2001, Washington, D.C., August, 31, 2005; Air Line Pilots' Association, "Court Upholds 'Whitlow Letter' 16-Hour Duty Limit," 2002, August 31, 2005.

70. F. P. Cappuccio et al., "Implementing a 48 h EWTD-Compliant Rota for Junior Doctors in the UK Does Not Compromise Patients' Safety: Assessor-Blind Pilot Comparison," *Q. J. Med.* 102 (2009): 271–82.

71. R. J. Blendon et al., "Common Concerns amid Diverse Systems: Health Care Experiences in Five Countries," *Health Aff.* (Millwood) 22 (2003): 106–21; C. Schoen et al., "Taking the Pulse of Health Care Systems: Experiences of Patients with Health Problems in Six Countries," *Health Aff.* (Millwood) (2005) Jul–Dec, Suppl Web Exclusives: W5–509–25.

72. D. E. Altman, C. Clancy, and R. J. Blendon, "Improving Patient Safety: Five Years after the IOM Report," *N. Engl. J. Med.* 351 (2004): 2041–43; C. Vincent et al., "Is Health Care Getting Safer?" *British Medical Journal* 337 (2008): a2426; L. L. Leape and D. M. Berwick, "Five Years after *To Err Is Human:* What Have We Learned?" *JAMA* 293 (2005): 2384–90.

73. Philibert, "Sleep Loss and Performance"; Arnedt et al., "Neurobehavioral Performance."

74. American Medical Association, "Medical Students and Residents Work-Hour Survey," July 14, 2005, http://www.ama-assn.org/; Accreditation Council for Graduate Medical Education, "Statement of Justification/Impact for the Final Approval of Common Standards Related to Resident Duty Hours," January 11, 2002, http://www.acgme.org/acWebsite/home/home.asp.

75. L. A. Petersen et al., "Does Housestaff Discontinuity of Care Increase the Risk for Preventable Adverse Events?" *Annals of Internal Medicine* 121 (1994): 866–72.

76. L. A. Petersen et al., "Using a Computerized Sign-Out Program to Improve Continuity of Inpatient Care and Prevent Adverse Events," *Joint Commission Journal on Quality Improvement* 24 (1998): 77–87.

77. R. Stickgold, "Sleep-Dependent Memory Consolidation," *Nature* 437 (October 27, 2005): 1272–78.

78. Institute of Medicine, *Resident Duty Hours: Enhancing Sleep, Supervision, and Safety* (Washington, D.C.: National Academies Press, 2008).

79. J. M. Rothschild et al., "Risks of Complications by Attending Physicians after Performing Nighttime Procedures," *JAMA* 302 (2009): 1565–72.

80. National Sleep Foundation, Executive Summary of the 2002 "Sleep in America" poll by WB&A Market Research, 4–2–2002 Washington, D.C., 2002, 1–43.

81. Kaiser Family Foundation, Agency for Healthcare Research and Quality, and Harvard School of Public Health, "National Survey on Consumers' Experiences with Patient Safety and Quality Information," Menlo Park, Calif., 2004.

82. R. J. Blendon et al., "Views of Practicing Physicians and the Public on Medical Errors," *N. Engl. J. Med.* 347 (2002): 1933–40.

83. Ibid.

84. A. D. Saxena and C. F. George, "Sleep and Motor Performance in On-Call Internal Medicine Residents," *Sleep* 28 (2005): 1386–91.

9. Sleep-deprived Nurses

1. K. A. Lee, "Self-Reported Sleep Disturbances in Employed Women," *Sleep* 15 (1992): 493–98.

2. Ibid.

3. U. M. Edéll-Gustafsson, E. I. Kritz, and I. K. Bogren, "Self-Reported Sleep Quality, Strain and Health in Relation to Perceived Working Conditions in Females," *Scandinavian Journal of Caring Sciences* 16 (2002): 179–87.

4. J. S. Ruggiero, "Correlates of Fatigue in Critical Care Nurses," *Research in Nursing and Health* 26 (2003): 434–44.

5. J. Geiger-Brown, A. M. Trinkoff, and V. E. Rogers, "The Impact of Work Schedules, Home, and Work Demands on Self-Reported Sleep in Registered Nurses," *Journal of Occupational and Environmental Medicine* 53 (2011): 303–7.

6. K. Heiler, "The 'Petty Pilfering of Minutes' or What Has Happened to the Length of the Working Day in Australia?" *International Journal of Manpower* 19 (1998): 266–80; A. E. Rogers, W. Hwang, L. D. Scott, L. H. Aiken, and D. F. Dinges, "The Working Hours of Hospital Staff Nurses and Patient Safety," *Health Affairs* 23 (2004): 202–12; L. D. Scott, W. Hwang, A. E. Rogers, T. Nysse, G. E. Dean, and D. F. Dinges, "The Relationship between Nurse Work Schedules, Sleep Duration, and Drowsy Driving," *Sleep* 30 (2007): 1801–7; A. M. Trinkoff, J. Geiger-Brown, B. Brady, J. Lipscomb, and C. Muntaner, "How Long and How Much Are Nurses Now Working? Too Long, Too Much, and without Enough Rest Between Shifts, a Study Finds," *American Journal of Nursing* 106 (2006): 60–71.

7. Trinkoff et al., "How Long and How Much Are Nurses Now Working?"

8. Ibid.

9. U.S. Health Resources and Service Administration, "The Registered Nurse Population: Findings from March 2004 National Sample Survey of Registered Nurses," ftp://ftp.hrsa.gov/bhpr/workforce/0306rnss.pdf (accessed May 20, 2009).

10. J. Geiger-Brown, V. E. Rogers, A. M. Trinkoff, R. B. Bausell, and S. Scharf, "Sleep, Sleepiness, Fatigue and Performance in 12-hour Shift Nurses," under review, 2011.

11. J. A. Lipscomb, A. M. Trinkoff, J. Geiger-Brown, and B. Brady, "Work-Schedule Characteristics and Reported Musculoskeletal Disorders of Registered

Nurses," *Scandinavian Journal of Work, Environment and Health* 28 (2002): 394–401; Trinkoff et al., "How Long and How Much Are Nurses Now Working?"; A.M. Trinkoff, J. A. Lipscomb, J. Geiger-Brown, C. L. Storr, and B. A. Brady, "Perceived Physical Demands and Reported Musculoskeletal Problems in Registered Nurses," *American Journal of Preventive Medicine* 24 (2003): 270–75; A.M. Trinkoff, C. L. Storr, and J. A. Lipscomb, "Physically Demanding Work and Inadequate Sleep, Pain Medication Use, and Absenteeism in Registered Nurses," *Journal of Occupational and Environmental Medicine* 43 (2001): 355–63.

12. S. Sonnentag and F. R. H. Zijlstra, "Job Characteristics and Off-Job Activities as Predictors of Need for Recovery, Well-Being, and Fatigue," *Journal of Applied Psychology* 91 (2006): 330–50.

13. A.M. Trinkoff, C. L. Storr, and J. A. Lipscomb, "Physically Demanding Work and Inadequate Sleep, Pain Medication Use, and Absenteeism in Registered Nurses," *Journal of Occupational and Environmental Medicine* 43 (2001): 355–63.

14. L. Knowlton, "Neurobehavioral Consequences of Sleep Dysfunction," *Psychiatric Times* 16 (1999): 99; L. Smith, S. Folkard, P. Tucker, and I. Macdonald, "Work Shift Duration: A Review Comparing Eight Hour and 12 Hour Shift Systems," *Occupational and Environmental Medicine* 55 (1998): 217–29; P. Tucker, J. Barton, and S. Folkard, "Comparison of Eight and 12 Hour Shifts: Impacts on Health, Wellbeing, and Alertness during the Shift," *Occupational and Environmental Medicine* 53 (1996): 767–72.

15. Geiger-Brown, Trinkoff, and Rogers, "The Impact of Work Schedules, Home, and Work Demands."

16. G. G. Kay and B. K. Logan, *Drugged Driving Expert Panel Report: A Consensus Protocol for Assessing the Potential of Drugs to Impair Driving* (Washington, D.C.: National Highway Traffic Safety Administration, 2011).

17. Scott et al., "Relationship between Nurse Work Schedules, Sleep Duration, and Drowsy Driving."

18. Geiger-Brown et al., "Sleep, Sleepiness, Fatigue and Performance in 12-hour Shift Nurses."

19. A.M. Trinkoff, R. Le, J. Geiger-Brown, and J. Lipscomb, "Work Schedule, Needle Use, and Needlestick Injuries among Registered Nurses," *Infection Control and Hospital Epidemiology* 28 (2007): 156–64.

20. M. A. Miller and F. P. Cappuccio, "Inflammation, Sleep, Obesity and Cardiovascular Disease," *Current Vascular Pharmacology* 5 (2007): 93–102.

21. D. F. Dinges, F. Pack, K. Williams, K. A. Gillen, J. W. Powell, G. E. Ott, C. Aptowicz, and A. I. Pack, "Cumulative Sleepiness, Mood Disturbance, and Psychomotor Vigilance Performance Decrements during a Week of Sleep Restricted to 4–5 Hours per Night," *Sleep* 20 (1997): 267–77; R. R. Rosa, "Extended Workshifts and Excessive Fatigue," *Journal of Sleep Research* 4 (1995): S51–S56; M. R. Rosekind, P. H. Gander, K. B. Gregory, R. M. Smith, D. L. Miller, R. Oyung, L. L. Webbon, and J. M. Johnson, "Managing Fatigue in Operational Settings I: Physiological Considerations and Countermeasures," *Behavioral Medicine* 21 (1996): 157–65; H. P. A. Van Dongen, G. Maislin, J. M. Mullington, and D. F. Dinges. "The Cumulative Cost of Additional Wakefulness: Dose-Response Effects on Neurobehavioral Functions and Sleep Physiology from Chronic Sleep Restriction and Total Sleep Deprivation," *Sleep* 26 (2003): 117–26.

22. Van Dongen, Maislin, Mullington, and Dinges, "Cumulative Cost of Additional Wakefulness."

23. G. Belenky, N. J. Wesensten, D. R. Thorne, M. L. Thomas, H. C. Sing, D. P. Redmond, M. B. Russo, and T. J. Balkin, "Patterns of Performance Degradation and Restoration during Sleep Restriction and Subsequent Recovery: A Sleep Dose Response Study," *Journal of Sleep Research* 12 (2003): 1–12.

24. D. F. Dinges and N. B. Kribbs, "Performing while Sleepy: Effects of Experimentally Induced Sleepiness," in *Sleep, Sleepiness and Performance: Human Performance and Cognition,* ed. T. H. Monk (Oxford: John Wiley and Sons, 1991), 97–128; J. Horne, *Why We Sleep: The Functions of Sleep in Humans and Other Mammals* (New York: Oxford University Press, 1988); A. Lubin, "Performance under Sleep Loss and Fatigue," *Research Publications–Association for Research in Nervous and Mental Disease* 45 (1967): 506–13; H. L. Williams, A. Lubin, and J. J. Goodnow, "Impaired Performance with Acute Sleep Loss," *Psychological Monographs* 73 (1959): 26.

25. J. T. Arnedt, J. Owens, M. Crouch, J. Stahl, and M. A. Carskadon, "Neurobehavioral Performance of Residents after Heavy Night Call vs after Alcohol Ingestion," *Journal of the American Medical Association* 294 (2005): 1025–33.

26. M. M. Halbach, C. O. Spann, and G. Egan, "Effect of Sleep Deprivation on Medical Resident and Student Cognitive Function: A Prospective Study," *American Journal of Obstetrics and Gynecology* 188 (2003): 1198–1201; National Institute for Occupational Safety and Health, "Overtime and Extended Work Shifts: Recent Findings on Illnesses, Injuries and Health Behaviors," 2004, www.cdc.gov/niosh/docs/2004–143/health.html (accessed May 20, 2009); D. C. Rollinson, N. K. Rathley, M. Moss, R. Killiany, K. C. Sassower, S. Auerbach, and S. S. Fish, "The Effects of Consecutive Night Shifts on Neuropsychological Performance of Interns in the Emergency Department: A Pilot Study," *Annals of Emergency Medicine* 41 (2003): 400–406; Smith, Folkard, Tucker, and Macdonald, "Work Shift Duration"; M. Van der Hulst, "Long Workhours and Health," *Scandinavian Journal of Work, Environment and Health* 29 (2003): 171–88.

27. E. O'Shea, "Factors Contributing to Medication Errors: A Literature Review," *Journal of Clinical Nursing* 8 (1999): 496–504.

28. A. L. Tucker and S. J. Spear, "Operational Failures and Interruptions in Hospital Nursing," *Health Services Research* 41 (2006): 643–62.

29. R. Jagsi and R. Surender, "Regulation of Junior Doctors' Work Hours: An Analysis of British and American Doctors' Experiences and Attitudes," *Social Science and Medicine* 58 (2004): 2181–91.

30. Trinkoff et al., "How Long and How Much Are Nurses Now Working?"

31. Scott et al., "Relationship between Nurse Work Schedules, Sleep Duration, and Drowsy Driving."

32. E. Atlantis, C. Chow, A. Kirby, and M. A. F. Singh, "Worksite Intervention Effects on Sleep Quality: A Randomized Controlled Trial," *Journal of Occupational Health Psychology* 11 (2006): 291–304.

33. Round-the-Clock Systems, "Shiftwork Education: The Saturn Strategy," http://www.roundtheclocksystems.com/library3_cs_01saturn.html (accessed May 20 2009).

34. R. Smith-Coggins, S. K. Howard, D. T. Mac, C. Wang, S. Kwan, M. R. Rosekind, Y. Sowb, R. Balise, J. Levis, and D. M. Gaba, "Improving Alertness and Performance in Emergency Department Physicians and Nurses: The Use of Planned Naps," *Annals of Emergency Medicine* 48 (2006): 596–604, e3.

35. D. E. McMillan, W. M. Fallis, M. P. Edwards, "Napping during Night Shift: Experiences of Critical Care Nurses," abstract 0372, *Sleep* 31 (2008): abstract supplement, A123.

36. W. A. Anthony and C. W. Anthony, "The Napping Company: Bringing Science to the Workplace," *Industrial Health* 43 (2005): 209–12.

37. M. Takahashi, H. Arito, and H. Fukuda, "Nurses' Workload Associated with 16 H Night Shifts II: Effects of a Nap Taken during the Shifts," *Psychiatry and Clinical Neurosciences* 53 (1999): 223–25.

38. American Nurses Association, "Assuring Patient Safety: The Employers' Role in Promoting Healthy Nursing Work Hours for Registered Nurses in All Roles and Settings," 2006, http://www.nursingworld.org/MainMenuCategories/The PracticeofProfessionalNursing/workplace/Workforce/NurseFatigue/Employers Role.aspx (accessed May 20, 2009); American Nurses Association, "Assuring Patient Safety: Registered Nurses' Responsibility in All Roles and Settings to Guard Against Working When Fatigued," 2006, http://www.nursingworld.org/MainMenu Categories/ThePracticeofProfessionalNursing/workplace/Workforce/Nurse Fatigue/Fatigue.aspx (accessed May 20, 2009).

39. American Nurses Association, "Assuring Patient Safety: The Employers' Role."

40. American Nurses Association, "Assuring Patient Safety: Registered Nurses' Responsibility."

41. J. Geiger-Brown, A. M. Trinkoff, K. Nielsen, S. Lirtmunlikaporn, B. Brady, and E. I. Vasquez, "Nurses' Perception of Their Work Environment, Health, and Well-Being," *AAOHN Journal* 52, no. 1 (January 2004): 20.

42. M. E. Foley, "American Nurses Association Denounces OSHA Ergonomics Plan" (Washington, D.C.: American Nurses Association Press, 2001).

43. American Association of Colleges of Nursing, "Nursing Shortage Fact Sheet 2009," http://www.aacn.nche.edu/Media/FactSheets/NursingShortage.htm (accessed May 20, 2009).

10. Wounds That Don't Heal

1. Institute of Medicine, *To Err Is Human: Building a Safer Health System* (Washington, D.C.: National Academies Press, 2000); Institute of Medicine, *Keeping Patients Safe: Transforming the Work Environment of Nurses* (Washington, D.C.: National Academies Press, 2004); L. L. Leape and D. M. Berwick, "Five Years after *To Err Is Human*: What Have We Learned?" *JAMA* 293 (19): 2384–90; Institute of Medicine, *Preventing Medication Errors: Quality Chasm Series* (Washington, D.C.: National Academies Press, 2007); T. E. Burroughs, A. D. Waterman et al., "Patients' Concerns about Medical Errors during Hospitalization," *Joint Commission Journal on Quality and Patient Safety / Joint Commission Resources* 33, no. 1 (2007): 5–14.

2. C. L. Bosk, *Forgive and Remember: Managing Medical Failure,* 2nd ed. (Chicago: University of Chicago Press, 2003).

3. A. W. Wu, "Medical Error: The Second Victim; The Doctor Who Makes the Mistake Needs Help, Too," *BMJ* 320 (March 18, 2000): 726–27; S. D. Scott, L. E. Hirschinger et al., "The Natural History of Recovery for the Healthcare Provider 'Second Victim' after Adverse Patient Events," *Quality and Safety in Health Care* 18, no. 5 (2009): 325–30.

4. Wu, "Medical Error"; Scott, Hirschinger et al., "The Natural History of Recovery for the Healthcare Provider"; N. J. Crigger, "Always Having to Say You're Sorry: An Ethical Response to Making Mistakes in Professional Practice," *Nursing Ethics* 11, no. 6 (2004): 568–76.

5. H. Cohen, E. S. Robinson et al., "Getting to the Root of Medication Errors: Survey Results," *Nursing* 33, no. 9 (2003): 36–45; A.M. Mayo and D. Duncan, "Nurse Perceptions of Medication Errors: What We Need to Know for Patient Safety," *Journal of Nursing Care Quality* 19, no. 3 (2004): 209–17; V. M. Ulanimo, C. O'Leary-Kelley et al., "Nurses' Perceptions of Causes of Medication Errors and Barriers to Reporting," *Journal of Nursing Care Quality* 22, no. 1 (2007): 28–33.

6. J. Osborne, K. Blais et al., "Nurses' Perceptions: When Is It a Medication Error?" *Journal of Nursing Administration* 29, no. 4 (1999): 33–38; Y.-K. Chang and B. A. Mark, "Antecedents of Severe and Nonsevere Medication Errors," *Journal of Nursing Scholarship* 41, no. 1 (2009): 70–78.

7. L. L. Leape, D. W. Bates et al., "Systems Analysis of Adverse Drug Events," *JAMA* 274, no. 1 (1995): 35–43; International Council of Nurses, "Nursing Matters Fact Sheet: Medication Errors," n.d., http://www.icn.ch/matters_errors_print.htm.

8. A. F. Cook, H. Hoas et al., "An Error by Any Other Name," *American Journal of Nursing* 104, no. 6 (2004): 32–43.

9. R. Koppel, T. Wetterneck et al., "Workarounds to Barcode Medication Administration Systems: Their Occurrences, Causes, and Threats to Patient Safety," *Journal of the American Medical Informatics Association* 15, no. 4 (2008): 408–23.

10. A. Musk, "Proficiency with Technology and the Expression of Caring: Can We Reconcile These Polarized Views?" *International Journal for Human Caring* 8, no. 2 (2004): 13–20; J. Novek, "IT, Gender, and Professional Practice: Or, Why an Automated Drug Distribution System Was Sent Back to the Manufacturer," *Science, Technology, and Human Values* 27, no. 3 (2002): 379–403.

11. K. Krichbaum, C. Diemert et al., "Complexity Compression: Nurses under Fire," *Nursing Forum* 42, no. 2 (2007): 86–94.

12. Koppel, Wetterneck et al., "Workarounds to Barcode Medication Administration Systems."

13. D. B. Weinberg, "When Little Things Are Big Things: The Importance of Relationships for Nurses' Professional Practice," in *The Complexities of Care: Nursing Reconsidered,* ed. S. Nelson and S. Gordon (Ithaca: Cornell University Press, 2006), 30–43.

14. Cohen, Robinson et al., "Getting to the Root of Medication Errors"; Crigger, "Always Having to Say You're Sorry"; H. Cohen and A.D. Shastay, "Getting to the Root of Medication Errors: Survey Report," *Nursing* 38, no. 12 (2008): 39–47.

15. R. Koppel, J. P. Metlay et al., "Role of Computerized Physician Order Entry Systems in Facilitating Medication Errors," *JAMA* 293, no. 19 (2005): 1197–1203.

16. S. Gordon and S. Nelson, "Moving beyond the Virtue Script in Nursing: Creating a Knowledge-Based Identity for Nurses," in Nelson and Gordon, *The Complexities of Care,* 13–29.

17. Weinberg, "When Little Things Are Big Things."

18. D. J. Mason, "Pride and Prejudice: Nurses' Struggle with Reasoned Debate," in Nelson and Gordon, *The Complexities of Care,* 44–49.

19. Wu, "Medical Error"; Scott, Hirschinger et al. "Natural History of Recovery for the Healthcare Provider."

20. M. A. Paget, *The Unity of Mistakes* (Philadelphia: Temple University Press, 2004).

21. J. B. McKinlay, "A Case for Refocusing Upstream: The Political Economy of Illness," in *The Sociology of Health and Illness: Critical Perspectives,* 7th ed., ed. P. Conrad (New York: Worth, 2005), 551–64.

11. On Teams, Teamwork, and Team Intelligence

1. Leonard Stein, "The Doctor-Nurse Game," *Archives of General Psychiatry* 16 (1967): 699–70; Leonard Stein, David Watts, and Timothy Howell, "The Doctor-Nurse Game Revisited," *New England Journal of Medicine* 322 (1990): 546–49.

2. T. M. Luhrmann, *Of Two Minds: The Growing Disorder in American Psychiatry* (New York: Alfred A. Knopf, 2000), 93.

3. Peter Pronovost, *Safe Patients, Smart Hospitals: How One Doctor's Checklist Is Transforming Health Care from the Inside Out* (New York: Hudson Street Press, 2010), 30–35.

4. John E. Heffner, "Letter from the MUSC Medical Director," in *The Many Faces of Nursing* (Charleston: MUSC Medical Center, 2002), 5.

5. Deborah M. Nadzam, "Nurses' Role in Communication and Patient Safety," *Journal of Nursing Care Quality* 24, no. 3 (2009): 185.

6. Joint Commission, "Behaviors That Undermine a Culture of Safety," Applicable Standards, July 9, 2008, http://www.jointcommission.org/NewsRoom/PressKits/Beha viors+that+Undermine+a+Culture+of+Safety/app_stds.htm (accessed July 19, 2010).

7. J. Richard Hackman, "Leading Teams," http://hbswk.hbs.edu/archive/2996. html (accessed June 14, 2010).

8. J. Richard Hackman, ed., *Groups That Work (and Those That Don't): Creating Conditions for Effective Teamwork* (San Francisco: Jossey-Bass, 1990), 6–7.

9. For an excellent discussion of how bullying or stereotyping impacts workers in health care, see Claude Steele, *Whistling Vivaldi and Other Cues about How Stereotypes Affect Us* (New York: W. W. Norton, 2010).

10. Suzanne Gordon, *Nursing against the Odds: How Health Care Cost-Cutting, Media Stereotypes, and Medical Hubris Undermine Nurses and Patient Care* (Ithaca: Cornell University Press, 2006).

11. Lorelei Lingard, "Rethinking Competence in the Context of Teamwork," in *Blind Spots: Health Professional Competence in the Twenty-first Century,* edited by Brian Hodges and Lorelei Lingard (Ithaca: Cornell University Press, forthcoming).

12. See Bernice Buresh and Suzanne Gordon, *From Silence to Voice: What Nurses Know and Must Communicate to the Public* (Ithaca: Cornell University Press, 2007).

13. Suzanne Gordon, observation of CRM curriculum, Airbus training center, Miami, March 2007.

14. See www.dynamicflight.com/avcfibook/glossary/.

15. J. S. Carroll and A. C. Edmondson, "Leading Organisational Learning in Health Care," *Quality and Safety in Health Care* 11 (2002): 51–56.

16. J. Richard Hackman, ed., *Groups That Work (and Those That Don't): Creating Conditions for Effective Teamwork* (San Francisco: Jossey-Bass, 1990), 6-7.

17. Janelle S. Taylor, "Confronting 'Culture' in Medicine's 'Culture of No Culture,'" *Academic Medicine* 78, no. 6 (2003): 555–59.

18. For an excellent example of this kind of study, see Earl L. Weiner, Barbara G. Kanki, and Robert L. Helmreich, eds., *Cockpit Resource Management* (Amsterdam: Academic Press, 1993).

19. Lingard, "Rethinking Competence," 20

20. Edwin Hutchins, *Cognition in the Wild* (Cambridge: MIT Press, 1995), 176.

21. Anita L. Tucker and Amy C. Edmondson, "Why Hospitals Don't Learn from Failures: Organizational and Psychological Dynamics That Inhibit System Change," Harvard Business School, November 6, 2002.

22. Chesley Sullenberger with Jeffrey Zaslow, *Highest Duty: My Search for What Really Matters* (New York: William Morrow, 2010).

CONTRIBUTORS

Joseph M. Bugajski, research vice president of Gartner, Inc., advises clients about IT governance; data management, integration, and business intelligence (BI); and application portfolio management. He co-chairs MIT's Information Quality Industry Symposium (IQIS) and Object Management Group's Finance Domain Task Force. Prior to joining Gartner, he was chief data officer at Visa, where he ensured the global interoperability and near-faultless operation of VisaNet, the world's largest payment system. Previously he was CEO of the BI software provider Triada. Before Triada, he managed prototype vehicle development for the Ford Motor Company. Bugajski holds four patents and has authored several dozen peer-reviewed publications.

Kathleen Burke, RN-BC, BSN, is a registered nurse at UCSF Medical Center in San Francisco. She holds a BS degree in nursing from the University of San Francisco and is ANCC board-certified in pain management. Her clinical experience over a decade and a half at UCSF includes having been a bedside nurse, charge nurse, preceptor, case manager, student health nurse, and nurse educator. Currently a staff nurse on the medical-surgical unit, she is chair of the UCSF Patient Safety Fellows. In 2007 she received the UCSF Department of Nursing Award for Excellence in Patient Safety.

Sean Clarke, RN, Ph.D., holds the RBC Chair in Cardiovascular Nursing Research at the University of Toronto and the University Health Network in Toronto. Clarke's research deals primarily with organizational aspects of acute care nursing (with a particular emphasis on staffing levels, work environment factors, patient outcomes, and nurses' occupational health) and nurse workforce issues. He has authored or co-authored some eighty articles and fifteen book chapters and co-edited a volume on medication safety for nurses. A fellow of the American Academy of Nursing, he holds adjunct appointments at the Université de Montréal and the University of Pennsylvania, and visiting appointments at University College, Dublin, and the University of Hong Kong.

Stephen M. Davidson, Ph.D., is a professor of health care management at Boston University's School of Management. He was director of the school's Health Care Management Program from 1985 to 1990. Before that, he served on the faculties of the University of Chicago (1971–1981) and the Kellogg Graduate School of Management at Northwestern University (1981–1985). In 2010 he published *Still Broken: Understanding the U.S. Health Care System*. His other books include *Remaking Medicaid: Managed Care for the Public Good*, co-edited with Stephen A. Somers; and *The Physician-Manager Alliance: Building the Healthy Health Care Organization*, written with Janelle Heineke and Marion McCollom. In addition to writing about health information technology, he has studied private health insurance claims both to develop new measures of quality of care and to compare utilization under managed care and indemnity insurance.

Jeanne Geiger-Brown, Ph.D., RN, is a nurse researcher with over ten years' experience studying nurses' health and safety. She received her Ph.D. in nursing from the University of Maryland, Baltimore, and her MSN in adult psychiatric nursing from Columbia University. She has been on the faculty of the University of Maryland School of Nursing since 2003 and is an associate professor and co-director of the Work and Health Research Center. She studies nurses' work schedules and occupational sleep deprivation with funding from the National Institute of Occupational Safety and Health. She is also a K–12 Multidisciplinary Clinical Research Scholar awardee from the University of Maryland School of Medicine under the NIH Roadmap program. Her research interest is at the intersection of occupational epidemiology, sleep medicine, and cognitive psychology.

Suzanne Gordon is a journalist and author who has been writing about health care for over twenty-five years. Co-editor of the Culture and Politics of Health Care Work series from Cornell University Press, she has written over four hundred articles for newspapers and magazines such as the *Atlantic*, the *Boston Globe*, the *New York Times*, the *Los Angeles Times*, the *Toronto Globe and Mail*, *Harper's*, and many others. She has written or edited thirteen books, of which eight are on health care. These include *Life Support: Three Nurses on the Front Lines; Nursing against the Odds: How Hospital Cost-Cutting, Media Stereotypes, and Medical Hubris Undermine Nurses and Patient Care; When Chicken Soup Isn't Enough: Stories of Nurses Standing Up for Themselves, Their Patients, and Their Profession;* and *Safety in Numbers: Nurse Staffing Ratios and the Future of Health Care*. Gordon is a visiting professor at the University of Maryland School of Nursing. Gordon served as a member of the National Advisory Committee on the Nursing Shortage for the Robert Wood Johnson Foundation and has been a project leader on a communication and safety grant for nurse managers that has been funded by the Robert Wood Johnson Foundation.

Jackie H. Jones, Ed.D., MSN, RN, is an associate professor of nursing at the WellStar School of Nursing, Kennesaw State University in Georgia. Clinical experience includes acute care, critical care, public health, long-term care, and home health. Her research and publications are eclectic, including such diverse topics as medication errors, development of critical thinking skills, health literacy, assessment, and concierge medicine. Additionally, she has contributed to a variety of nursing texts on topics such as fluid and electrolyte balance and nutrition, and served as a reviewer for texts on critical thinking and pharmacology.

Ross Koppel, Ph.D., is a faculty member of the University of Pennsylvania's Sociology Department; principal investigator at the Center for Clinical Epidemiology and Biostatistics, School of Medicine, University of Pennsylvania; faculty member at the Rand Corporation; evaluator of the Harvard Medical School project to restructure HIT architecture; and president of the Social Research Corporation.

Koppel's work in medical informatics reflects his long career as a researcher and professor of the sociology of work and organizations, statistics, ethnographic research, survey research, and medical sociology. He is the principal investigator of the University of Pennsylvania's study on hospital workplace culture and medication errors. In the past several years Koppel has published over twenty-five articles and book chapters on health care IT in *JAMA, Health Affairs, JAMIA, Journal of Biomedical Informatics, Journal of Clinical Care, Journal of the American Geriatrics Society, Journal of Managed Care, AHRQ-M&M,* and *Infection Control and Hospital Epidemiology,* as well as two books.

His work generally combines statistical analyses with survey research and ethnographic research, focusing on the use of HIT *in situ.* Koppel is Co-PI of an AHRQ-funded project to develop a guide to implementing HIT while mitigating unintended consequences. The recipient of Distinguished Career Awards in the Practice of Sociology from the American Sociological Association (ASA) and the Society for Applied Sociology, Koppel has also been honored with the William Foote Whyte Award from the ASA's section on public sociology and the Robert E. Park Award from the Association for Applied and Clinical Sociology.

Christopher P. Landrigan, MD, MPH, is an assistant professor of pediatrics and medicine at Harvard Medical School and a practicing pediatric hospitalist. He has over a decade's experience studying the quality and safety of hospital care. He was a founding member of the Harvard Work Hours, Health, and Safety Group, and has led a series of studies investigating the effects of provider sleep deprivation and work schedule redesign on patient safety. In addition, he studies communication and handoffs of care in hospitals. His goal is to identify safer models of care delivery and help to translate these models into policy and practice.

Peter Lazes, Ph.D., is the founder and director of Programs for Economic Transitions and the Healthcare Transformation Project at Cornell University's School of Industrial and Labor Relations. These institutes provide labor unions and management with customized consultation, training, research, and educational programs to implement strategic worker participation programs and new work systems. His current activities in hospitals and nursing homes involve methods of improving patient care and reducing costs as a result of frontline staff participation. He works with health care unions, hospitals, and employers to ensure that delivery system changes are coupled with payment reform legislation.

Bonnie O'Connor, Ph.D., is a folklorist, ethnographer, and medical educator whose areas of expertise are cultural and cross-cultural issues in health care; health belief and behavior; bioethics across multiple perspectives; and health professional-to-patient and interprofessional communications. She received her Ph.D. from the University of Pennsylvania and was Lois Mattox Miller Fellow in Medical Humanities at the Medical College of Pennsylvania, where she subsequently served on the faculty in community and preventive medicine for ten years before moving to the Warren Alpert School of Medicine at Brown University in early 2000. She is assistant director of the Brown pediatric residency program and associate professor (clinical) in the Division of Pediatric Ambulatory Medicine at Rhode Island Hospital/Hasbro Children's Hospital.

Sameh Samy, MB.B.CH, MSA, CPHQ, has been working in the field of performance improvement for over a decade and is the director of quality outcomes in the Organizational Performance Department at Maimonides Medical Center. He leads and facilitates patient safety and quality projects focusing on strategic integration of best practice models and outcomes. With regard to CQI (continuous quality improvement) concepts and methodology, he serves as a consultant to clinical and nonclinical staff. Sameh received his MD in Egypt in 1985 and came to the United States in 1991. He holds an MSA in health service administration and also is a certified professional in health care quality.

Christine A. Sinsky, MD, is a general internist in Dubuque, Iowa. A frequent invited lecturer on practice innovation, redesign, and the patient-centered medical home (PCMH), she has given over fifty workshops on practice redesign at professional society meetings, as well as private and academic medical centers. Sinsky serves on the physician advisory panel for the National Committee for Quality Assurance (NCQA) physician recognition programs, has presented at the Patient-Centered Primary Care Collaborative Stakeholder meeting, and has testified for the Office of the National Coordinator for Health Information Technology on the role of the electronic health record in care coordination.

Rosalind Stanwell-Smith, MB, B.Ch., M.Sc., FRCOG, FFPH, HonFRSPH, qualified as a physician at the University of Wales and then specialized in obstetrics and gynecology, later also training in epidemiology and public health and organizational behavior. Working in district, national, and academic posts in the UK, she conducted research studies, particularly in obstetrics and gynecology, infectious disease, and water-related disease. For over ten years she has worked independently in public health with a focus on hygiene and water. She has published and lectured on a broad range of topics, from applied epidemiology to public health history. In 2011, Stanwell-Smith's dissertation on the history of London's public toilets was awarded the Maccabean Prize from the Worshipful Society of Apothecaries, London. Her current posts are scientific adviser to the Royal Society for Public Health; honorary senior lecturer at the London School of Hygiene and Tropical Medicine; and public health adviser to four water companies. She is a past president of the Section of Epidemiology and Public Health at the Royal Society of Medicine and is the honorary secretary of the John Snow Society, commemorating the work of the nineteenth-century pioneer of anesthesia and epidemiology Dr. John Snow.

Joel Leon Telles, M. Phil., Ph.D., is system director of data management and analysis at Main Line Health System in Philadelphia, where he leads efforts to achieve data-driven improvement in patient care quality and safety. He conducts analysis of medical informatics systems such as smart IV pumps, barcode medication administration, and infection monitoring and alerting systems, and uses data from his analyses to provide feedback and performance improvement. He was previously at the Delaware Valley Healthcare Council, where he was responsible for compiling, managing, and reporting data on regional hospital utilization, quality indicators, managed care plan characteristics, multihospital systems, payment downgrade and denial, emergency preparedness, and other topics. He received his doctorate in sociology from Columbia University and has been on the faculty of UCLA and the University of Virginia, where he taught and published in the areas of statistics and methods, medical sociology, workforce, sociological theory, and other topics.

Linda A. Treiber, Ph.D., RN, is an associate professor of sociology at Kennesaw State University. Her clinical experience includes medical-surgical, addictions, and cardiac nursing as well as working as a house supervisor and nurse manager. Her research centers on the unintended consequences of rational action and the social sources of premature death and illness including medical errors and the mass marketing of prescription medications. She investigates the social construction of medication administration errors and their emotional impact on registered nurses. Other projects include in-depth interviews with patients and families of patients who have been the victims of medical mistakes.

Alison M. Trinkoff is an epidemiologist with over twenty years of experience, whose research has focused on nurses since 1991. She received her doctorate in psychiatric epidemiology from Johns Hopkins University, as a National Institute for Mental Health fellow, and with an NRSA from the National Institute for Nursing Research. She has been on the faculty of the University of Maryland School of Nursing since 1988 and is a professor in the Work and Health Research Center. She has been studying nurses' work schedules, job demands, practice environments, and related outcomes, including musculoskeletal problems and needle-stick injuries using complex survey designs and administrative data, while serving as principal investigator on four major externally funded studies.

Robert L. Wears, MD, MS, Ph.D., is a professor in the Department of Emergency Medicine at the University of Florida and a visiting professor in the Clinical Safety Research Unit at Imperial College, London. His interests lie in technical work studies, joint cognitive systems, and particularly the impact of information technology on safety and resilient performance.

INDEX

Note: Italic page numbers refer to figures.

nurses and physicians, 8, 57, 180–81, 183–93; and individual versus systems approach to safety, 125–28, 132–33; learning from, 58, 221, 232–33; management of, 222; and multiple small failures paradigm, 154–55; secrecy involving, 125, 133, 147, 184, 231, 235; and situational awareness, 213; and sleep deprivation, 60, 151, 152, 154, 161, 162, 164, 166–67, 168, 174. *See also* medication errors

Europe: and nurse working hours, 175; physicians' work hours, 152; and physician working hours, 163–64; rapid response teams, 136; and unions, 111

evidence-based medicine (EBM): and cleaning, 26–27; and clinical decision support systems, 76, 77; and errors, 58; and health care information technology, 66; and individual versus systems approach to safety, 133; patient safety dependent on, 230–31; and sleep deprivation, 166, 176–77; and teamwork, 58–59; and top-down modifications in nursing practice, 127; and workload, 60

5 Million Lives campaign, 100
Foley, Mary, 179
Food and Drug Administration (FDA), 241, 243
Fox, Renee, 244–45
Fracastoro, Girolamo, 23
Francis, Robert T., 43, 57
Franklin, Benjamin, 23
Freire, Paolo, 205
Friedman, R. C., 160
frontline workers: and design of patient safety initiatives, 97, 110, 111; and fear of reprisals, 106–7; and individual versus systems approach to safety, 133; and infection control techniques, 97; involvement in patient safety initiatives, 6, 93–94, 108, 115–20, 122; knowledge of work processes, 95–102, 119, 121, 246; reasons for lack of involvement in patient safety initiatives, 108–14, 121; and teamwork, 104; and unions, 106

Gardner, Howard, 217
Gawande, Atul, 3, 216
Geiger-Brown, Jeanne, 5, 7, 114, 155, 169, 171, 172
germ theory, 22–23, 24, 38
Goffman, Erving, 96, 103

Goleman, Daniel, 217
Gordon, Suzanne, 4, 5, 7, 8, 45, 58, 97, 98, 111, 124
Groopman, Jerome, 50

Hackman, J. Richard, 201, 204, 205, 209, 210, 211, 215–16
Hagy, Keith, 105–6
Han, Y., 73, 75
hand washing, 24, 27–29, 31, 37–38, 96, 98, 110, 119
Harrison, Michael, 75, 131
Harvard Work Hours, Health, and Safety (HWHHS) Group, 161–62, 163, 165
Healthcare Information and Management Systems Society (HIMSS), 66
health care information technology (HIT): complexity of, 9, 62; costs of, 84, 86–87, 88; data models of, 15–17, 19, 20, 248n5; design problems in, 18; government funding of, 240–41; homegrown systems, 69; interoperability of, 84, 240; market forces influencing, 64, 66–67, 84, 88, 89, 245; and "meaningful use" criterion, 66–67; and medication errors, 6, 62–63, 168, 183, 184, 188–89, 193; pace of improvement of, 81–86; and patient safety, 3, 5, 6, 65, 86, 87, 88, 89, 102, 104–5, 240–41, 245; promotion of, 65–66, 87, 88, 89, 130–31; recommendations for improvement of, 86–89; roles within health care systems, 64, 88–89, 146; rules for, 9; social costs of use of, 85; standards for, 9, 17, 19, 248n8; and unreliable information, 17–18. *See also* clinical decision support systems (CDSSs); computerized physician/provider order entry (CPOE) systems; electronic health records (EHRs); software and software vendors
health care management: and cleaning, 24, 25, 26, 31, 32, 33, 37, 99, 117–18; and health care information technology, 1–2, 84; individual versus systems approach to safety, 125, 126, 128–30, 133–34, 146–49; and interprofessional hierarchy, 121, 202–3; and patient safety initiatives, 4–5, 6, 93–94, 95, 96, 97, 101, 103–4, 106, 107–16, 117, 121–22; and sleep deprivation, 178; and status and hierarchy, 52, 55, 56; and Taylorism, 120; and teamwork, 56, 57, 101, 104; and workload, 93, 118
health care systems: application of industrial model to, 233–34; and applications